Concise
Neurology

Concise Neurology

Alberto J. Espay, MD, MSc
Assistant Professor
Department of Neurology
University of Cincinnati
Neuroscience Institute
Cincinnati, Ohio

José Biller, MD, FACP, FAAN, FAHA
Professor and Chairman
Department of Neurology
Loyola University Chicago
Stritch School of Medicine
Maywood, Illinois

Wolters Kluwer | Lippincott Williams & Wilkins
Health
Philadelphia · Baltimore · New York · London
Buenos Aires · Hong Kong · Sydney · Tokyo

Acquisitions Editor: Frances Destefano
Product Manager: Tom Gibbons
Production Manager: Bridgett Dougherty
Senior Manufacturing Manager: Benjamin Rivera
Marketing Manager: Brian Freiland
Design Coordinator: Terry Mallon
Production Service: Aptara, Inc.

Library of Congress Cataloging-in-Publication Data
Espay, Alberto J., author.
   Concise neurology / Alberto J. Espay, MD, MSc, Assistant Professor, Department of Neurology, University of
Cincinnati, Neuroscience Institute, Cincinnati, Ohio, José Biller, MD, FACP, FAAN, FAHA, Professor and Chair-
man, Department of Neurology, Loyola University Chicago, Stritch School of Medicine, Maywood, Illinois.
      p. ; cm.
   Includes bibliographical references and index.
   Summary: "Concise Neurology is to be used as a reference by neurologists and neurology trainees who
have already learned about a topic, but want a quick yet thoughtful summary of key points. It can be par-
ticularly useful for novice or experienced neurologists held to time pressures"—Provided by publisher.
   ISBN-13: 978-1-4511-1360-0 (pbk. : alk. paper)
   ISBN-10: 1-4511-1360-9 (pbk. : alk. paper)
   1. Neurology—Handbooks, manual, etc.   2. Nervous system—Diseases—Handbooks, manuals, etc.
I. Biller, José, 1948- author.   II. Title.
   [DNLM: 1. Nervous System Diseases—diagnosis—Handbooks.   2. Nervous System Diseases—therapy—
Handbooks.   WL 39]
   RC355.E87 2011
   616.8–dc22
                                                                                               2010052676

CCS0211

Dedication

To my parents, Italo and Patricia. He steered me from my journalistic dreams of adolescence into a life of service in medicine, secretly knowing that I was to never dissolve my allegiance to the two. She nurtured the certainty of these passions, always keeping me focused on what was at the core: people.

AJE

To the memory of my parents Osías and Elena.

JB

Preface

Throughout our training and subsequent practice in Neurology, everyone stumbles upon an enormous amount of information using many different outfits: review articles, landmark papers, course handouts, conference notes, online cases, and crowning it all, textbooks of every imaginable kind. In a few years, these sources morph into an impressive but hopelessly scattered collection of highlighted sentences, asterisked paragraphs, and handwritten footnotes. It would seem a Herculean task to revisit these sources if only to retrieve what was felt to be the four-line jest of any 20-page manuscript prior to a test, preparing for a conference, or just for the sheer pleasure of remembering the data, whenever one can bask under such joy.

What follows is the account of our trip to the fountainhead. Every curricular subject matter in neurology has been identified, insightfully stripped to the core, and collected into what might be thought of as the essential body of neurological knowledge. Here they are, just about in their original spirit: lean facts devoid of rhetorical discussions but also unshackled by the oppression of bullet-fed handouts. The scope of this vade mecum of sorts is deliberately designed to lie halfway between the encyclopedic coverage of a textbook and the shallow doctrinal tidbits found in all-you-need-to-know-to-pass review books, which rely excessively on "grocery lists" for comprehensive topical coverage.

Traces of biochemical reactions or glances at ultrastructural cellular organelles are shown in a fragmentary yet systematic fashion only to help engrave in memory a critical piece of data that draws on the scholarship of neurology. Those with specialized interests within our field will exercise their frustration muscles, as the outline of the text is not bound to satisfy the need for an expanded overview of specific areas of basic science progress, however exciting they have become. Risking a pedantic style, it will soon become evident a round-oriented factual collection of the basic but comprehensive neurologic knowledge we have come to learn as essential for the day-to-day practice survival and for the certification procedures leading to it.

The units are organized in arbitrary sequence and hierarchy to satisfy both systematic review and random reading. Each section stands independent from each other. Cross-references are used seldomly and only to prevent needless repetition when the subject is approached elsewhere, but an effort is made to preserve the continuity whenever possible. We aimed at maintaining a thematic unity on a page-by-page basis, a goal easier to attain in this dual-authored effort. This allows casual reading to be almost as fruitful as the progressive, planned review. Should the book be serendipitously opened in "anticoagulation," for instance, the reader will access a capsulized review of the heparin, warfarin, and thrombolysis stroke trials as well as current therapeutic guidelines. Flipping through neighboring pages will rapidly refresh the position of the clinically relevant thrombophilias in relationship to the coagulation pathway, indications for lifelong anticoagulation, causes of hyperhomocysteinemia, and the bare bones of the most important etiologies of strokes in the young. None of the topics are meant to be held as evidence-based literature but rather generally accepted knowledge.

In such light, the authors have attempted to present a concise but representative, comprehensive, and accurate review of the primary literature on each topic. Brevity was one of our primary goals, and, to this end, we have chosen to provide only select references for anyone wishing to complement the reading experience. This book should be viewed as "our take" on the subject, and we assume full responsibility for any unforeseen interpretative errors. We welcome any comments from readers who take issue with any of the content, and we will do our best to make appropriate revisions in future editions.

Thus, *Concise Neurology* is most likely to be used as a reference by neurologists and neurology trainees who have already learned about a topic but want a quick yet thoughtful summary of key points. It can be particularly useful for novice or experienced neurologists held to time pressures. Creative licenses are only restricted to the preamble of each unit. A topic whose intention is to draft an outline of the upcoming chapters or connect them in some way has been chosen to elicit interest for the text it introduces. These page-long bloviating exercises can be disposed of for the benefit of time as they tend to indulge upon, but do not replace, concepts covered later in a less stylized fashion. Reacting to Will Durant's paradox, who said "sixty years ago I knew everything; now I know nothing: education is a progressive discovery of our own ignorance," may this book expedite that discovery but assist in restraining the anxiety that comes with its realization.

ALBERTO J. ESPAY

JOSÉ BILLER

Acknowledgments

The authors kindly recognize the contribution of Dr. Biagio Azzarelli, who generously gave us all the neuropathology figures he collected over a lifetime of teaching at Indiana University, before his retirement in 2004. We especially thank Frances DeStefano, Acquisitions Editor, and Tom Gibbons, Senior Production Editor, both at Lippincott Williams & Wilkins/Wolters Kluwer Health, for their encouragement and professionalism. Our gratitude is also extensive to Samir Roy, the project manager from Aptara Corporation, who provided excellent editorial and typesetting services, and Martha Headworth, from the University of Cincinnati Neuroscience Institute, who enhanced important concepts through a number of the book illustrations. Finally, we thank our patients for continuously teaching and inspiring us.

List of Abbreviations

TGA .... Transient Global Amnesia
5-HT .... Serotonin
ACA .... Anterior cerebral artery
Ach .... Acetylcholine
AChR .... Acetylcholine receptors
AD .... Alzheimer's disease
AD .... Autosomal dominant
ADC .... Apparent diffusion coefficient sequence
ADEM .... Acute disseminated encephalomyelitis
ADHD .... Attention-deficit hyperactivity disorder
AdoCbl .... Adenosylcobalamin
ADR .... Acute dystonic reaction
AEDs .... Antiepileptic drugs
AION .... Anterior ischemic optic neuropathy
ALD .... Adrenoleukodystrophy
ALS .... Amyotrophic lateral sclerosis
APP .... Amyloid precursor protein
AOA1 .... Ataxia-ocular motor apraxia 1
AOA2 .... Ataxia-ocular motor apraxia 2
APP .... Amyloid precursor protein
AR .... Autosomal recessive
ARAS .... Ascending reticular activating system
ASO .... Antistreptolysin O (ASO)
AT .... Ataxia-telangiectasia
ATM .... Acute transverse myelopathy
AVM .... Arteriovenous malformations

BAEP .... Brainstem auditory evoked potentials
BPPV .... Benign paroxysmal positional vertigo
BZDs .... Benzodiazepines

CAA .... Cerebral amyloid angiopathy
CADASIL .... Cerebral autosomal dominant arteriopathy with subcortical infarcts and leukoencephalopathy
Cbl .... Cobalamin
CBZ .... Carbamazepine
CDMS .... Clinically definite multiple sclerosis
CEA .... Carotid endarterectomy
CIDP .... Chronic inflammatory demyelinating polyneuropathy
CIS .... Clinically isolated syndrome
CJD .... Creutzfeldt-Jakob disease
CK .... Creatine kinase
CMAP .... Compound muscle action potential
CMT .... Charcot-Marie-Tooth
CMT1 .... Charcot-Marie-Tooth type 1

CMV .... Cytomegalovirus
CN III .... Oculomotor (third cranial nerve)
CN IV .... Trochlear (fourth cranial nerve)
CN VI .... Abducens (sixth cranial nerve)
CNS .... Central nervous system
CO .... Carbon monoxide
COPD .... Chronic obstructive pulmonary disease
Corneal .... Corneal reflexes
COX .... Cytochrome oxidase
Cp .... Ceruloplasmin
CPEO .... Chronic progressive external ophthalmoplegia
CPM .... Central pontine myelinolysis
CRAO .... Central retinal artery occlusion
CRP .... C-reactive protein
CRPS .... Complex regional pain syndrome
CSD .... Cortical spreading depression
CSF .... Cerebrospinal fluid
CTS .... Carpal tunnel syndrome

DIC .... Disseminated intravascular coagulation
DLB .... Dementia with Lewy bodies
DM .... Myotonic dystrophy
DMD .... Duchenne muscular dystrophy
DMSA .... Meso-2,3-dimercaptosuccinic acid
DRBA .... Dopamine receptor blocking agents
DWI .... Diffusion-weighted MRI sequence

EBV .... Epstein Barr virus
EDTA .... Ethylene-diamine-tetra-acetic acid
EOM .... Extra-ocular muscles
ESM .... Ethosuximide
ESR .... Erythrocyte sedimentation rate
ET .... Essential tremor

FAB .... Frontal Assessment Battery
FAS .... Fetal alcohol syndrome
FBM .... Felbamate
FSHD .... Facioscapulohumeral dystrophy
FVL .... Factor V Leiden mutation
FXTAS .... Fragile X-associated tremor/ataxia syndrome

GBP .... Gabapentin
GBS .... Guillain-Barré syndrome
GCA .... Giant-cell arteritis
GEFS+ .... Generalized epilepsy with febrile seizures plus
GHB .... Gamma-hydroxybutyric acid
GluR3 .... Glutamate receptor 3
GP .... Globus pallidus
GPe .... Globus pallidus pars externa
GPi .... Globus pallidus pars interna

HARP .... Hypoprebetalipoproteinemia, acanthocytosis, retinitis pigmentosa and pallidal degeneration
HPE .... Holoprosencephaly
HSE .... Herpes simplex encephalitis
HSP .... Hereditary spastic paraparesis
HSV .... Herpes simplex virus
HyperKPP .... Hyperkalemic periodic paralysis
HypoKPP .... Hypokalemic periodic paralysis type 1
HZV .... Herpes zoster virus

ICA .... Internal carotid artery
ICH .... Intracerebral hemorrhage
IM .... Intramuscular
INO .... Internuclear ophthalmoplegia
IV .... Intravenous
IVIG .... Intravenous immunoglobulin

JME .... Juvenile myoclonic epilepsy

KS .... Korsakoff syndrome

LEMS .... Lambert-Eaton myasthenic syndrome
LHON .... Leber hereditary optic neuropathy
LMN .... Lower motor neuron
LS .... Leigh syndrome
LTG .... Lamotrigine
LTR .... Levetiracetam

MAO .... Monoamine oxidase
MCA .... Middle cerebral artery
MCP .... Middle cerebellar peduncle
MDMA 3,4-methylenedioxy-methamphetamine
MeCbl .... Methylcobalamin
MELAS .... Mitochondrial encephalomyopathy, lactic acidosis, and stroke-like episodes
MERRF .... Myoclonus epilepsy with ragged-red fibers
MGUS .... Monoclonal gammopathy of unknown significance
MLD .... Metachromatic leukodystrophy
MLF .... Medial longitudinal fasciculus
MM .... Multiple myeloma
MND .... Motor neuron disease
MS .... Multiple sclerosis
MSUD .... Maple syrup urine disease
mtDNA .... Mitochondrial DNA
MTHFR .... 5,10-methylenetetrahydrofolate reductase
MuSK .... Muscle-specific kinase

NARP .... Neuropathy, ataxia, and retinitis pigmentosa
NBIA-1 .... Neurodegeneration with brain iron accumulation type 1
NBIA-2 .... Neuroferritinopathy or Neurodegeneration with brain iron accumulation type 2

NCL...Neuronal ceroid lipofuscinosis
NCV...Nerve conduction velocities
nDNA ....Nuclear DNA
NFT...Neurofibrillary tangles
NKH ....Nonketotic hyperglycinemia
NMJ...Neuromuscular junction
NMO..Neuromyelitis optica
NMS..Neuroleptic malignant syndrome
NO..Nitrous oxide
NSAIDs ....Nonsteroidal anti-inflammatory drugs

OCB..Oligoclonal bands
OH..Orthostatic hypotension
ON..Optic neuritis
OPMD ....Oculopharyngeal muscular dystrophy
OT ....Orthostatic tremor
OXZ..Oxcarbazepine

PB ....Phenobarbital
PCA...Posterior cerebral artery
PCP...Phencyclidine
PDHC ....Pyruvate dehydrogenase complex
PEO ....Progressive external ophthalmoplegia
PFO ....Patent foramen ovale
PHF...Paired helical filaments
PHT ....Phenytoin
PKD ....Paroxysmal kinesigenic dyskinesia
PLE ....Paraneoplastic limbic encephalitis
PLMS...Periodic limb movements of sleep
PLMW..Periodic limb movements while awake
PLS...Primary lateral sclerosis
PMC..Paramyotonia congenita
PME ....Progressive myoclonic encephalopathies
PML ....Progressive multifocal leukoencephalopathy
PNKD ....Paroxysmal nonkinesigenic dyskinesia
PNS...Peripheral nervous system
PPRF..Paramedian pontine reticular formation
PRES ....Posterior reversible encephalopathy syndrome
PRM ....Primidone
PS1...Presenilin 1
PS2...Presenilin 2
PSG...Polysomnography
PSP ....Progressive supranuclear palsy

RAPD..Relative afferent pupillary defect
RBD ....REM sleep behavior disorder
riMLF...Rostral interstitial nucleus of the medial longitudinal fasciculus
RIP ....Nucleus raphe interpositus
RLS...Restless leg syndrome
RRF ....Ragged-red fibers
rRNA ....Ribosomal RNAs

SAH ....Subarachnoid hemorrhage
SCLC ....Small-cell lung cancer
SLE..St. Louis encephalitis
SN ....Substantia nigra
SNRI..Serotonin norepinephrine reuptake inhibitors
SP...Amyloid plaques
SQ..Subcutaneous
SSRI ....Selective serotonin reuptake inhibitors
STN..Subthalamic nucleus

T1W...T1-weighted magnetic resonance imaging
T2W...T2-weighted magnetic resonance imaging
Tau ....Tau protein
TCA ....Tricyclic antidepressants
TGB..Tiagabine
TIA...Transient ischemic attack
TM ....Transverse myelitis
TPM..Topiramate
TPN ....Total parenteral nutrition
tRNA ....Transfer RNA

UMN ....Upper motor neuron

VaD...Vascular dementia
VAMP...Vesicle-associated membrane protein
VGB..Vigabatrin
VGCC ....Voltage-gated calcium channels
VGKC ....Voltage-gated potassium channels
VLCFA..Very-long-chain fatty acids
VPA...Valproic acid

WNV...West Nile virus encephalitis

ZNM ....Zonisamide

Contents

Preface   vii

Acknowledgments   ix

List of Abbreviations   xi

1 Basics of Metabolism and Pediatric Neurology..1

Spectrum of Vitamin B_{12}-Requiring Disorders   2
Carbohydrate Metabolism: Inherited Muscle Glycogenosis   3
Mitochondrial Metabolism   4
Lipid Metabolism   5
Purine Metabolism Disorders   6
Peroxisomal Disorders   11
Lysosomal Disorders: Sphingolipidoses   12
Lysosomal Disorders: Mucopolysaccharidoses   14
Porphyrias   15
Dopamine and Catecholamine Metabolic Disorders   16
Norepinephrine System   17
Serotonin System   18
Electrolyte Derangements   19
Voltage-Gated Channels (Ionic Interaction)   24
Gamma-Aminobutyric Acid   27
Glutamate Receptors   28
Autism Spectrum Disorders   29
Attention-Deficit Hyperactivity Disorder   30
Floppy Infant Syndrome   31
Microcephaly   33
Macrocephaly   35
Glutaric Aciduria Type I   36
Biotinidase Deficiency   37
Mitochondrial Diseases   38
Mitochondrial Encephalomyopathy Syndromes   39
Maternally Inherited Leigh Syndrome and Related Disorders   40
Primary White Matter Disorders   41
Primary Gray Matter Disorders   43
Symmetrical Bilateral Signal Abnormalities within the Basal Ganglia   44
Angelman Syndrome   45
Neurocutaneous Syndromes (Phakomatoses)   46

2 Stroke, Migraine, and Epilepsy..48

Stroke   49
Emergency Treatment of Ischemic Stroke   53
Antiplatelet Drugs   54
Carotid Endarterectomy   56
Transient Ischemic Attack   57
Subarachnoid Hemorrhage   58
Intracerebral Hemorrhage   59
Increased Intracranial Pressure   60
Patent Foramen Ovale   61

Neurovascular Syndromes   62
Thalamic Syndromes   64
CADASIL   70
Important Stroke Mimickers   72
Thrombotic Microangiopathies   74
Disseminated Intravascular Coagulation   75
Epilepsy   76
Generalized Frontally Dominant Slow (3.5 Hz) Spike and Wave   77
Centrotemporal Spikes and Waves   77
Febrile Seizures   78
Antiepileptic Agents   79
Mechanisms of Action of AEDs   80
Surgery for Epilepsy   82
Status Epilepticus   83
Epilepsy in Women   84
Neonatal and Pediatric EEG   85
Brainstem Auditory Evoked Potentials 87
Visual Evoked Potentials   88
Somatosensory Evoked Potentials   88
Myoclonic Encephalopathies   90
Atypical Progressive Myoclonic Encephalopathy   91
Myoclonus and Renal Failure   92
Epileptic Encephalopathies with Myoclonus   93
Sleep Disorders   94
Coma   98
Persistent Vegetative State 99
Brain Death   100
Migraine and Other Headaches   101
Selected Secondary Headaches   107

3   Infectious Diseases 108

Cerebrospinal Fluid   109
Viral Encephalitis   111
Imaging of Viral Encephalitis   112
Aseptic Meningitis Syndrome   115
Postencephalitic Parkinsonism   116
HIV/AIDS-Related Infectious Disorders   117
Neuroimaging of Abscesses   119
Neurosyphilis   120
Lyme Disease (Neuroborreliosis)   121
Progressive Multifocal Leukoencephalopathy   122
Parasitic Diseases of the Nervous System   123
Neurosarcoidosis   125
Whipple Disease   126
Subacute Sclerosing Panencephalitis   127
Prion Diseases   128
Pathology of Infectious Diseases   130
Pathology of Fungal Infections   131
Pathology of Prion Diseases   133

4   Neurotoxicology 134

Manganese Toxicity   135
Botulism   136
Nonbotulism Causes of Toxic Weakness   137
Envenomations   138

Lead Poisoning   139
Mercury Intoxication   140
Toxic Gases   142
Toxic Solvents and Other Chemicals   143
Marine Biotoxins   144
Substance Abuse Disorders   145
Alcohol and Sedatives Abuse and Withdrawal   146
Alcoholism   147
Psychostimulants: Cocaine and Amphetamine   150
Marijuana, Hallucinogens, and PCP   151
Opioids Intoxication and Withdrawal   152
Toxic Leukoencephalopathies   153
Neuroleptic Malignant Syndrome   154

5 Movement Disorders 155

Cerebellar ataxias   155
Inherited Ataxias with Identifiable Biochemical Errors   156
Hereditary Ataxias: Autosomal Dominant Inheritance   157
Episodic Ataxias   159
Hereditary Ataxias: Autosomal Recessive Inheritance   160
Hereditary Ataxias: X-Linked Inheritance   164
Congenital Ataxic Disorders   166
Acquired Ataxias: Selected Disorders   168
Neurodegeneration with Brain Iron Accumulation   169
Acanthocytosis-Related Neurologic Disorders   170
Dystonia   171
Parkinson Disease   178
Imaging in Parkinson's Disease and Other Parkinsonisms   180
Levodopa-induced Dyskinesias   183
Tremor in Conditions Other Than PD   187
Progressive Supranuclear Palsy   189
Multiple System Atrophy   191
Autonomic Dysfunction in Neurodegenerative Diseases   193
Corticobasal Degeneration   194
Machado-Joseph Disease   195
Other Parkinsonian Disorders   196
Pathology of Tauopathies   198
Pathology of Synucleinopathies   199
Chorea   200
Huntington Disease   201
Sydenham Disease   202
Restless Leg Syndrome (Ekbom Syndrome)   203
Paroxysmal Dyskinesias   204
Selected Facial Disorders   206
Myoclonus   207
Wilson Disease   208
Tourette Syndrome   209

6 Behavioral Neurology 210

Behavioral Neuroanatomy   211
Amnesia   213
Memory Primer   214
Agnosias   215
Apraxias   216
Aphasias   217

Acquired Dyslexia and Peripheral Dyslexia   218
Neglect   219
Delirium or Acute Confusional State   220
Alzheimer's Disease   221
Mild Cognitive Impairment   224
Vascular Dementia   225
Dementia with Lewy Bodies (DLB)   226
Frontotemporal Lobar Degeneration   227
Focal Atrophy Syndromes in Dementias   229
Frontal Assessment Battery (FAB): Office Assessment of Frontal Function   230

7   Neuro-ophthalmology and Neuro-otology **231**

Transient Monocular Visual Loss   232
Permanent Monocular Visual Loss   233
Binocular Visual Loss   235
Cerebral Visual Loss   236
Anisocoria   237
Diplopia   239
Disorders of Saccades   241
Nystagmus   242
Selected Cerebellar, Pontine, and Midbrain Oculomotor Syndromes   244
Giant-Cell Arteritis   245
Tolosa-Hunt Syndrome   246
Dizziness: Vertigo and Lightheadedness   247
Benign Paroxysmal Positional Vertigo   248
Ménière's Disease   250
Cerebellar Ataxia with Bilateral Vestibulopathy   251

**8   Demyelinating Diseases, Neuro-oncology and Disorders of
     Neural Tube Closure and Other Congenital Malformations**......................**252**

Multiple Sclerosis   253
Posterior Reversible Encephalopathy Syndrome   261
Autoimmune Channelopathies   263
Autoimmune Encephalopathies   264
Brain Tumors   265
Circumscribed Astrocytomas   266
Diffuse Astrocytomas   267
Oligodendrogliomas   268
Ependymal Tumors   269
Neuronal Tumors   270
Mixed Ganglioneuronal Tumors   271
Primitive Neuroectodermal Tumors   272
Meningeal and Mesenchymal Tumors   273
Primary Central Nervous System Lymphoma   274
Pineal Tumors and Keratin-Containing Masses   275
Paraneoplastic Syndromes of the CNS   277
Paraneoplastic Syndromes of the PNS   278
Disorders of Neural Tube Closure and Other Congenital Malformations   280

9   Neuromuscular Disorders **283**

Brachial Plexopathies   284
Brachial Neuropathies   285
Assessment of Hand Weakness   287

Lumbar Plexus   288
Sacral Plexus   288
Tibial Nerve   289
Peroneal Nerve   289
Assessment of Foot Drop   290
Guillain-Barré Syndrome   291
Chronic Inflammatory Demyelinating Polyneuropathy   292
Myasthenia Gravis   293
Amyotrophic Lateral Sclerosis (Motor Neuron Disease)   294
Spinal Cord Pathologies per Compartment   297
Neurogenic Bladder   299
Axonal Polyneuropathies   301
Complex Regional Pain Syndrome   303
Neurogenic Orthostatic Hypotension   304
Autosomal Dominant Recurrent Hereditary Neuropathies   305
Paraproteinemic Neuropathies   308
Multiple Myeloma   310
Amyloid Neuropathies   311
Peripheral Nerve Tumors   312
Muscular Dystrophies: X-Linked Dystrophinopathies   313
Limb-Girdle Muscular Dystrophies   314
Congenital Muscular Dystrophies   315
Distal Myopathies   316
Myotonic Dystrophy   317
Facioscapulohumeral Dystrophy   318
Scapuloperoneal Dystrophy   318
Oculopharyngeal Muscular Dystrophy   318
Inflammatory Myopathies   319
Metabolic Myopathies   321
Episodic Muscle Weakness   322
Familial Periodic Paralysis: Clinical Recognition   323
Progressive or Stable Muscle Weakness   324
Mitochondrial Myopathies   325
Other Myogenic Causes of Cramps and Myalgia   326
Neurogenic Causes of Cramps and Myalgia   327
Congenital Myopathies   328
Malignant Hyperthermia Syndrome   329
Critical Illness-Related Neuropathy and Myopathy   330

10   Psychiatry...**331**

Depression   332
Bipolar Disorder   335
Anxiety Disorders   336
Obsessive-Compulsive Disorder   338
Personality Disorders   339
Eating Disorders   340
Schizophrenia and Other Psychoses   341
Delusions   343
Neuroleptic-Induced Movement Disorders   344
Somatoform Disorders   345
Dissociative Disorders   347

Suggested References for Further Reading   348
Index   359

Concise
Neurology

Basics of Metabolism and Pediatric Neurology

1

The complexity and fascination for metabolic diseases can be introduced by unfolding the story of vitamin B_{12} (cobalamin [Cbl]). While its deficiency in adults is widely suspected in the presence of megaloblastic anemia and ataxic paraparesis (subacute combined degeneration), the deeper plot rises in children with inborn errors of B_{12} metabolism. Their failure to convert Cbl into its two active forms, methylcobalamin (MeCbl) and adenosylcobalamin (AdoCbl), which are essential cofactors for methionine synthase (MS) and methylmalonyl CoA mutase, respectively, leads to hyperhomocysteinemia with hypomethioninemia (**HC**) and methylmalonic acidemia (**MMA**). Hyperhomocysteinemia leads to vascular diseases, especially in the hyperhomocysteinemia of cystathionine synthase (CS), and the hypomethioninemia keeps folate building as 5-methyl-tetrahydrofolate (MTHF), which renders it useless for the synthesis of purine and, therefore, DNA. The resulting gastrointestinal (glossitis and diarrhea) and hematologic (anemia) deficits are reversed by folate replacement.

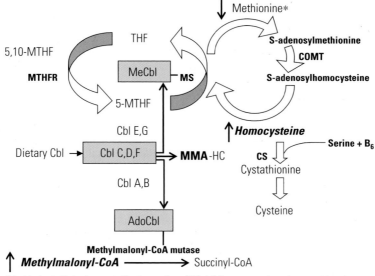

*Methionine is high when cystathionine synthase (CS) deficiency causes hyperhomocysteinemia.

However, the neurologic deficits are independent of purine synthesis and dissociated from the hematologic signs and inversely correlate with the degree of anemia and macrocytosis. Abnormal myelination presumably results from either a deficiency of S-adenosylmethionine or the accumulation of methylmalonate and methylpropionate into branched-chain fatty acids. When the combined hepatic synthesis of MeCbl and AdoCbl is impaired, both methionine synthase and methylmalonic-CoA mutase are affected and a different phenotypic expression, **MMA-HC,** arises.

Spectrum of Vitamin B$_{12}$-Requiring Disorders

Subacute combined degeneration (SCD)	Methylmalonic aciduria (MMA)	Homocystinuria (HC)	MMA-HC
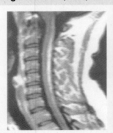	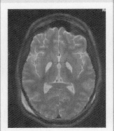	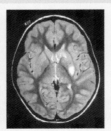	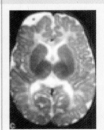
Symmetric spastic **paraparesis**, dorsal (sensory ataxia due to loss of vibration sense) and lateral (corticospinal tracts) column loss with peripheral neuropathy	Profound ketotic **hyperglycinemic encephalopathy** and intermittent lethargy, vomiting, tachypnea, and coma with early death or severe developmental retardation in survivors*	Marfanoid habitus, lens dislocation, livedo reticularis, **mental retardation**, brittle hair, and thromboembolic strokes from homocysteine-induced endothelial injury	Dysmorphic face, hypotonia, ataxia, seizures, optic atrophy, psychomotor delay, and hemolytic-uremic syndrome (**HUS**): azotemia, thrombocytopenia microangiopathic hemolytic anemia, transient callosal splenium edema

*Selective necrosis of the globus pallidus** is an important MRI finding in MMA. Differential diagnoses include propionic acidemia, pyruvate dehydrogenase deficiency, kernicterus, and carbon monoxide poisoning.

Diagnosis of Vitamin B$_{12}$ Deficiency

In profound vitamin B$_{12}$ deficiency, there is pancytopenia with hypoproliferative anemia characterized by macrocytosis, hypersegmentation of neutrophils, and signs of ineffective erythropoiesis (elevated lactate dehydrogenase and indirect bilirubin). When the vitamin B$_{12}$ deficiency is milder, the following algorithm (*NEJM* 2004;351:1333–1341) replaces the Schilling test and the antibodies against parietal cells (nonspecific) and against intrinsic factor (insensitive).

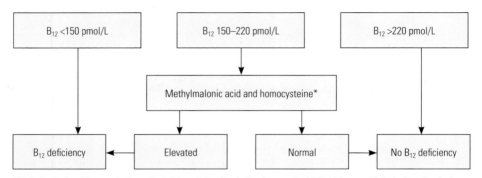

*Methylmalonic acid concentration reflects intracellular vitamin B$_{12}$ stores and exhibits higher specificity for low vitamin B$_{12}$ status than any other metabolite including homocysteine.

Carbohydrate Metabolism: Inherited Muscle Glycogenosis

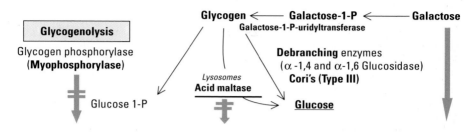

McArdle's (Type V)	Pompe's (Type II)	Galactosemia
AR, Chromosome 11	AR, Chromosome 17q	AR
Exercise-induced **cramps** and **myoglobinuria**, with "second wind." Progressive proximal weakness occurs in one third or patients. Forearm ischemic test: lactate increases <5 mg/dL above baseline. Biopsy: **subsarcolemmal blebs**. No phosphorylase activity.	Profound generalized **hypotonia** and **CHF** in neonates. **Proximal arm and distal leg weakness** (scapuloperoneal pattern) in young adults. **Encephalopathy** from accumulation of glycogen in the brain. Biopsy: large **PAS-positive vacuoles**. No acid maltase activity in fibroblasts.	Newborn: failure to thrive, white matter disease, **cataracts**, and **megalencephaly**. Later: **Hepatosplenomegaly** (with coagulopathy) and ovarian failure.

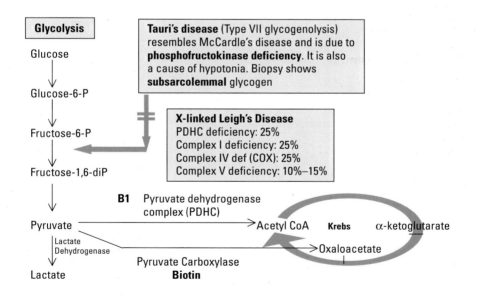

Mitochondrial Metabolism

(See also *Mitochondrial diseases, Glutaric aciduria type I, Mitochondrial encephalomyopathy syndromes, and Mitochondrial myopathies.*)

Mitochondrial DNA (mtDNA) is a small circular molecule that possesses its own genetic material, is inherited from the mother, and has no introns. Each mtDNA encodes 22 transfer RNAs (tRNA), 13 polypeptides, and 2 ribosomal RNAs (rRNA). The mtDNA-encoded genes supply crucial components of the respiratory or electron transport chain. However, the vast majority of the mitochondrial proteins are encoded in the nuclear DNA (nDNA), which can cause diseases with varying heritability patterns:

- *Autosomal recessive*: Krebs cycle disorders such as **fumarase deficiency** (**microcephaly,** neutropenia, and thrombocytopenia) and α-**ketoglutarate dehydrogenase complex deficiency** (B_1-dependent microcephaly and hypertrophic cardiomyopathy)
- *X-linked recessive*: **intermittent ataxia with lactic acidosis** due to PDHC deficiency (B_1-dependent myopathy, lactic acidosis, **corpus callosum agenesis,** and facial dysmorphism), and **ornithine transcarbamylase deficiency** (See *Urea cycle defects*)

Disorders of Oxidative Phosphorylation (Electron Transport Chain)

Complex I NADH/CoQ red	Complex II SDH/CoQ red	Complex III RedCoQ/CytoC red	Complex IV COX	Complex V ATP synthase
MELAS	Encephalo-myelopathy	Myopathies	**MELAS**	Leigh
MERRF		Cardiomyopathy	**MERRF**	**NARP**
Alper's			Alper's	**Kearns-Sayre**
Kerns-Sayre		**Kerns-Sayre**	Kearns-Sayre	
Leigh			Leigh	
Parkinson			Menkes'	
Leber (LHON)	**SDH**: succinate dehydrogenase; **COX**: cytochrome C oxidase **CoQ**: coenzyme Q		Alzheimer's	
MPTP Haloperidol Rotenone	Malonate	Antimycin A	Cyanide Sodium azide	Selective mitochondrial poisons

In addition to the above toxins, mitochondrial disease can also be acquired such as in Reye's syndrome and zidovudine treatment.

Tissues with high oxidative metabolism have a relatively low threshold for, and are especially vulnerable to, mtDNA mutation. Thus, most mtDNA disorders are **encephalomyopathies,** disorders where brain and muscle are primarily affected (see *Mitochondrial diseases*).

Lipid Metabolism

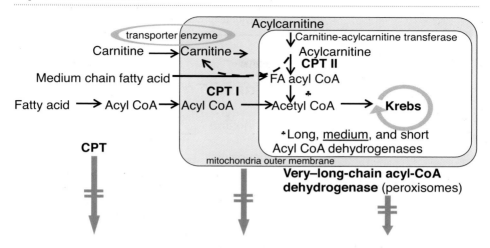

Carnitine Palmitoyl Transferase Deficiency	Medium Chain Acyl-CoA (MCAD) Deficiency	X-Linked Adrenoleukodystrophy
AR, chromosome 1	AR, chromosome 1	X-linked, *ALDP* gene
Intolerance to **sustained exercise** (muscle pain, and swelling) without cramps. **Long fasting** may trigger symptoms **without generating ketones.** High CK and myoglobinuria during attacks. Biopsy: **lipid droplets** in muscle fibers	**Recurrent coma** or vomiting, confusion, and lethargy. **Low or absent ketones** during attacks. **Cardiomyopathy** may be present. It is the main cause of **carnitine deficiency** (carnitine is <20 μmol/mg). L-carnitine replacement is indicated.	**Posterior demyelination** and **Addison disease** in males associated with progressive quadri- or paraparesis (spinal form: adrenomyeloneuropathy). High level of **very long chain fatty acids** in plasma, RBCs, WBCs, or fibroblasts is diagnostic.

Primary Carnitine Deficiency	Secondary Carnitine Deficiency
Carnitine transporter deficiency, MCAD	Excessive production of Acyl-CoA
Recurrent acute encephalopathy, lactic acidosis, **high ammonia**, hypoglycemia, and liver dysfunction with variable **hypotonia** and **cardiac myopathy**. Episodes are triggered by infection or starvation. Rx: L-carnitine 60 mg/kg/d (IV), or 200 mg PO	Free carnitine is trapped in acyl-carnitine esters subsequently lost in urine. **Organic acidurias are the major cause**. Also seen in Reye's syndrome, valproate hepatotoxicity, malnutrition, pregnancy, liver failure, TPN, and renal tubular disease
Acylcarnitine:carnitine ratio >0.4, low free carnitine (<10 μmol/mg)	Acylcarnitine:carnitine ratio >0.4, low free carnitine (<20 μmol/mg)

Purine Metabolism Disorders

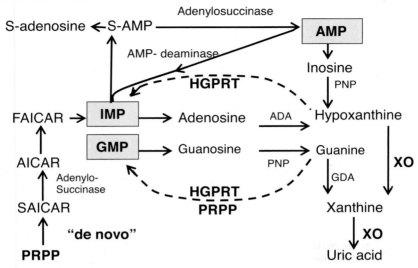

PRPP, Phosphoribosyl pyrophosphate; AICAR, aminoimidazole carboxamide ribotide; SAICAR, succinyl AICAR; FAICAR, formyl AICAR; S-AMP, adenylosuccinate; AMP, GMP, and IMP, adenosine, guanosine, and inosine monophosphate; ADA, adenosine deaminase; GDA, guanine deaminase; PNP, purine nucleoside phosphorylase; **HGPRT**, hypoxanthine-guanine phosphoribosyltransferase; **XO**, xanthine oxidase.

HGPRT Deficiency: Lesch-Nyhan Syndrome	PRPP Synthetase Superactivity	Adenylosuccinase Deficiency
X-linked	X-linked	AR, chromosome 22
Choreoathetosis with MR, dystonia, **hypotonia**, leg **spasticity**, **self-mutilation** (biting)*, and **hyperuricemia**. Renal but not CNS damage is prevented by allopurinol (xanthine oxidase inhibitor)	**Sensorineural deafness** +/− **ataxia** or hypotonia. Tophaceous gout alone is found in heterozygotic female carriers. Uric acid is increased in affected males. **Xanthine** and **hypoxanthine** levels are high in plasma and CSF	**Autism**, abnormal movements, growth and **psychomotor delay**, **seizures**, amaurosis, hypotonia, and **vermal cerebellar hypoplasia**. S-adenosine and SAICAR are elevated in plasma and CSF.

*The oromandibular and lingual dystonia of Lesch-Nyhan syndrome, including the common self-injurious tongue biting, is similar to that seen in chorea-acanthocytosis and tardive dyskinesia.

Uric acid should be elevated in both plasma *and* urine: HGPRT deficiency in Lesch-Nyhan syndrome (LNS) and the *de novo* synthetic disorder PRPP superactivity. Children with LNS may have normal uric acid because of higher renal clearance. They are classified as CP until renal complications or gout discloses the etiology.

Immunodeficiency disorders are common with ADA and PNP deficiencies. The latter may present with *spastic diplegia*, as in LNS, because HGPRT, although not defective, lacks the substrates normally provided by PNP.

Urea Cycle Defects

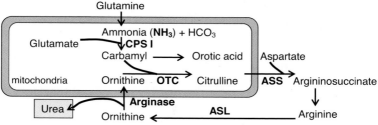

ASS and **ASL**, argininosuccinate synthase and lyase, respectively; **CPS**, Carbamyl phosphate synthetase; **OTC**, Ornithine transcarbamylase deficiency.

Hyperammonemia from Selected Urea Cycle Disorders

OTC Deficiency (Type II)	CPS Deficiency (Type I)	Arginase Deficiency
X-linked dominant	AR	AR
Neonatal encephalopathy and death or mental retardation. Variant: **episodic headache** and **ataxia**, also occurring in females in association with **ophthalmoplegia**.	Neonatal encephalopathy or **recurrent vomiting**, and lethargy with unusual **eye movements**. Hyperventilation may cause respiratory alkalosis.	Later childhood onset as **progressive spastic paraparesis**, seizures, and **MR** with **recurrent vomiting**. Respiratory alkalosis from hyperventilation.
↑ NH_3, orotic aciduria, ↓ plasma citrulline	↑ NH_3, ↓ plasma citrulline	↑ NH_3, ↑ plasma arginine

ASS and ASL Deficiencies
AR
Neonatal encephalopathy or chronic **ataxia**, MR, seizures, **recurrent vomiting**, and **trichorrhexis nodosa**
↑ NH_3, Orotic aciduria, ↑ citrulline, citrullinuria

Hyperammonemia from Other Causes
- Valproate therapy
- Reye syndrome
- Hyperornithinemia, hyperammonemia, homocitrullinuria (HHH) syndrome
- Lysinuric protein intolerance
- Glycine encephalopathy
- Herpes simplex infection
- Asparaginase treatment
- Organic acidurias

Neonatal hyperammonemia algorithm

Respiratory ↑pH

1. ↑ **Urine Organic Acids** (metabolic ↓pH): Congenital lactic acidosis, organic aciduria, and fatty acid oxidation defects; If normal → citrulline
2. ↑↑↑ **Citrulline** (>1,000 µM): ASS deficiency; ↑↑ (100–300 µM): ASL deficiency; If normal (6–20 µM) → plasma/CSF glycine
3. ↑↑↑ **Glycine**: Nonketotic hyperglycinemia; Normal → transient neonatal hyperammonemia; Absent/trace → Urinary orotic acid
4. ↑↑ **Orotic acid**: OTC deficiency; ↓: CPS deficiency

Aminoacid metabolism

Hyperphenylalaninemia

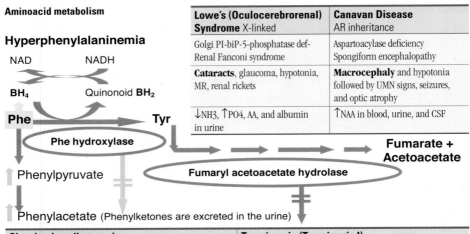

Lowe's (Oculocerebrorenal) Syndrome X-linked	Canavan Disease AR inheritance
Golgi PI-biP-5-phosphatase def-Renal Fanconi syndrome	Aspartoacylase deficiency Spongiform encephalopathy
Cataracts, glaucoma, hypotonia, MR, renal rickets	**Macrocephaly** and hypotonia followed by UMN signs, seizures, and optic atrophy
↓NH3, ↑PO4, AA, and albumin in urine	↑NAA in blood, urine, and CSF

Classic phenylketonuria AR inheritance	Tyrosinemia (Tyrosinosis I) AR inheritance
Phenylalanine hydroxylase deficiency	Fumaryl acetoacetate hydrolase deficiency
MR (dysmyelination), persistent vomiting, **microcephaly**, **hypopigmentation**, **eczematoid** skin, and abnormal behavior. There is **musty** odor in urine. **Tremor**, hypertonia, and hyperactivity may be present. Infantile spasms and GTC seizures may occur in childhood.	Acute **encephalopathy**, **liver failure**, and renal tubular Fanconi's syndrome. **Painful disesthesias** from acute motor **axonal neuropathy** are most common. **Acute intermittent porphyria** with **GBS-like picture** can develop from inhibition of δ-ALA by succinylacetone. A **rotten cabbage** odor is noted.
↑ Phe (>20 mg/dL), ↓ Tyr, urinary excretion of phenylketones	↑ Tyr (>3 mg/dL), ↑ α-fetoprotein, ↑ δ-ALA, ↑ succinylacetone

Dihydropteridine (BH_2) reductase deficiency is also known as atypical phenylketonuria or phenylketonuria type 2, which impairs resynthesis of tetrahydrobiopterin (BH_4), the cofactor of phenylalanine, tyrosine and tryptophan hydroxylases, causes a global reduction of biogenic monoamines (serotonin, dopamine, epinephrine and norepinephrine).

Sulfur-containing aminoacids

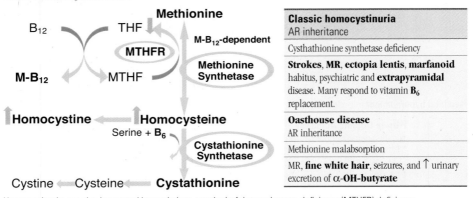

Classic homocystinuria AR inheritance
Cysthathionine synthetase deficiency
Strokes, **MR**, **ectopia lentis**, **marfanoid** habitus, psychiatric and **extrapyramidal** disease. Many respond to vitamin B_6 replacement.
Oasthouse disease AR inheritance
Methionine malabsorption
MR, **fine white hair**, seizures, and ↑ urinary excretion of α-**OH-butyrate**

Homocystinuria can also be caused by methylene tetrahydrofolate reductase deficiency (MTHFR) deficiency.

Organic Acidurias

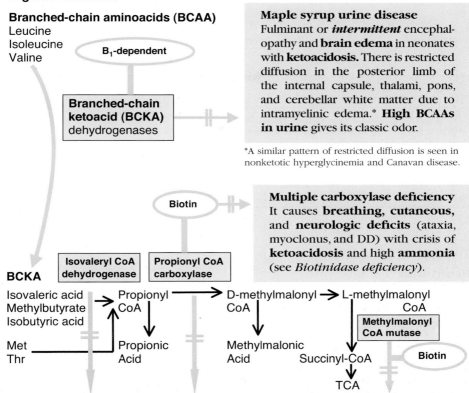

Branched-chain aminoacids (BCAA)
Leucine
Isoleucine
Valine

B_1-dependent

Branched-chain
ketoacid (BCKA)
dehydrogenases

Maple syrup urine disease
Fulminant or *intermittent* encephalopathy and **brain edema** in neonates with **ketoacidosis.** There is restricted diffusion in the posterior limb of the internal capsule, thalami, pons, and cerebellar white matter due to intramyelinic edema.* **High BCAAs in urine** gives its classic odor.

*A similar pattern of restricted diffusion is seen in nonketotic hyperglycinemia and Canavan disease.

Biotin

Multiple carboxylase deficiency
It causes **breathing, cutaneous, and neurologic deficits** (ataxia, myoclonus, and DD) with crisis of **ketoacidosis** and high **ammonia** (see *Biotinidase deficiency*).

Isovaleryl CoA
dehydrogenase

Propionyl CoA
carboxylase

BCKA

Isovaleric acid
Methylbutyrate
Isobutyric acid

Propionyl → D-methylmalonyl → L-methylmalonyl
CoA   CoA   CoA

Methylmalonyl
CoA mutase

Met
Thr

Propionic
Acid

Methylmalonic
Acid

Succinyl-CoA

Biotin

TCA

Isovaleric Acidemia	Propionic Acidemia	Methylmalonic Acidemia
AR	AR, **Biotin-dependent**	AR, B_{12}-**dependent**
Neonatal **MSUD-like** presentation. There is a chronic infantile form. "**Sweaty feet**" smell in urine is characteristic.	**Episodic ketotic hyperglycinemia** with acidosis and **hyperammonemia**. A **bleeding diathesis** (with tendency for ICH) and sepsis-like picture are effects from **pancytopenia**. Recurrent acidosis, growth retardation, seizures, dystonia, or chorea in survivors.	
	↑ **T2W MRI signal** in the **caudate and putamen**	↑ **T2W MRI signal** in the **globus pallidus**
Isovaleryl-lysine in urine, ↓ isovaleryl CoA dehydrogenase activity in fibroblasts	↑ **Propionate**, ↑ glycine, ↑β-hydroxypropionate, ↑ methylcitrate, ↓ propionyl CoA activity in fibroblasts	↑ **Methylmalonate**, ↑ propionyl CoA, ↑ propionate, ↑glycine, ↑ ammonia.
Treatment: Glycine dexotifies isovaleryl CoA, ↓ leucine intake	**Biotin**, protein restriction, carnitine, metronidazole reduces propionate by gut bacteria	**Cobalamin**, protein restriction, carnitine, betaine for associated homocystinuria

General treatment for all organic acidurias: Carnitine, peritoneal dialysis

Hyperglycinemias

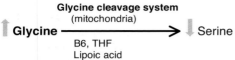

Glycine cleavage system
(mitochondria)

⬆ Glycine ———————————➤ ⬇ Serine

B6, THF
Lipoic acid

Nonketotic Hyperglycinemia: Glycine Encephalopathy	Ketotic Hyperglycinemia: Inborn Errors of Metabolism
AR	AR; See *Organic acidurias*, above
Progressive neonatal encephalopathy after protein feedings is initiated. **Hypotonia** and **myoclonic** seizures. **Hiccups** should suggest the diagnosis.	Propionic acidemia Methylmalonic acidemia Isovaleric acidemia Acquired: valproic acid
Abnormal **myelination** and abnormal or **absent corpus callosum**. No GCS activity. ↑Glycine	**Organic acids** accumulate, ↑ammonia, ketoacidosis, hypoglycemia, lactic acidosis

Tryptophan Disorders

Renal transport

Reabsorption

Tryptophan ➤ Formylkynurenine ➤ Hydroxykynurenine ➤ Glutaryl CoA

Kynurinase

Hartnup's Disease	Hypertryptophanemia	Hydroxykynurenuria
Photosensitive rash, *episodic* **personality changes**, depression, psychosis, headache, and **ataxia**. Treatment: Nicotinamide 50–300 mg/d	Pellagra-like rash, mental retardation, **ataxia**	Mental retardation, migraine-like **headaches**
	Rash with neurological disease are seen in other vitamin deficiencies: **thiamine** and **biotinidase**.	
Tryptophanuria	↑ Tryptophan	↑ Tryptophan

Renal/Intestinal
Dibasic AA uptake

Acetoacetate ⬅ Acetoacetyl CoA ⬅ Glutaryl CoA

Lysine ————————————————————➤ Lysine
Arginine
Ornithine

Lysinuric intolerance	Hyperlysinemia	Glutaric Aciduria I
↓ **Ornithine** → secondary **urea cycle dysfunction**. Post-prandial encephalopathy, DD, MR, psychosis, and seizures. Treatment: citrulline.	MR, poor growth, variable neurologic deficits.	Deficiency of glutaryl CoA dehydrogenase. See *Glutaric Aciduria I.*

Peroxisomal Disorders

Peroxisomes are 40 times more abundant in oligodendrocytes than neurons or astrocytes. Their main function is H_2O_2 metabolism, phospholipid biosynthesis, fatty acids β-oxidation for **very-long-chain fatty acids (VLCFA),** cholesterol and dolichol synthesis, and pipecolic and phytanic acid degradation.

Disorders of Peroxisome Assembly (Group 1: Common features are **hepatic disease, retinopathy, deafness,** and developmental delay)	Disorders of Single Protein Function (Group 2)
Zellweger syndrome	Refsum disease (HMSN type 4)
Neonatal adrenoleukodystrophy	X-linked adrenoleukodystrophy (ALD)
Infantile Refsum disease	Glutaric aciduria type III
Rhizomelic chondrodysplasia punctata	Hyperoxaluria type I

Any patient presenting with retinal pigmentation and peripheral neuropathy and recurrent encephalopathy should be screened for VLCFA, phytanic acid, and pristanic acid. Central cerebellar and posterior brain white matter disease may be seen in these patients.

Zellweger syndrome (cerebro-hepato-renal syndrome) consists of psychomotor arrest, seizures, **hypotonia** with **arthrogryposis** (camptodactyly, knee and ankle deformities), **facial dysmorphism** (high forehead with flat facies), and brain malformations, including hypoplastic corpus callosum and migration abnormalities (**pachygyria** and **polymicrogyria**). VLCFA and **pipecolic acid** are high; RBC plasmalogen is low.

Infantile Refsum disease patients have mental retardation, pigmentary retinopathy, deafness, dysmorphic features, hepatomegaly, and neuropathy.

Rhizomelic chondrodysplasia punctata (3-oxoacyl-CoA thiolase deficiency) presents with short (rhizomelic) proximal limbs, microcephaly, mental retardation, **cataracts,** dysmorphic face, and ichthyosis. X-ray shows "stippled" epiphyses. **Low plasmalogen and increased phytanic acid** are the biochemical findings.

Refsum disease (HMSN type 4, phytanoyl-CoA hydroxylase deficiency, *PAHX* gene mutations) presents with **cataracts, retinitis pigmentosa, deafness, chronic hypertrophic neuropathy,** and **ataxia,** with or without miosis, anosmia, cardiac, and skin involvement. **Phytanic acid** and **pipecolic acid** are increased.

X-linked ALD (peroxisomal ATPase) binding cassette protein [*ABCD1*] gene, lignoceroyl CoA synthetase deficiency, Xq28) cause cerebral inflammatory demyelination in the parieto-occipital (85%) or frontal (15%) regions with garland of contrast enhancement, beginning at 4–10 years, and progressing rapidly, over a mean of 2 years, to a vegetative state. It affects myelin, adrenal cortex, and the Leydig cells of the testes. Adrenal insufficiency occurs in 85% or cases. Adrenomyeloneuropathy with spastic paraparesis and distal sensory loss and Addison disease are alternative phenotypes in young adults. Serum and fibroblasts show high VLCFA. Heterozygotes have a 20% false-negative rate.

Lysosomal Disorders: Sphingolipidoses

Gaucher Disease (β-Glucosidase or Glucocerebrosidase Deficiency)

Glucocerebrosidase (or, rarely, saposin C) deficiency leads to the accumulation of glucocerebroside (glucosylceramide). *Type I* is most common but does not affect the central nervous system. *Type II,* a rapidly progressive developmental regression form, expresses with choreoathetosis, **horizontal supranuclear gaze palsy**, and initial hypotonia evolving into spasticity. *Type III* is the slower juvenile form, heralded by **hepatosplenomegaly** and followed by **myoclonic seizures, bone pain,** trismus, strabismus, **horizontal supranuclear gaze palsy, spasticity,** ataxia, and dementia. **Gaucher cells** (macrophages filled with insoluble glycolipids) can be identified in spleen, lymph nodes, and bone marrow.

GM$_1$ Gangliosidosis (β-Galactosidase Deficiency)

The infantile and late infantile/juvenile forms show developmental regression with epileptic encephalopathy and spasticity, but only the infantile form exhibit skeletal dysplasia, dysmorphism ("pseudo-Hurler"), and **cherry-red spot.** The adult form manifests progressive dysarthria, dystonia, spasticity, and cerebellar ataxia. A **juvenile parkinsonian phenotype** has been reported. Brain MRI shows T2W **thalamic hypointensity** with or without putaminal hyperintensity. Bone marrow biopsy reveals vacuolated Gaucher-like cells and **foamy histiocytes.**

GM$_2$ Gangliosidosis (Hexosaminidase Deficiency)

Accumulation of GM$_2$ ganglioside in the brain occurs disproportionately more commonly among Ashkenazi Jews due to deficiency of hexosaminidase A in Tay-Sachs disease and of both hexosaminidase A and B in Sandhoff's disease. The classic infantile form of **Tay-Sachs disease** begins with an **abnormal startle response** followed by spastic motor regression, **cherry-red spot,** progressive blindness, deafness, **macrocephaly,** and epileptic encephalopathy. The late-infantile and juvenile forms present with psychiatric features, ataxia, and (upper or lower) **motor neuron disease** and progress into dementia and non-cherry-spot visual loss. Adult picture may mimic slowly progressive motor neuron disease, spinal muscular atrophy, or spinocerebellar degeneration. **Sandhoff's disease** displays a Tay-Sachs phenotype but with visceromegaly. Biopsy outcome is similar to GM$_1$ gangliosidosis.

Fabry Disease (Galactosidase A Deficiency, Anderson-Fabry Disease)

This X-linked recessive disorder (only non-AR sphingolipidosis) is due to deficiency of galactosidase A, which leads to the infarction-causing deposition of globotriaosylceramide (ceramide trihexoside) in vascular endothelium. It may present with episodic neuropathic pain crises with **chronic acroparesthesias,** early-onset **strokes,** myocardial infarction, nephropathy, **hypohydrosis,** lower-trunk **angiokeratomas,** cataracts, and **corneal whorls** on slit-lamp. Ceramide trihexoside is measurable in urine. Electron microscopy shows tightly packed **lamellated inclusions** in the cytoplasm of the cell bodies on specimens of spinal ganglia, vasa nervorum, and perineurium of peripheral nerves.

Niemann-Pick Disease (Sphingomyelinase Deficiency) (*NPC1* and *NPC2*)

Type A is the severe neurovisceral form of infants associated with **cherry-red spot,** progressive **hepatosplenomegaly, psychomotor regression, hypotonia,** and **seizures.** *Type B* may have some of the above systemic deficits without neurologic impairment. Types A and B appear most often in Jewish families. *Type C* affects all ethnic groups and is the most common. Ataxia and dystonia are followed by **supranuclear vertical gaze palsy,** seizures, and dementia. **Hepatosplenomegaly** often coexists. Foamy (lipid-laden) cells or **"sea-blue histiocytes"** in the liver and bone marrow are diagnostic.

Metachromatic Leukodystrophy (Arylsulfatase A or Saposin B Deficiency)

Deficiency of arylsulfatase A or its activator, saposin B, leads to accumulation of cerebroside sulfate, which causes progressive (frontal-predominant) **central and peripheral demyelination.** The NCV are <30 m/s even when reflexes are brisk. Progressive **spastic quadriparesis** may be associated with **blindness, seizures, dementia,** and **peripheral neuropathy.** Increased urinary sulfatides with normal arylsulfatase A levels are seen in MLD due to saposin B deficiency. **Ballooned macrophages** with "metachromatic" (brown-purple) sulfatide deposits with cresyl violet staining are diagnostic on brain and nerve specimens.

Krabbe Disease (Galactocerebroside β-Galactosidase Deficiency)

Deficiency of β-galactocerebrosidase or its activator, saposin A (in late onset cases), leads to accumulation of globoid cells (altered macrophages), which causes astrocytic gliosis and (parieto-occipital) **central and peripheral demyelination.** Features are **spasticity with areflexia,** ataxia, dementia, and optic atrophy with vision loss. Isolated spastic paraparesis may occur in adult onset cases. Perivascular PAS-positive **ballooned or globoid multinucleated macrophages** due to cerebroside accumulation are diagnostic.

Galactosialidosis (β-Galactosidase *and* Neuraminidase Deficiencies)

Types I and II are also known as **sialidosis** and develop only with neuraminidase deficiency. The adult, type I, form presents in the fourth decade with gait impairment, myoclonus (with or without seizures), and **decreased color vision** with night blindness. Key findings include **cherry-red spot,** nystagmus, and hyperreflexia. The infantile or type II form has a classic mucopolysaccharidosis phenotype with developmental regression, hepatosplenomegaly, severe dysostosis multiplex, deafness, ataxia, and **cherry-red spot.** The juvenile or type III form, common in Japan, shows skeletal dysplasia, dysmorphism, corneal clouding, cherry-red spots, and **angiokeratomatous rash in the buttocks** and inguinal regions. **Urinary oligosaccharides** are increased.

> **Cherry-red spot in order of frequency:** (1) sialidosis (cherry-red spot-myoclonus); (2) Tay-Sachs disease (GM_2 gangliosidosis); (3) β-galactosidosis (GM_1 gangliosidosis); (4) Niemann-Pick disease; (5) Gaucher disease, infantile; and (6) metachromatic leukodystrophy.

Lysosomal Disorders: Mucopolysaccharidoses

Lysosomal storage disorders are due to a deficiency of enzymes needed to break down glycosaminoglycans, which include heparan sulfate, dermatan sulfate, keratan sulfate, chondroitin sulfate, and hyaluronan. Quantitative glycosaminoglycans in urine with electrophoresis is preferred for diagnosis over the low sensitive screening for urinary mucopolysaccharides. Radiologic findings of dysostosis multiplex are characteristic.

Mucopolysaccharidosis Type I (Hurler Syndrome)

Deficiency of α-L-iduronidase causes accumulation and excretion of dermatan sulfate and heparan sulfate in the cornea, collagen, and leptomeninges. After a normal birth, slow developmental regression occurs after 2 years of age. The **Hurler phenotype** consists of dwarfism, macroglossia, coarse facial features, **corneal clouding,** deafness, dysostosis multiplex, psychomotor retardation, abdominal hernia, stiff joints, and visceromegaly. There may be **macrocephaly** with **prominent perivascular or Virchow-Robin spaces** and communicating hydrocephalus likely related to a **thick dura. Scheie's syndrome** is an allelic disorder with a mild Hurler's phenotype.

Mucopolysaccharidosis Type II (Hunter Syndrome)

The only **X-linked mucopolysaccharidosis** is due to deficiency of iduronate-2--sulfatase and begins in childhood rather than infancy and progresses slower than Hurler syndrome. Blindness is due to **retinal degeneration instead of corneal clouding.**

Mucopolysaccharidosis Type III (Sanfilippo Syndrome)

Deficiency of α-N-acetyl-glucosaminidase causes only visceral accumulation of heparan sulfate. Despite profound mental retardation, aggressiveness, and hyperactivity, there are **relatively mild or no somatic features** other than hirsutism and synophrys. Deafness and seizures may occur.

Mucopolysaccharidosis Type IV (Morquio Syndrome)

Deficiency of α-N-acetyl-glucosamine-6-sulfatase causes visceral accumulation of keratan sulfate. Unlike other mucopolysaccharidoses, intelligence is preserved and short stature is caused by short-trunk dwarfism. The source of visual loss is **corneal clouding. Cervical cord compression** is the most severe complication: hypoplasia of the odontoid causes **atlantoaxial subluxation and instability.**

Mucopolysaccharidosis Type VI (Maroteaux-Lamy Syndrome)

Deficiency of **arylsulfatase B** causes accumulation and excretion of dermatan sulfate. Patients have the typical Hurler phenotype but with normal intelligence. **Hydrocephalus** may result from **pachymeningitis** and **myelopathy** from dural thickening or vertebral abnormalities.

> **Dysostosis multiplex** of certain storage disorders (mucopolysaccharidoses, mannosidosis, mucolipidosis, fucosidosis, sialidosis type II, galactosialidosis) consists of thickened calvarium, large skull, abnormally shaped teeth, anterior breaking of the lumbar vertebrae, enlarged diaphysis of long bones, thick clavicles, oar-shaped ribs, among other skeletal defects.

Porphyrias

The porphyrias are a group of disorders with **defects in heme biosynthesis** that result in cutaneous signs, neuropsychiatric signs, or both. Heme causes feedback inhibition of δ-**aminolevulinic acid (ALA) synthetase,** the first enzyme in the heme synthetic pathway.

Acute intermittent porphyria (AIP), inherited in an autosomal dominant fashion, is caused by **mutations in the porphobilinogen deaminase gene** (PBG-D, 11q), limiting the enzyme activity by at least 50%. However, 90% of individuals with the enzyme deficiency never have any clinical symptoms. **ALA and PBG** are highly excreted in urine.

Symptoms of AIP can be similar to those of lead poisoning (lead is an inhibitor of δ-aminolevulinic acid dehydratase), in which ALA excretion increases without comparable excretion of PBG. Symptoms include a predominantly axonal motor peripheral neuropathy, which may mimic the **Guillain-Barré syndrome** (without much protein elevation in CSF) also affecting the radial and peroneal nerves, and autonomic abnormalities, particularly hypertension and tachycardia. **Epilepsy** may occur and treatment with AED may worsen the picture. **Psychiatric** symptoms may range from delirium, mood change, anxiety, depression, or an acute or chronic psychosis, which can lead to the misdiagnosis of conversion disorder. Gastrointestinal symptoms due to **autonomic neuropathy** include abdominal pain (which may lead to unnecessary abdominal surgeries), vomiting, constipation, and diarrhea. These may occur alone or in combination with neurologic or psychiatric symptoms. A number of inductors and triggers of AIP are known, among them:

Inductors of ALA synthetase	Environmental triggers
Barbiturates	Menses
Antiepileptic drugs	Pregnancy
Analgesics	Starvation
Sulfonamides	Emotional stress
Sedatives	Intercurrent infections
Birth control pills	Smoking

Screening is facilitated by qualitative urinary PBG measurement and diagnosis is established using the **Watson-Schwartz** test for quantitative measurement of urinary PBG and ALA. The most reliable test is assay of PBG-deaminase in RBC membranes. Pathologically, demyelinating lesions of central and peripheral nervous system may be found. **Treatment** consists of a combination of **propranolol** (up to 100 mg every 4 hours may be needed), which may reverse autonomic manifestations, **hematin,** used for neuropathy and abdominal symptoms, **diazepam** (perhaps GBP) as the only AED that does not worsen or trigger AIP attacks, **codeine** and **meperidine** for pain, and **chlorpromazine** for psychotic bouts.

Dopamine and Catecholamine Metabolic Disorders

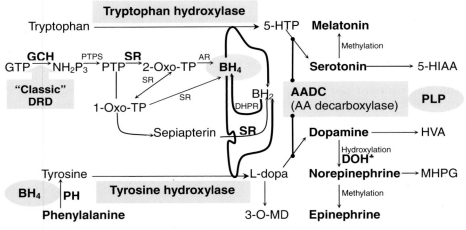

BH$_4$, tetrahydro**biopterin**; GCH-1, GTP cyclohydrolase; NH$_2$P$_3$, dihydro**neopterin** triphosphate; PTP, 6-Pyruvoyl-tetrahydropterin; PTPS, PTP synthase (deficiency: high neopterin to biopterin ratios); SR, sepiapterin reductase; AR, aldose reductase. DHPR, dihydropteridin reductase (deficiency: high BH$_2$, low BH$_4$); PH, phenylalanine hydroxylase; PLP, pyridoxal phosphate or pyridoxine (B$_6$), cofactor of AADC. **Residual tyrosine hydroxylase** (TH) activity is predictive of the predominance of dystonia (high TH activity) or parkinsonism (low TH activity) in biogenic amine disorders.
   ⁺DOH, dopamine hydroxylase deficiency causes disabling orthostatic hypotension and congenital ptosis.

Inborn errors in biopterin synthesis and AADC produce both serotonin and catecholamine deficiencies. Tetrahydrobiopterin (BH$_4$) production is important as it serves as a cofactor for tyrosine, tryptophan, and phenylalanine hydroxylases.

- **GCH1 deficiency:** low CSF biopterin and neopterin, low HVA and HIAA
- **Tyrosine hydroxylase deficiency:** low CSF HVA, normal HIAA and biopterin
- **Tryptophan hydroxylase deficiency:** low HIAA, normal HVA and biopterin
- **AADC deficiency:** low HVA/HIAA, high 3-O-MD/5-HTP, normal biopterin
- **Parkin gene mutation:** low CSF biopterin, normal neopterin

The first four are dopamine-responsive disorders of biogenic amines (*DRD*, often with a dystonia phenotype). The latter can masquerade as DRD.

Catecholamine Deficiency	Dopamine Deficiency (mostly from GCH-1 mutation or TH deficiency)
Ptosis and miosis	*Oculogyric crises*
BP liability and postural hypotension	Parkinsonism, dystonia, and tremor
Paroxysmal diaphoresis, salivation, and temperature instability	Axial hypotonia with limb hypertonia with paroxysmal dystonia (mostly in AADC)

Other causes of oculogyric crisis (besides biopterin disorders) are postencephalitic parkinsonism, Japanese B encephalitis, Wilson's disease, iatrogenic (phenothiazines, organophosphates, and antiepileptic drugs such as carbamazepine), Chediak-Higashi syndrome, putaminal hemorrhage, and pantothenate kinase-associated neurodegeneration.

Norepinephrine System

The locus ceruleus (LC), in the dorsolateral pontine tegmentum, is the major cluster of norepinephrine (NE)-synthesizing neurons, projecting diffusely to throughout the CNS. The NE system has a major role in arousal, attention, and stress response. In the brain, NE also contributes to long-term potentiation, pain modulation, and control of local blood flow.

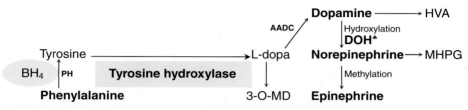

BH4, tetrahydro**biopterin**; PH, phenylalanine hydroxylase; AADC, aminoacid decarboxylase.
  *DOH, dopamine hydroxylase deficiency causes disabling orthostatic hypotension and congenital ptosis.

The main mechanism of NE inactivation is its presynaptic reuptake via a selective NE transporter, followed by metabolism by monoamine oxidase A (MAO-A) and catechol-O-methyltransferase (COMT), with formation of 3-methoxy-4-hydroxyphenylglycol (MHPG), measurable in CSF.

Mechanisms to Increase NE	Examples
Decrease presynaptic reuptake	Cocaine, tricyclics, amphetamines
Decrease postsynaptic reuptake (COMT)	Tolcapone, entacapone
Inhibit MAO-A	Clorgyline
Inhibit MAO-B	Selegiline (Deprenyl)
Inhibit both MAO-A and -B (nonselective)	Pargyline
Block NE vesicle storage	Reserpine, tetrabenazine
Block tyrosine hydroxylase	α-methyltyrosine

Adrenergic Receptors (and Blockers)

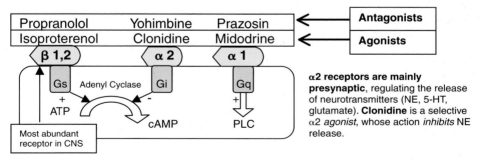

α2 receptors are mainly presynaptic, regulating the release of neurotransmitters (NE, 5-HT, glutamate). **Clonidine** is a selective α2 agonist, whose action inhibits NE release.

The striatum contains high concentrations of **α2c receptors** in dopaminergic terminals. Idazoxan, an α2c antagonist, may reduce L-dopa-induced dyskinesias in Parkinson's disease.

Serotonin System

Serotonin (5-hydroxytryptamine, 5-HT) has an important neuromodulatory action mediated by a large variety of 5-HT receptor subtypes. The central serotonergic system has been implicated in cognition, emotion, impulse control, circadian and sleep-wake cycle regulation, and pain modulation. The raphe nuclei provide 5-HT inputs to the **basal ganglia circuits** and prefrontal cortex. 5-HT is degraded by **MAO-A** to 5-hydroxy indole acetic acid (**5-HIAA**).

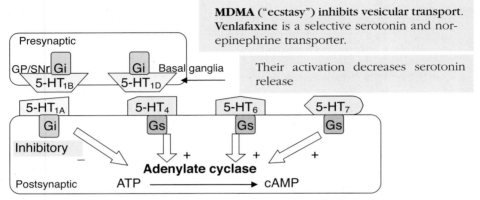

MDMA ("ecstasy") inhibits vesicular transport. Venlafaxine is a selective serotonin and norepinephrine transporter.

Their activation decreases serotonin release

5-HT_{1B-1D} receptors inhibit glutamate and GABA release in all basal ganglia circuits.

Receptors	Location	Agonist	Antagonist
5-HT_{1A}	Hippocampus Raphe nucleus	Buspirone (partial) Sarizotan (full)	
5-HT_{1B-1D}		Sumatriptan	
5-HT_{1C}	Choroid plexus Limbic system		
5-HT_{2A-2C}	Frontal cortex Hippocampus	Lysergic acid diethylamide (LSD)	Trazodone Nefazodone Mirtazapine Risperidone Quetiapine Olanzapine
In animal models, **5-HT_{2c} receptor antagonists** potentiate the antiparkinsonian action of D2 agonists and improve the related dyskinesias.			
5-HT_3	Area postrema Entorhinal cortex	Dopamine agonists	Ondansetron Granisetron Antiemetics

With the exception of 5-HT_3-receptors, which are cation channels that elicit fast depolarization, all 5-HT-receptor families are members of the G protein-coupled receptor superfamily. The most abundant are the 5-HT_1 and 5-HT_2 receptors.

Combined treatment with 5-HT_{1A} and 5-HT_{1B} receptors receptor agonists or mixed 5-HT_{2A-2C} antagonists synergistically reduces dyskinesia induced by chronic L-dopa in animal models.

Electrolyte Derangements

Hypernatremia (Serum Na$^+$ >145 mmol/L)

The hypertonic hyperosmolality of hypernatremia causes cellular dehydration. Extreme ages are most vulnerable. Encephalopathy ranges from drowsiness to coma, and may include seizures, *hyper*reflexia, rigidity (even opisthotonos), tremor, chorea, or myoclonus.

Pure Water Loss	Hypotonic Fluid Loss	Hypertonic Na$^+$ Gain
Diabetes insipidus Neurogenic (TB, hystiocytosis, tumors sarcoidosis, trauma)▲ Nephrogenic (renal disease or drugs)▲	Diuretic excess Vomiting, diarrhea NG drainage enterocutaneous fistula Excessive sweating Burns	Na+ bicarbonate infusion Hypertonic feedings Hypertonic saline enemas Na$^+$ chloride Primary hyperaldosteronism Cushing's syndrome
Changes in the intra- and extra-cellular fluid compartments		
Equal extra- and intracellular fluid loss	Relatively larger extracellular fluid loss	Increase in extracellular fluid, decrease in intracellular fluid

▲Nephrogenic DI can be induced by hypercalcemia, hypokalemia, lithium, demeclocycline, foscarnet, methoxyflurane, and amphotericin B. Neurogenic DI can be caused by Guillain-Barré syndrome, ethanol ingestion, meningitis, encephalitis, and aneurysms.

Brain shrinkage induced by hypernatremia can cause hemorrhagic events (ICH, SDH, or SAH; intraventricular hemorrhage in neonates). The brain adaptive response, or "osmoprotection," includes the accumulation of electrolytes (rapid adaptation, hours) and organic osmolytes, such as taurine and glutamine (slow adaptation, days) that do not reverse the hyperosmolality. **Rapid correction of the hypertonic state may lead to cerebral edema** (and seizures, coma, and death) as the accumulated electrolytes and solutes cannot be rapidly dissipated. Slow correction of hypernatremia (0.5 mmol/L/h or 10 mmol/L/d) is preferred.▲

Rapid correction of hyponatremic patients may lead to brain shrinkage and **central pontine myelinolysis** (CPM). To maintain cell volume, brain cells take up Na$^+$, K$^+$, and Cl$^-$ first, and then organic osmolytes, such as myoinositol and amino acids. These organic osmolytes are protective against damages to proteins or DNA from increased ion strength within cells. The regions with the least ability to reaccumulate organic osmolytes, such as the central pons, the basal ganglia, and cerebellum, are the areas most vulnerable to developing the oligodendrocyte and myelin loss with relative preservation of neurons typical of CPM. The more severe and chronic the hyponatremia, and the faster the correction rate, the likelier it becomes that CPM may develop. It rarely occurs when Na$^+$ >120 mmol/L and the hyponatremia is acute in onset.

▲Hypotonic fluids are used (Na$^+$ per infusate in parenthesis): 5% dextrose (0), 0.2% NaCl (34), 0.45% NaCl (77), and Ringer's lactate (130). Each infusate changes the serum Na$^+$ according to the following formula: Na$^+$ change = ([infusate Na$^+$ - serum Na$^+$] ÷ [total body water + 1])

Hyponatremia (Serum Na$^+$ <136 mmol/L)

Hyponatremia, mainly caused by the nonosmotic release of vasopressin, induces **brain edema and secondary intracranial hypertension.** The chronic adaptive response includes releasing intracellular K$^+$ (rapid adaptation) and organic osmolytes (slow adaptation), which do not reverse the hypotonic hypo-osmolality. Rapid correction of the hypotonic state may lead to brain shrinkage and osmotic demyelination or myelinolysis of pontine or extrapontine neurons that can cause quadriplegia, pseudobulbar palsy, seizures, coma, and death. Slow correction of hyponatremia (8–10 mmol/L/d) is always preferred.[♦] Too slow a correction, however, may lead to death from brain edema. Unlike hypernatremia, *hypo*reflexia and muscle cramps are often present.

Impaired Renal Water Excretion		Excessive Water Intake
Extracellular Fluid Loss	**Normovolemic**	Psychogenic polydipsia
Diuretic excess	**SIADH**: cancer, CNS infections,	Dilute infant formula
Adrenal insufficiency	surgery, trauma, stroke, drugs	Exercise-induced (EIH):
Renal tubular acidosis	(desmopressin, oxytocin, tricyclics	excessive water intake
Diarrhea, vomiting	phenothiazines, SSRIs, opiates, CBZ,	
Third spacing	vincristine, cyclophosphamide)	**Hypertonic Hyponatremia**
Excessive vomiting	Hypothyroidism	
	Adrenal insufficiency	**Hyperglycemia**
Extracellular Fluid Gain	Thiazide diuretics	Hypertonic mannitol
		Hyperlipidemia (lab artifact[*])
CHF, **cirrhosis, nephrotic**		Hyperproteinemia (lab artifact[*])
syndrome, renal failure,		[*]:'pseudohyponatremia'
pregnancy		

Hyperglycemia: an increase of 100 mg/dL in serum glucose decreases serum Na$^+$ by about 1.7 mmol/L with a rise in serum osmolality of ~2.0 mOsm/kg water; **SIADH**: syndrome of inappropriate secretion of antidiuretic hormone is a common cause of hyponatremia (other common causes in bold, above).

- Water restriction is indicated in patients with symptomatic hyponatremia *and* dilute urine (osmolality <200 mOsm/kg water).
- Hypertonic fluids (and furosemide) are used when symptoms are severe or when urine is concentrated *and* the patient is eu- or hypervolemic.
- Demeclocycline (600-1,200 mg/d) helps in chronic SIADH by inducing a nephrogenic DI in those who fail increased Na$^+$ intake and furosemide.
- Conivaptan is a vasopressin receptor antagonist recommended for euvolemic hyponatremia.

SIADH results from failure to suppress the secretion of antidiuretic hormone (ADH), arginine vasopressin, and from the neurohypophysis, despite normal or increased plasma volume. Anorexia, nausea, and vomiting are followed by headache, blurred vision, lethargy, disorientation, irritability, and muscle cramps. There may be *hypo*reflexia, abnormal sensorium, and seizures. Natriuresis without maximally diluted urine (250-1,400 mOsm/kg) develops.

[♦]Fluids are used depending on tonicity (Na$^+$ per infusate in parenthesis): 5% NaCl (855), 3% NaCl (513), 0.9% NaCl (154), Ringer's lactate (130), 0.45% NaCl (77), 0.2% NaCl (34), and 5% dextrose (0). The same formula applies for calculations. Hypertonic saline is usually combined with furosemide diuresis (equivalent to one-half isotonic saline solution) to avoid treatment-induced expansion of the extracellular volume.

Hypokalemia

Generalized weakness, predominantly **proximal,** is the common outcome of hypokalemia that results from gastrointestinal or renal loss, often induced by drugs. An **ascending paralysis** with respiratory involvement that **spares facial muscles and muscle stretch reflexes** occurs when K^+ is <2.0 mmol/L. **CK** begins to increase when the K^+ level falls below 3.0 mmol/L (rhabdomyolysis). Digoxin toxicity is increased by hypokalemia. **Tetany is seen during alkalosis,** which decreases ionized calcium by binding calcium to proteins. Paradoxically, when hypocalcemia is present, hypokalemia protects against tetany. **Correction of hypokalemia can precipitate hypocalcemic tetany. Magnesium** deficiency causes reduced intracellular K^+ (impaired Na^+/K^+-ATPase) and renal K^+ wasting.

Transcellular Shift	Increased Renal Loss
β2-sympathomimetics (albuterol, terbutaline, metaproterenol, ephedrine, pseudoephedrine, phenylpropanolamine) **xanthines** (theophylline, caffeine), verapamil intoxication, chloroquine intoxication, **insulin overdose**	**Diuretics** (acetazolamide, thiazides, furosemide), mineralocorticoids (fludrocortisone), high-dose penicillin and **glucocorticoids** **Through Mg^+ depletion:** cisplatin, aminoglycosides, amphotericin B
Disorders: **hyperthyroidism**, familial hypokalemic periodic paralysis, high-epinephrine conditions	**Metabolic alkalosis** due to vomiting, hyperaldosteronism, and Cushing's distal renal tubular acidosis

K^+ replacement should be given at a rate ≤20 mmol/h in glucose-free solutions with cardiac monitoring. **Potassium chloride (KCl)** is the most suitable salt for repletion of the common forms of hypokalemia, but K^+ bicarbonate ($KHCO_3$) and K^+ phosphate (KPO_4) are used in acidosis and hypophosphatemia, respectively. KPO_4 may lead to phosphorus intoxication, which reduces calcium and causes **hypocalcemic tetany. Mg^+ replacement** alone may correct hypokalemia.

Hyperkalemia

Weakness, either episodic or progressive, almost universally occurs when K^+ exceeds 9 mmol/L, associated with a sensation of **burning paresthesias.** Even when **flaccid quadriplegia** with respiratory involvement develops, the cranial nerves are spared. **Hyporeflexia** is common. Neurologic deficits without cardiac conduction defects only occur when hypercalcemia (antidysrhythmic) is present. Hyperkalemia results from **metabolic acidosis,** renal failure, **insulin deficiency** (diabetic ketoacidosis), **adrenal insufficiency,** crush injuries (rhabdomyolysis), and drugs (K^+-sparing diuretics, NSAIDs, beta-blockers, and digoxin intoxication).

Calcium chloride or **calcium gluconate** prevents cardiac arrhythmias, whereas alkalinizing agents such as **sodium bicarbonate** are used to shift K^+ from the extra- to the intracellular compartment. **Insulin with glucose** is administered to facilitate the cellular uptake of K^+. **Sodium polystyrene sulfonate (Kayexalate)** and other binding resins promote exchange of potassium for sodium in the GI system. In mild hyperkalemia, **furosemide** is used to enhance excretion.

Hypocalcemia

The manifestations are both peripheral in the form of **tetany** (from carpopedal spasm and trismus to opisthotonos and respiratory compromise) and central as **encephalopathy** with **seizures** from **intracranial hypertension. Chvostek's sign** (facial contraction after facial nerve percussion) and **Trousseau's sign** (tetany induced by inflating the blood pressure cuff 20 mm Hg above systolic pressure) demonstrate hypocalcemia-induced peripheral nerve irritability.

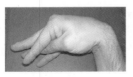

Carpopedal spasm

Tetany applies to painful finger contractions resulting in thumb adduction, metacarpophalangeal flexion, and interphalangeal finger extension, which may be confused with dystonia. It is associated with **hypocalcemia** as well as **hypomagnesemia, hypokalemic alkalosis,** and **respiratory alkalosis.**

In **hypomagnesemia,** magnesium should be replaced before calcium, and the underlying cause of the low magnesium explored (in the presence of metabolic acidosis, conversely, calcium must be corrected before correcting the acidosis). In the absence of hypomagnesemia, parathyroid hormone (PTH) must be checked. If PTH is low or inappropriately normal, the patient has **hypoparathyroidism** (autoimmune [polyglandular failure syndrome], surgical, or congenital [DiGeorge syndrome], which may include **basal ganglia calcification**). If PTH is high, serum phosphorus should be checked next: if low, **vitamin D deficiency or resistance** (rickets) is suspected; if high, **pseudohypoparathyroidism** (sporadic or autosomal dominant [Albright's osteodystrophy]), rhabdomyolysis, tumor lysis syndrome, renal insufficiency, and phosphate ingestion must be investigated. For acute cases, **calcium gluconate** 10–30 mL of 10% IV can be given over 10 minutes. After 2 hours continuous IV infusion should be started if the ionized calcium level is low, at 0.5 mg/kg/h (moderate) or 1–1.5 mg/kg/h (severe hypocalcemia). Calcium administration may precipitate digitalis toxicity in patients on digoxin whose digitalis level are high. Other causes are **hypoalbuminemia,*** acute pancreatitis, and drugs: **phenobarbital,** alcohol, **phenytoin,** carbamazepine, foscarnet, cimetidine, and aluminum.

Hypercalcemia

A wide range of **changes in consciousness** (from drowsiness to coma) with associated depression or anxiety and myoclonus and rigidity can be seen in hypercalcemia. **Proximal weakness** and **hyperreflexia** are features of chronic hypercalcemia. Vasospasm may induce **strokes.** The usual etiologies are primary hyperparathyroidism, hyperthyroidism, **malignancy, sarcoidosis,** adrenal insufficiency, and vitamin D intoxication. Drugs capable of increasing calcium are thiazides, calcium carbonate (antacid), lithium, and theophylline.

Biphosphonates (pamidronate, etidronate) prevent osteoclast recruitment and viability; **calcitonin** inhibits bone resorption and enhances calcium excretion.

---

* In **hypoalbuminemia**, the most common cause of hypocalcemia, calcium levels may appear normal. Corrected calcium (mg/dL) = measured total Ca (mg/dL) + 0.8 (4.4 – serum albumin [g/dL]). EKG may reveal prolonged QT interval. False hypocalcemia can be seen with heparin, oxalate, citrate, or hyperbilirubinemia.

Hypomagnesemia

Tetany with Chvostek's and Trousseau's signs occur either directly or by reducing ionized calcium levels. CNS effects are mainly **seizures,** confusion, delirium, or coma. **Hyperreflexia,** tremor, chorea, and **startle responses with myoclonus** have been described. Common etiologies are **parenteral nutrition,** acute tubular necrosis, hypoparathyroidism, hyperthyroidism, and hyperaldosteronism.

Hypermagnesemia

Weakness and hyporeflexia are seen between levels of 7-9 mmol/L and **areflexia** is the hallmark of $Mg^+ \geq 9$ mmol/L. The **decreased neuromuscular excitability** is due to displacement of calcium by magnesium at the NMJ. Respiratory failure is a potential development. **There are no CNS effects,** confirmed by the lack of epileptic or cognitive symptoms. **Iatrogenic magnesium,** contained in **antacids** and **laxatives** or given during the **treatment of eclampsia,** is required for the neurologic deficits to appear. Hypermagnesemia may worsen neuromuscular diseases such as Lambert-Eaton myasthenic syndrome and myasthenia gravis.

> **Acute flaccid areflexic paralysis with respiratory insufficiency** can occur in **hypermagnesemia and hypophosphatemia**. Untreated **hyperkalemia** may cause chronic flaccid quadriplegia. (Hypokalemia and hypercalcemia lead to hyperreflexic weakness.)

Hypophosphatemia

Peripheral neurologic symptoms of hypophosphatemia begin when the levels fall below 1 mg/dL (**acute areflexic paralysis** with diaphragmatic, pharyngeal, facial, and extraocular weakness preceded by perioral paresthesias) and central deficits are added when phosphate is <0.5 mg/dL (**hypophosphatemic encephalopathy can mimic Wernicke's encephalopathy:** seizures, tremor, ataxia, nystagmus, bilateral abducens palsy). Myonecrosis and **rhabdomyolysis** are felt to be the basis of alcoholic myopathy. As iatrogenic as hypermagnesemia, low phosphate arises in the setting of **hyperalimentation,** hemodialysis, **hyperparathyroidism,** respiratory alkalosis, aluminum-containing antacids, and **glucose load** in alcoholic or starved patients.

Hyperphosphatemia is invariably associated with the clinical features of hypocalcemia. Other pathways leading to ↓Ca are summarized as follows (derangements in potassium and hypermagnesemia do not affect the CNS):

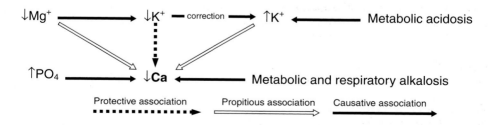

Voltage-Gated Channels (Ionic Interaction)

Channels open in response to alterations of the membrane permeability or conductance, which depends on transmembrane potential. In the resting state, all voltage-gated sodium channels (VGNC) are closed and permeability is very low, with a slight inward leak extruded by the Na^+/K^+ ATPase pump. Since enough voltage-gated potassium channels (VGKC) are open, the resting permeability is greater to potassium (K^+) than to sodium (Na^+) by a factor of 50–100. Hence, the equilibrium potential for K^+ determines the resting potential.

Sodium channels allow quick Na^+ influx to depolarize the membrane to reach a new equilibrium potential of about +60 mV. Its closing begins the end of depolarization and begins the refractory period. **Tetrodotoxin** (from puffer fish) and **saxitoxin** (from shellfish) block the Na^+ channels.

> **Related channelopathies:** Hyperkalemic periodic paralysis (HyperPP) and paramyotonia congenital (PMC).

Potassium channels open later than the Na^+ channels but remain open longer (VGKC activation/deactivation is ~10 times slower than VGNC). K^+ efflux repolarizes and hyperpolarizes at the end of the action potential. The Ca^+-activated K^+ channels are both voltage- and ligand-gated and open when Ca^+ ions bind to the cytoplasmic side. Acetylcholine controls neuronal excitability via regulation of the Kv7 potassium channels. **Tetraethyl ammonium chloride** blocks the slow K^+ channels, and **4-aminopyridine** blocks the fast K^+ channels.

> **Related channelopathy:** Episodic ataxia type 1. VGKC are functionally blocked by antibodies (paraneoplastic neuromyotonia) and by **dendrotoxin** (eastern green mamba snake venom peptide).

Calcium channels exist in three types: **T** (low threshold), in the inferior olive for oscillatory behavior; **L** (high threshold), slowly inactivating (site of action of calcium channel blocker drugs); and **N** (high threshold), transient. The **α-2-δ subunit (A2d) of the voltage-gated calcium channels** (VGCC), which regulates release of nociceptive neurotransmitters at the dorsal root entry zone, is antagonized by **conotoxin,** from venomous marine cone snails, and its synthetic derivative **ziconotide,** helping control neuropathic pain. This A2d antagonism is part of the mechanism of action of **gabapentin and pregabalin.**

> **Related channelopathies:** Hypokalemic periodic paralysis (HypoPP) and episodic ataxia type 2.

Depolarization spreads *electrotonically* (passively) in the dendrites and soma but by *saltatory* conduction after the axon hillock (where the action potential is most likely to begin its course down the axon due to the high density of voltage-gated Na^+ channels present there).

Channelopathies in Muscle Disease

Skeletal muscle was the first tissue on which hereditary diseases caused by ion channel defects, the periodic paralysis (PP), and myotonias were described. Several other diseases are now included in the classification of channelopathies.

Sodium Channels (Autosomal Dominant; SCN4A, 17q)

- **Hyperkalemic periodic paralysis (HyperKPP)** manifests in the first decade of life as frequent but brief attacks of weakness for 15-60 minutes, often precipitated by resting after vigorous exercise, potassium intake, and stress. **Myotonia of eyelids and limbs** is present between attacks. Progressive vacuolar myopathy develops over time. Respiratory muscles are spared.
- **Paramyotonia congenita (PMC)** is characterized by myotonia during or after exercise or exposure to cold. Interictally, **facial, eyelid, and pharyngeal myotonia** may be present. EMG shows myotonic activity and decreased CMAP amplitudes with muscle cooling.
- **Potassium-aggravated myotonia** is not affected by cold exposure.

Chloride Channels (Autosomal Dominant and Recessive; CLCN1, 7q)

- **Myotonia congenita** (AD: **Thomsen disease;** AR: **Becker myotonia**) results in attacks of myotonia triggered by forceful muscle contraction after a period of rest. With repeated contractions (**warm-up phenomenon**) the myotonia is reduced. **Mexiletine** is the treatment of choice.

Calcium Channels (Autosomal Dominant; CACNL1A3, 1q)

- **Hypokalemic periodic paralysis type 1 (HypoKPP),** the most common PP (~1:100,000), leads to transient flaccid weakness in voluntary muscles except facial and respiratory. Attacks of hours (up to days) occur on awakening after vigorous exercise or a carbohydrate-rich meal. Onset is always before the age of 30 years. **Suspect thyrotoxicosis if onset is after age 30.** Symptoms can be **induced by glucose,** glucagon, or epinephrine challenges. Permanent proximal weakness eventually develops due to vacuolar myopathy.
- **Malignant hyperthermia (ryanodine receptor 1 [RyR1], 19q)** consists of extreme muscle rigidity, rhabdomyolysis, and hyperthermia caused by halogenated volatile anesthetics and depolarizing muscle relaxants.
- **Central core disease (RyR1, allelic to, and may evolve into, MH)** causes nonprogressive muscular weakness and a floppy-infant syndrome with hip displacement and scoliosis. Central cores are seen on muscle biopsy.

> K^+ **and glucose** have opposite effects in the PP: K^+ **triggers a hyperKPP attack** and glucose administration is the remedy; **glucose triggers a hypoKPP attack** and K^+ administration is the remedy.

Andersen-Tawil syndrome (ATS, KCNJ2, 17q) presents in the first decade of life with the triad of PP, ventricular ectopy (including long QT interval), and skeletal abnormalities (hypertelorism, small mandible, clinodactyly, low-set ears).

Channelopathies in Epilepsy

Potassium Channels

Benign familial neonatal seizures (BFNS) arise in previously normal neonates on the **second or third day of life** and **remit spontaneously by 6 weeks.** These are focal motor seizures that secondarily generalize, associated with apnea, cyanosis, and staring. Development and intellectual outcome is usually normal, but there is a small risk for later epilepsy with good response to AEDs. BFNS show **autosomal dominant inheritance with high penetrance.** Slow K$^+$ channel dysfunction is the pathogenic mechanism, due to mutations in **KCNQ2 (20q)** and **KCNQ3 (8q)** encoding the voltage-gated potassium channel subunits Kv7.2 and Kv7.3. These form the heteromeric channel responsible for the slow M current, which regulates subthreshold electrical excitability of neurons. **KCNQ2 and KCNQ3 are brain-specific; KCNQ1 is heart-specific** (long QT syndrome; Jervell and Lang-Nielsen syndrome applies to congenital deafness and long QT interval).

Sodium Channels

Generalized epilepsy with febrile seizures plus (GEFS+), also termed autosomal dominant epilepsy with febrile seizure plus (ADEFS+), applies to **febrile seizures occurring *after* age 6 years** or afebrile generalized seizures of tonic-clonic, absence, myoclonic, and atonic types. Most children have benign, spontaneously remitting epilepsies and normal development, but some may have more severe phenotypes such as myoclonic-astatic epilepsy or Dravet syndrome. GEFS+ results from mutations in *SCN1B* (encodes β_1-subunit of the voltage-gated sodium channel), *SCN1A* (the α_1-subunit), or *GABRG2* (the γ_2-subunit of the GABA$_A$ receptor).

Severe myoclonic epilepsy in infancy (SMEI, Dravet syndrome) is a rare epileptic syndrome affecting 1 in 40,000 children **before 1 year of age,** consisting of generalized or unilateral febrile clonic, evolving into myoclonic, seizures and subsequent psychomotor retardation and ataxia. Interictal EEG is initially normal, but over time it shows generalized (poly)spike-and-waves, focal abnormalities, and photosensitivity. VPA and TPM may be helpful, whereas **LTG and CBZ may exacerbate seizures**. About 70%–80% of children with Dravet syndrome have *SCN1A* loss-of-function mutations (deletions), mostly *de novo*. The same voltage-gated sodium channel subunit, *SCN1A,* can express as clinically distinct syndromes in GEFS+ and SMEI.

Nicotinic Channel

Autosomal dominant nocturnal frontal lobe epilepsy (ADNFLE) is characterized by clusters of brief tonic and hyperkinetic motor seizures occurring mostly during non-REM sleep in childhood. ADNFLE is frequently misdiagnosed as sleep disorder, paroxysmal nocturnal dystonia, or night terror. Secondary generalization can occur, but most patients remain conscious throughout their seizures. Response to antiepileptic drugs for partial epilepsy is positive. ADNFLE is associated with mutations in *CHRNA4* (α4-subunit) and *CHRNB2* (β2-subunit). These subunits are components of a common neuronal nicotinic acetylcholine receptor.

Gamma-Aminobutyric Acid (GABA)

GABA is the most abundant inhibitory neurotransmitter in the brain and major *presynaptic* inhibitor in the spinal cord (main *postsynaptic* inhibitor is **glycine**).

- **GABA$_A$ receptors** are pentameric ionotropic channels that cause **fast inhibitory postsynaptic potential by the influx of Cl$^-$ ions** (fast IPSP). They are activated by *muscinol* and inhibited by *bicuculline* and *picrotoxin* (which cause seizures). **Benzodiazepines** and **steroids** bind to the α subunit, whereas **barbiturates** bind to the β subunit.

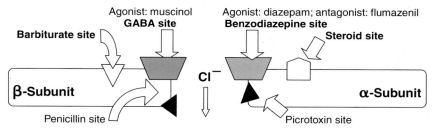

GABA$_A$ receptors are in the hippocampus, striatum, spinal cord, and cerebellar granular layers. GABA$_A$ receptor-dependent inhibition is enhanced in thalamocortical neurons in absence seizures.

- **GABA$_B$ receptors** are metabotropic G-protein channels that cause **slow postsynaptic inhibition by closing Ca$^+$ and opening of K$^+$ channels** (slow IPSP), akin to α-2 adrenergic and D$_2$ dopamine receptors. **Baclofen and gamma-hydroxybutyric** acid bind to **presynaptic** GABA$_B$ receptors.
- **GABA$_C$ receptors** are metabotropic G-protein Cl$^-$ channel restricted to the retina, hippocampus, and neocortex. **Glutamate and 5-HT** bind to **GABA$_C$ receptors,** activate phospholipase C, and result in inhibition of Cl$^-$ influx.

GABA and glutamate are both synthesized and broken down in pathways linked to the citric acid cycle (Krebs cycle). The metabolism and regeneration of the principal inhibitory and excitatory neurotransmitters are intimately linked:

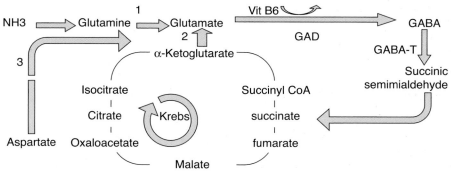

GAD: Glutamic acid decarboxylase
GABA-T: GABA transaminase
1. Glutaminase 2. Glutamate dehydrogenase
3. Aspartate aminotransferase

Anti-GAD antibodies are found in stiff person syndrome. Spasticity is treated with GABA$_B$ agonists, such as baclofen. Valproate (VPA) enhances GABA synthesis and decreases degradation. Vigabatrin and VPA block GABA-T to decrease GABA degradation. Gabatril blocks GABA transporter, involved in reuptake. GABA does not cross the BBB.

Glutamate Receptors

The most abundant CNS excitatory neurotransmitter, glutamate, acts on both **iono-tropic** receptors (NMDA, AMPA, and kainate), which have an intrinsic or directly gated ion channel, and **metabotropic** receptors (mGluR 1–8), which are coupled to G proteins (α, β, and γ subunits).

The NMDA receptor is a high-conductance **cation-channel receptor,** permeable to Na^+/Ca^{2+} (in) and K^+ (out). Mg^{2+}, **Zn, H$^+$,** and **dizolcipine,** all of which have their binding sites, block the channel. Other antagonists include **phencyclidine (PCP),** MK801, and **ketamine.**

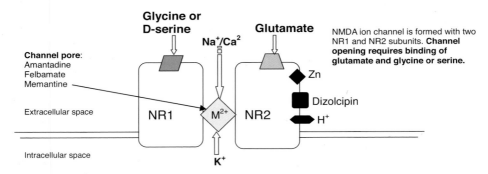

NMDA ion channel is formed with two NR1 and NR2 subunits. **Channel opening requires binding of glutamate and glycine or serine.**

NMDA receptors are ubiquitous but present in amygdala, hypothalamus, prefrontal cortex, and hippocampus in highest densities. The greater permeability of this channel to Ca^{2+} mediates long-term potentiation (LTP), important for learning and memory. **NMDA receptor overstimulation** results in cell death due to excessive intracellular Ca^{2+}. This occurs in the setting of high extracellular glutamate concentration during epilepsy, hypoxemia (stroke, hypotension), and some neurodegenerative conditions (ALS, Huntington's disease). **NMDA receptor understimulation** (such as with PCP or due to anti-NMDA receptor encephalitis) produces psychotic behavior, abnormal movements (rigidity, dystonia, orofacial movements), and autonomic dysfunction (cardiac dysrhythmia, hypertension, hypersalivation).

Kainate-quisqualate-A (AMPA) are cation-channel receptors permeable to Na+ and K+, typical of fast excitatory synapses, which mediate precise information (where, what, and when). They are located mainly in the forebrain and are the main source of EPSPs in the CNS (seizurogenic). AMPA receptors agonized by β-N-oxalyl amino-L-alanine (BOAA) can lead to lathyrism (spastic paraparesis caused by chronic chickpeas ingestion). **The kainate receptors** are localized in primary afferent C-fibers in the spinal cord.

The indirectly gated (metabotropic) mGluR1-8 receptors, coupled to second messengers cAMP and PLC, are involved in synaptic plasticity, learning, memory, and neuroprotection.

Autism Spectrum Disorders

Autism spectrum disorders (ASD) are complex neurodevelopmental disorders characterized by **social impairment** (low empathy, eye-to-eye contact, failure to develop peer relationships), communication or **language delay,** and behavioral deficits in the form of **restricted range of activities** with repetitive and obsessive interests and possibly stereotypies or mannerisms. Key red flags include no babble talk and hand gestures by 12 months, no single words by 16 months, no two-word phrases by 24 months, and any loss of social or language skills. There may be severe attention, anxiety, and depressive symptoms. ASD typically begins before the age of 3 years and comprises the following subtypes:

- **Autistic disorder** represents the most debilitating subtype within ASD.
- **High-functioning autism** (HFA) meets autistic disorder criteria but has an IQ in the average or above-average range of functioning. **Asperger syndrome** is a subgroup of HFA whereby IQ is at or above average, there is less overall symptomatic impairment, and there is no history of language delay.
- **Pervasive developmental disorder not otherwise specified** (PDD-NOS) applies to children who either meet the criteria for autistic disorder with onset of symptoms after the age of 3 years or have less-impairing social, communication, and behavioral deficits, or atypical symptomatology.

ASD affect significantly **more males than females** by a 4:1 ratio with an overall prevalence of almost 60 per 10,000. **PDD-NOS is the most frequent subtype** within ASD. Asperger syndrome occurs less frequently than the two other subtypes. The sibling risk rate for autism is ~4.5%, ten times that of the general population. Monozygotic twins of the same sex are 60% concordant for autism.

Functional neuroimaging studies have shown **increased activity in primary sensory areas** and decreased activity in areas associated with higher cognitive processing, including the orbitofrontal and medial frontal cortex hypofunction. Brain volumes are larger than average by 2–4 years of age (**transient postnatal macrocephaly**), reflecting an enlargement of cerebellar and cerebral white matter and cerebral gray matter. The overgrowth is anteroposterior, with the frontal lobes being the largest, and may reflect a failure of synaptic pruning or an excess of synaptogenesis. There is thinning of the internal capsule and corpus callosum (especially posterior). The **amygdala is enlarged and hyperactive** and the **Purkinje cell count and dendritic branching are low,** which disinhibit the cerebellar deep nuclei and overexcite the thalamus and cerebral cortex.

SSRIs are recommended for social interactions, ritualistic behaviors, aggression and obsessive-compulsive tendencies. Atypical antipsychotics may target depression, irritability, and repetitive, stereotypical behaviors. Stimulants may improve hyperactivity. Mood stabilizers can target affective instability, impulsivity, and aggressive behaviors.

Attention-Deficit Hyperactivity Disorder (ADHD)

ADHD is defined as **developmentally atypical levels of inattention, hyperactivity, and impulsiveness,** starting **prior to 7 years of age.** Many children are restless, inattentive, and impulsive in some settings but do not meet the criteria for ADHD. ADHD applies only when these symptoms are (1) **persistent over time,** (2) present **both at home and at school,** and (3) **impair social, family, or school performance.** ADHD affects about 5% of school-aged children worldwide, predominantly males (3:1 to 8:1). About one-third of ADHD cases have at least one ADHD parent. The risk to first-degree relatives of affected individual is 8-10 times that of the general population. ADHD persists into adolescence in about 30%–50% of affected individuals.

The *DSM-IV-TR* distinguishes two dimensions in the behavior of individuals with ADHD: inattention and hyperactivity/impulsivity. Based on these two dimensions, **three behavioral subtypes are identified:**
- Primarily inattentive
- Primarily hyperactive/impulsive
- Combined inattentive and hyperactive/impulsive

> **For a diagnosis of ADHD,** the patient must present with six or more symptoms of inattention, six or more symptoms of hyperactivity/impulsivity, or both for an inattentive, hyperactive/impulsive, or combined subtype diagnosis.

Associated psychiatric disorders are identified in most children with ADHD. **Conduct disorder** (persistent lying, stealing, or other societal transgressions), and a milder variant, **oppositional defiant disorder** (argumentativeness, stubbornness, and temper outbursts), occur in about 20%–25% of cases. Other comorbidities include anxiety, depression, Tourette's, and learning disabilities. Compared to non-ADHD peers, ADHD children have higher rates of motor vehicle accidents, smoking, and alcohol and drug abuse. **Secondary ADHD** may occur in the setting of traumatic brain injury, autism spectrum disorder, and genetic syndromes such as velocardiofacial syndrome (22q11 deletion).

Stimulant drugs improve concentration and reduce hyperactivity. The commonly used drugs are methylphenidate, dextroamphetamine, and more recently atomoxetine (Strattera) and a mixture of amphetamine and dextroamphetamine (Adderall). **Atomoxetine** has emerged as the treatment of choice for patients who fail to benefit from either methylphenidate or dextroamphetamine or for those with some contraindication to stimulants. **Clonidine,** an α-2 agonist, reduces behavioral symptoms of ADHD and improves the sleep disturbance that may arise with stimulant treatment. **Guanfacine** causes less sedation and hypotension than clonidine and may be effective for children with ADHD and comorbid tic disorder. **Bupropion** is used in treatment-resistant patient but is generally less effective than methylphenidate in improving attention and is contraindicated in patients with a comorbid seizure disorder.

Floppy Infant Syndrome

Due to *supraspinal hypotonia (normoreflexic)*:
- **Prader-Willi syndrome** (1:15,000) is characterized by hypotonia, obesity, minor facial dysmorphism, short stature, mental retardation, and cryptorchidism or hypogonadism. Fluorescence *in situ* hybridization (FISH) detects (70%) a **deletion in paternally derived chromosome 15q** (implying maternal disomy).
- **Oculocerebrorenal syndrome (Lowe syndrome)** is an **X-linked** hypotonic and demyelinating disorder associated with congenital **cataracts and glaucoma** that progresses to mental retardation and renal tubular acidosis, aminoaciduria, and proteinuria.
- **GM$_2$ gangliosidosis**

Peroxisomal disorders
- **Zellweger syndrome (cerebro-hepato-renal syndrome)** is recognized by facial dysmorphism (high forehead with flat facies), **arthrogryposis** (especially camptodactyly and flexion deformities of the knee and ankle), and hepatomegaly. **Cerebral malformations** include hypoplastic corpus callosum, migration abnormalities, pachygyria, and polymicrogyria. Serum studies show **pipecolic acidemia and increased VLCFA**
- **Neonatal adrenoleukodystrophy** (AR inheritance instead of X-linked in the infantile form) is part of the "Zellweger spectrum" with invariable hepatomegaly, retinitis pigmentosa, and psychomotor retardation.

Due to *motor unit hypotonia (hyporeflexic)* (excluding SMAs):
- **Polyneuropathies** (congenital hypomyelinating neuropathy, giant axonal neuropathy, hereditary motor-sensory neuropathies [HMSN])

Neuromuscular junction disorders
- **Infantile botulism** occurs between 2–26 weeks of age and is announced by severe **constipation** and poor feeding, which progresses to bulbar weakness (with **ptosis and mydriasis**) and generalized **areflexia.**
- **Familial infantile myasthenia** is a pre- and postsynaptic AChR antibody negative areflexic disorder presenting at birth with **ptosis** (normal ocular motility) and apnea. Thymectomy and immunosuppression do not help.
- **Transitory myasthenia gravis** (lasting <20 days) occurs from passive transfer of AChR antibodies to 15% of offspring of myasthenic mothers

Metabolic myopathies include myophosphorylase deficiency (McArdle disease), phosphofructokinase deficiency (Tarui's disease), acid maltase deficiency (Pompe's disease), and myoadenylate deaminase (MAD) deficiency.

Muscular dystrophies include congenital muscular dystrophies (laminin α2 chain deficiency and Fukuyama disease along with other cerebro-ocular dysplasia syndromes) and congenital myotonic dystrophy.

Congenital myopathies, also called **fiber-type disproportion myopathies,** encompass nemaline rod, centronuclear, and central core myopathies.

Spinal Muscular Atrophy (Anterior-Horn-Cell Floppy Infant)

Spinal muscular atrophy (SMA, 5q) is a nonprogressive hereditary motor **neuronopathy** caused by anterior horn cell damage that results in generalized weakness with normal cognition and sensation. The identified genes are the ***survival motor neuron* gene** (deleted in 95% of SMAs I–III) and the ***neuronal apoptosis inhibitory protein* gene** (deleted in nearly 70% of SMA I patients). The gene carrier frequency has been estimated to be 1 in 50–80 and the incidence 1 in 6,000-10,000 live births. Scoliosis, contractures, and pneumonia are common complications in those who live long enough (SMA II and III).

Severe spinal muscular atrophy (Werdnig-Hoffmann disease, SMA I) begins before 6 months of age in a poorly sucking infant that never sits without support and has a high likelihood of dying before the age of 2 years. The infant lies in a frog-like position and has pectus excavatum and a chest bell-shaped deformity. Abdominal breathing within the first few months forewarns poor prognosis.

Chronic spinal muscular atrophy (SMA II) begins between 6–18 months in patients with motor delay who achieve independent sitting and whose lifespan usually extends into adolescence. A postural **finger tremor** (*minipolymyoclonus*) is a constant feature.

Juvenile spinal muscular atrophy (Kugelberg-Welander disease, SMA III) becomes symptomatic after 18 months of age and all patients ultimately walk independently and have a nearly normal life expectancy. **Proximal weakness** (legs greater than arms) justifies the differential confusion with Duchenne and limb-girdle muscular dystrophies.

Adult spinal muscular atrophy (SMA IV), indistinguishable from SMA III, overlaps with some forms of MND also linked to chromosome 5.

Muscle biopsy shows small **round muscle fiber grouping** (instead of the usual checkerboard pattern), involving both fiber types, with occasional predominance of very large type 1 fibers. Angulated fibers, present in other denervating conditions, are rare in SMA.

SMA variants associated with deletion of the *survival motor neuron* gene:
- Arthrogryposis multiplex congenita (severe joint deformities)
- Congenital axonal neuropathy

SMA may be mimicked by the following conditions:
- **Kennedy's disease** (X-linked spinobulbar muscular atrophy): **gynecomastia,** congenital fractures, joint contractures, and **sensory neuropathy**
- **Fazio-Londe disease** is a MND limited to lower cranial nerves that start in the second decade of life and progresses to death in 1–5 years
- **Hexosaminidase A deficiency** (adult onset GM_2 gangliosidosis)

Microcephaly

The mean full-term infant OFC is **35 cm.** During the first year, the OFC increases at the rate of **1 cm/m** (faster in the first semester), reaching **46–48 cm** at one year. Two standard deviations below the mean OFC define microcephaly.

Acquired Causes (Secondary Microcephaly)

Prenatal or perinatal anoxic, toxic, inflammatory, or teratogenic insults may occur in a genetically normal brain. The common lesions are porencephaly, ventriculitis, and cortical laminar necrosis or periventricular leukomalacia.

> **Microcephaly with calcifications** suggests tuberous sclerosis, congenital cytomegalovirus (CMV) and toxoplasmosis, Cockayne's syndrome, AIDS, hyperthyroidism, and familial calcification of the basal ganglia.

Some distinct causes of acquired microcephaly are:

- **Fetal alcohol syndrome,** recognized in a microcephalic child by the short palpebral fissures, short and upturned nose, short fourth and fifth metacarpals, and thin upper lip.
- **Untreated maternal phenylketonuria (PKU)** where OFC is inversely correlated with phenylalanine levels.
- **Congenital infections** (**TORCH** [*C*: CMV and Coxsackie], syphilis, AIDS):
  - **Toxoplasmosis** more commonly causes **hydrocephalus** with or without **calcification** of the basal ganglia and periventricular regions. Chorioretinitis and sensorineural deafness may occur. Pyrimethamine-sulfadiazine improves outcome in newborns.
  - **Rubella** causes **micro-ophthalmia, cataracts,** and **pigmentary retinopathy** with, less frequently, hepatomegaly and congenital cardiac malformations. Deafness is the most common sequelae. It causes the highest rate of behavioral abnormalities and **autism.**
  - **CMV** has high affinity for the germinal matrix and causes periventricular tissue necrosis with subsequent **calcification.** Other findings are hepatomegaly, **chorioretinitis,** and thrombocytopenia. There is a high risk of sensorineural deafness. **Schizencephaly,** pachygyria and other **teratogenic** disorders can be seen with CMV.
  - **Herpes virus,** especially HSV-2, may causes **vesicles and bullae,** encephalitis, or disseminated disease (hepatitis, chorioretinitis, DIC). Hydranencephaly or polycystic encephalomalacia may occur.
  - **Syphilis** leads to **meningoencephalitis** early on. **Periostitis** and **osteochondritis** of long bones are clinical hallmarks. Combined use of VDRL and FTA-ABS in CSF facilitates the diagnosis.

Developmental regression disorders, such as Angelman syndrome, Rett syndrome, and neuronal ceroid lipofuscinosis, can simulate acquired microcephaly since the OCF begins to decrease after birth.

Genetic Forms (Primary Microcephaly)

Brain malformations such as lissencephaly and holoprosencephaly with or without macro- or microgyria, migratory disturbances, or agenesis of the corpus callosum are common indications of its prenatal origin.

- **Angelman syndrome:** severe mental retardation and multiple-type seizures associated with "puppet-like" gait, paroxysms of laughter, and large mouth. Angelman may be caused by maternal deletion, paternal uniparental disomy, or imprinting of chromosome 15q11. The deleted *GABRB3* gene codes for a GABA subunit receptor.

- **Miller-Dieker syndrome (lissencephaly type I,** 17p13 deletion) also causes mental retardation and epilepsy (infantile spasms) and results from a migrational arrest between weeks 12–16 of gestation. The pachygyric cortex has four instead of six layers. The dysmorphic features include **high forehead with vertical soft tissue ridging,** narrow bitemporal diameter, furrowing when crying, anteverted nostrils, and micrognathia.

- **Smith-Lemli-Opitz syndrome** is a disorder of the cholesterol biosynthetic pathway that leads to microcephalic developmental delay and facial and body dysmorphism (anteverted nostril, eyelid ptosis, inner epicanthal folds, micrognathia, **syndactyly of second and third toes,** and hypospadias and cryptorchidism). It is diagnosed by finding **low serum cholesterol and high cholesterol precursor 7-dehydrocholesterol (7DHC).** Its birth prevalence of 1 in 20,000 makes it the third most common genetic disorder behind cystic fibrosis and phenylketonuria.

- **Rubinstein-Taybi syndrome** (16p) is recognized by the presence of broad thumbs and toes along with slanted palpebral fissures, low anterior hairline, and hypoplastic maxilla with overcrowding of the teeth.

- **X-linked dominant disorders**
  - **Rett syndrome (MeCP2)** is a developmental regression disorder following early normal life until 7-18 months of life whereby there is loss of purposeful hand movements followed by gait apraxia, truncal ataxia, and hyperventilation.
  - **Aicardi syndrome** is characterized by infantile spasms, agenesis of the corpus callosum, microphthalmos, and chorioretinal lacunae.

- **Cockayne's syndrome** (defective DNA repair) results in photosensitivity, cachectic appearance, dwarfism, ataxia, **retinal degeneration,** and basal ganglia calcification. It physically resembles bird-headed Seckel syndrome.

- **Trisomies:** Down syndrome and trisomy 18; **Deletion:** Cri-du-chat syndrome (deletion 5p)

- Carbohydrate-deficient glycoprotein syndrome

- Dubowitz syndrome (infantile eczema)

- Neuronal ceroid lipofuscinosis

- Pelizaeus-Merzbacher disease

- Mitochondrial disorders

- Organic acidurias

Macrocephaly

Macrocephaly without megalencephaly

- **Hydrocephalus:** *Noncommunicating* includes Chiari II, Dandy-Walker malformation, Walker-Warburg syndrome (lissencephaly type II); *communicating* includes dural sinus thrombosis, vein of Galen aneurysm, and incontinentia pigmenti
- Subdural fluid (*"external hydrocephalus:"* hematoma, hygroma, empyema)

Macrocephaly with megalencephaly

- **Fragile X syndrome**
- Neurocutaneous syndromes such as **neurofibromatosis,** Sturge-Weber syndrome and Klippel-Trenaunay-Weber syndrome (unilateral)
- **Overgrowth syndromes:**
  - **Sotos syndrome:** Cerebral gigantism with acromegalic features, mental and motor retardation, **poor coordination,** large ventricles, high forehead from **dolichocephaly,** and rapid growth and skeletal maturation. MRI may show **agenesis of the corpus callosum,** cerebellar **vermian hypoplasia,** and **large cisterna magna.**
  - **Weaver syndrome:** Sporadic macrosomia with faster osseous maturation, developmental delay, progressive spasticity, **camptodactyly,** broad thumbs, and dysmorphism (hypertelorism, epicanthal folds, large ears, relative micrognathia, inverted nipples)
  - **Simpson-Golabi syndrome:** X-linked recessive disorder of mental retardation, hypotonia, coarse facies, hypertelorism, and broad flat nose, caused by a mutation in the gene that encodes glypican 3.
- **Leukodystrophies:**
  - **Canavan** disease
  - **Alexander** disease
  - Megalencephalic leukoencephalopathy with subcortical cysts in the anterior temporal region due to *MLC1* gene mutations
- Lysosomal storage diseases, especially GM_2 gangliosidosis (**Tay-Sachs**)
- **Mucopolysaccharidoses**
- **Glutaric aciduria**
- Benign (familial) anatomic megalencephaly

Brain Edema

- Toxic: **lead intoxication,** galactosemia
- Idiopathic intracranial hypertension (pseudotumor cerebri) from hypoadrenocorticism, hypoparathyroidism, and hypervitaminosis A

Thick Skull

- Cranioskeletal dysplasia (rickets, osteopetrosis, osteogenesis imperfecta, hyperphosphatemia, achondroplasia)
- Anemia (extramedullary hematopoiesis)
- Myotonic dystrophy (cranial hyperostosis)

Glutaric Aciduria Type I

Glutaric aciduria type I is the most common identifiable autosomal recessive inborn error of metabolism of **lysine, hydroxylysine, and tryptophan.** It is associated with progressive or nonprogressive **extrapyramidal disease** resulting from a **deficiency of glutaryl-CoA dehydrogenase** (mitochondrial electron transport enzyme). This condition may be the cause of misdiagnosed "cerebral palsy" in some children.

> **Cerebral palsy** can be mimicked by metabolic disorders such as Lesch-Nyhan syndrome, pyruvate dehydrogenase deficiency, argininemia, cytochrome oxidase deficiency, and female carriers of ornithine transcarbamylase deficiency.

At birth, besides possibly hypotonia (without dystonia yet), patients may manifest **macrocephaly** and their neuroimaging studies show **relative frontotemporal atrophy and increased subarachnoid spaces.**

The first febrile illness (or any catabolic process) leads to **acute coma** and a number of other sequential deficits, namely:

- **Acute onset of extrapyramidal symptoms** (choreoathetosis or dystonia, dysarthria, and dysphagia), which may become **recurrent**
- **Bulging fontanels,** acutely, mimicking meningitis
- **Bilateral subarachnoid cysts** in temporal fossae
- **Widely open opercula,** possibly secondary to the cysts
- **High T2W MRI signal in caudate head and putamen**
- **Chronic subdural fluid collections** may erroneously lead to entertaining the diagnosis of nonaccidental trauma
- **Dystonic spasms** are common and may be confused with epileptic events, which are uncommon

Diagnosis of glutaric aciduria type I is suggested by the following tests:

- Increased urinary glutaric acid and **3-hydroxyglutaric acid**
- Decreased **glutaryl-CoA dehydrogenase** in cultured fibroblasts
- **Glutaric acid** or **glutaryl carnitine** in amniotic fluid (prenatal)
- Urine for **glutaryl carnitine** by mass spectroscopy (newborn screen)

Differential diagnosis should consider the maternally inherited Leigh syndrome as well as selected **organic acidurias** such as propionic acidemia, methylmalonic aciduria, L-2-hydroxyglutaric aciduria, multiple acyl-CoA dehydrogenase deficiency (GA type II), glutaryl-CoA oxidase deficiency, and 3-methylglutaconic aciduria. There is large excretion of 2-hydroxyglutarate (>500 mg/g creatinine) in the latter three.

Treatment is based on a low-protein diet with avoidance of dietary lysine and tryptophan and of fasting and catabolic states, supported by high fluid intake and urine alkalinization.

Biotinidase Deficiency

Biotinidase is a ubiquitous cell enzyme (encoded at **3p**) that ensures the breakdown of biocytin into biotin, a water-soluble B-complex coenzyme for four **carboxylase enzymes** crucial in gluconeogenesis, fatty acid synthesis, and the catabolism of branched-chain amino acids. Its deficiency, which affects one of every 70,000 births, causes **multiple carboxylase deficiency:**

- **Pyruvate carboxylase,** converts pyruvate to oxaloacetate, the initial step in gluconeogenesis, to which **Acetyl-CoA carboxylase** belongs
- **Propionyl-CoA carboxylase** catabolizes several branched-chain amino acids and odd-chain fatty acids (see *Propionic acidemia*)
- **Beta-methylcrotonyl-CoA carboxylase** is involved in the catabolism of leucine, one of the branched-chain amino acids

Defects in the latter two cause organic aciduria (disorder in the metabolism of branched-chain amino acids leucine, isoleucine, and valine). Acquired biotin deficiency may occur from consumption of raw eggs (which contain **avidin,** a glycoprotein antagonist of biotin), biotin-free long-term parenteral nutrition, and **prolonged use of the AEDs, phenytoin, primidone,** and **carbamazepine.** High urine concentration of β-hydroxyisovalerate is a marker of early biotin deficiency.

The clinical picture consists of **myoclonic or tonic-clonic seizure disorder,** motor delay, hypotonia, **ataxia, hearing loss** and **optic atrophy,** or other ophthalmologic problems, accompanied by:

- **Breathing abnormalities:** hyperventilation, laryngeal **stridor,** and apnea
- **Cutaneous abnormalities:** skin rash and **alopecia**
- Cellular immunologic abnormalities: fungal opportunistic infections

> **Skin rash or alopecia** may also be seen in zinc or essential fatty acids deficiency, thiamine deficiencies, and tryptophanemia.

Laboratory support for biotinidase deficiency relies on:

- **Anion gap metabolic ketoacidosis,** due to the accumulation of abnormal organic acid metabolites of **propionate and lactate in blood** and hydroxyisovalerate, propionate, methylbutyrate, and isobutyrate in urine (see *Organic acidurias*)
- **Hyperammonemia** with elevated pyruvate
- Elevated lactate first in CSF, then peripherally in chronic biotin deficiency

Treatment is based on lifelong **biotin supplementation,** 5–10 mg/d. Seizures and the biochemical disturbances resolve faster than the cutaneous abnormalities. It may take weeks to months for hair growth to replace alopecia. Optic atrophy and hearing loss may not improve at all if a long period has elapsed between onset of symptoms and therapy.

Mitochondrial Diseases

Mitochondrial DNA is a double-stranded, closed circular 16.5-kb molecule that contains 37 genes arranged in two strands, a guanine-rich heavy (made of coding regions or exons, only) and a cytosine-rich light strand. Since the egg supplies all the mtDNA, its **inheritance is exclusively maternal.** Boys and girls receive mtDNA mutations, but only mothers can pass them on to their offspring.

	Mitochondrial Genetics
Polyplasmy	Mitochondria do not distribute evenly during cell division; the ratio of mutant to wild type mtDNA can vary substantially among successive generations of cells over time
Holoplasmy	When all mtDNA within a cell are identical
Heteroplasmy	Normal and mutated mtDNA coexist within every cell
Mutation accumulation	Heteroplasmic cells can become homoplasmic with mutant mtDNA over many generations given the lack of both repair mechanisms and recombination
Mitotic segregation	Normal and mutated mtDNA proportions can shift during cell division altering pathologic threshold for particular tissues and changing phenotypes from normal to diseased or vice versa
Threshold effect	Critical number of mutated mtDNA needed to cause disease, which varies among individuals, systems, and tissues

Tissues with high oxidative metabolism have a relatively low threshold for, and are especially vulnerable to, mtDNA mutation. Thus, most mtDNA disorders are **encephalomyopathies,** disorders where brain and muscle are primarily affected.

Multiorgan involvement is an important clue to the diagnosis. **Overlapping clinical presentations or changing phenotype** results from the phenomenon of mitotic segregation. For instance, children with Pearson's syndrome (mtDNA deletions in blood), showing sideroblastic anemia and exocrine pancreatic insufficiency, who survive into the second decade often develop Kearns-Sayre syndrome (mtDNA deletions accumulating in muscle and other tissues).

MAJOR DISTINCTIVE FEATURES OF THE FIVE MAJOR MITOCHONDRIAL DISORDERS

Defects in protein-synthesis genes			Defects in protein-coding genes	
KSS/CPEO	**MELAS**	**MERRF**	**LHON**	**NARP**
Ophthalmoplegia, retinopathy, heart block	Seizures, episodic vomiting, cortical blindness	Myoclonus, ataxia	Optic atrophy, dystonia	Neuropathy, retinitis pigmentosa
RRF in muscle in 90% of KSS, single large mtDNA deletion in 50% of CPEO	RRF in muscle and point mutations in the **tRNA$^{Leu(UUR)}$ gene** nucleotide in 80%	RRF in muscle and point mutations in the **tRNA^{Lys} gene** nucleotide in 80%	*No RRF in muscle;* **mtDNA point mutations** in ND1, ND4 and ND6 genes	*No RRF in muscle;* **mtDNA point mutations** in the ATPase 6 gene

Diseases from defects in protein-coding genes (LHON and NARP, shaded boxes) are *not* accompanied by RRF on muscle biopsy. Polymerase chain reaction (PCR) is the molecular diagnostic testing of choice to identify mutations in the mtDNA on all of the above except KSS/CPEO in which Southern blot is used.

Mitochondrial Encephalomyopathy Syndromes

Kearns-Sayre Syndrome (KSS)

KSS is a childhood-onset (age <20 years) disorder defined as the combination of **chronic progressive external ophthalmoplegia** (CPEO), **atypical pigmentary retinopathy,** and **mitochondrial myopathy** with one of the following: cardiac conduction defect, ataxia, or a CSF protein above 100 mg/dL. Other potential deficits are **dementia, deafness, depressed ventilatory drive,** episodic coma, and **multiple endocrine abnormalities** such as hypothyroidism, diabetes mellitus, hypoparathyroidism, hyperaldosteronism, and growth hormone deficiency. **Pearson's syndrome** survivors may develop KSS. Brain MRI shows increased T2W signal in the thalamus and subcortical white matter with **sparing of the periventricular region.**

- Most cases are **sporadic** and have a **single large mtDNA deletion.**
- Complexes I, III, IV, and V may be defective

Mitochondrial Encephalopathy with Lactic Acidosis and Stroke-Like Episodes (MELAS)

Children with **MELAS** present with episodic seizures, vomiting, and recurrent hemiparesis and hemianopsia often associated with severe migrainous attacks. Strokes occur in nonvascular distributions, especially in the **occipital lobes.** Dementia develops eventually. MELAS may first occur in adults with stroke, diabetes mellitus, and possibly deafness or intracranial calcification.

- Most cases result from a **point mutation in the tRNA$^{leu(UUR)}$ gene**
- Complexes I (common) and IV may have partial defects
- MELAS is the single most common mitochondrial disorder

Myoclonus Epilepsy with Ragged-Red Fibers (MERRF)

MERRF is recognized in individuals with myoclonic epilepsy, ataxia, and myopathic weakness with or without sensorimotor polyneuropathy (with pes cavus) and widespread mitochondrial dysfunction, expressing as deafness, optic atrophy, ataxia, spasticity, dementia, or even recurrent stroke-like events. **Multiple symmetric lipomatosis** and **cardiomyopathy** with conduction block and CHF may occur.

- Most cases result from a **point mutation in the tRNA^{lys} gene**
- Complexes I and IV have partial defects

Leber Hereditary Optic Neuropathy (LHON)

Painless blindness develops acutely and sequentially in a young man who may also have ataxia, spasticity, psychiatric disorders, peripheral neuropathy, variable myopathic features, and cardiac conduction defects. Tobacco and alcohol may precipitate visual loss. It may cause bilateral striatal necrosis.

- Most cases result from **several mtDNA point mutations**
- Complex I is most often defective as a result of these mutations

Neuropathy, Ataxia, and Retinitis Pigmentosa (NARP)

NARP presents with Leigh syndrome when the percentage of mutated mtDNA is very high.

Maternally Inherited Leigh Syndrome (LS) and Related Disorders

LS applies to the subacute necrotizing encephalomyelopathy that causes episodic neurologic decline or developmental regression especially evident at the time of intercurrent infection. The typical picture consists of dystonia and choreoathetosis in a child with **acquired microcephaly** and poor feeding. Ataxia, cerebellar tremor, breathing (**apnea,** gasping, periodic hyperventilation, sighing) and **visual (optic atrophy,** nystagmus, **oculomotor palsies**) abnormalities are reported. In addition, the following clinical phenotypes are recognized:

- **Neuropathy, ataxia, and retinitis pigmentosa (NARP syndrome)** is the variant present in 10%-15% of Leigh syndrome with white matter abnormalities suggesting leukodystrophy. Complex V deficiency from ATP synthase deficiency leads most often to the NARP phenotype. Seizures and recurrent polyneuropathy are common. The larger the causal mtDNA mutation the more typical the NARP phenotype.

- **Episodic lactic acidosis and fasting hypoglycemia** in severely retarded and spastic epileptic children should suggest **pyruvate carboxylase deficiency** (resulting from **biotinidase deficiency,** biotin deficiency, or holocarboxylase synthetase deficiency).

- **Stridor or apnea, skin rash, seizures, hypotonia, ataxia,** and anion-gap metabolic acidosis are more specific to **biotin deficiency.**

- **Athetoid cerebral palsy phenotype with corpus callosum agenesis and cystic lesions** in the basal ganglia, cerebellum, and brainstem on MRI is the X-linked phenotype in 25% of LD because of **pyruvate dehydrogenase complex (PDHC)** deficiency. A **spinocerebellar degeneration** with lactic and pyruvic acidosis is another potential manifestation of PDHC deficiency.

- **Ataxia, ophthalmoplegia,** neuropathy, and pyramidal signs are the manifestations of **complex IV** due to **COX** deficiency.

The neuropathologic features are similar to those of thiamine or B_1 deficiency (Wernicke encephalopathy-like disorder; B_1 is a cofactor for PDHC) except for the **lack of involvement of the mammillary bodies.** Inheritance can be autosomal recessive and maternal due to complex I and IV deficiencies and the NARP mutations.

The blood lactate to pyruvate ratio may be helpful as enzymatic defects closer to the glycolytic pathway (PDHC deficiency) have a ratio <20, whereas **electron transport chain defects** (complex V deficiency) **have ratios >20.** Lactate and pyruvate concentrations are usually mildly elevated but increase in response to an oral glucose load. The management is based on a combination of thiamine (B_1), 100-600 mg/d, carnitine, coenzyme Q_{10}, and antioxidants along with high-fat low-carbohydrate diet. B_1 is especially helpful in PDHC deficiency. **Biotin** supplementation is indicated in biotin/biotinidase deficiency. Dichloroacetate remains experimental.

Primary White Matter Disorders

Leukodystrophies		Deficiency	Features (Pathology, MRI)
MLD (AR) See *Lysosomal disorders*	*Frontal*	Arylsulfatase A (22q), ↑ cerebroside sulfatide	**Frontal-predominant** demyelination* with U-fiber sparing; peripheral neuropathy is not seen in juvenile onset.*
X-linked ALD See *Peroxisomal disorders*	*Occipital*	Peroxisomal defect in acyl-CoA synthetase (↑ VLCFA)	**Posterior** (parieto-occipital) demyelination with splenium of corpus callosum affected and rim **contrast enhancement.**
Krabbe globoid cell (AR) See *Lysosomal disorders*	*Thalami*	Galactocerebroside-β-galactosidase (14q)	**Posterior** (parieto-occipital) demyelination with multinucleated globoid cells, hyperdense basal ganglia (BG).
Alexander disease (Sporadic)	*Macro-cephaly*	GFAP gene mutation Infantile ≈ death by 3 y Juv ≈ bulbar weakness Adult AD ≈ MS	**Frontal** lobe and BG involved. U-fibers and posterior capsule preserved. Biopsy: low myelin and Rosenthal fibers.
Canavan disease (AR)	*Least myelination* · *Macro-cephaly*	Aspartoacylase gene♦ ↑ Urine and CSF NAA (*N*-acetylaspartic acid)	**Subcortical** spongiform degeneration, affected U-fibers, hypotonia → spasticity, optic atrophy.
Pelizaeus-Merzbacher (X-linked)	*Least myelination* · *Micro-*	Myelin PLP gene mutation (Xq28)	Immature myelination for age, generalized myelin islands or **tigroid myelination** may be present.

* Stripes of normal signal within abnormal white matter may be seen in lysosomal storage disorders.

♠**Peripheral neuropathy can be seen in three leukodystrophies**: **Krabbe** disease, **MLD**, and Cockayne disease.

♦ Only two mutations are the basis for Canavan disease among 98% of individuals of Ashkenazi Jewish ancestry. Screening programs are therefore feasible in this population. The carrier frequency for the mutations is very high, 1:37.

Congenital metabolic disorders may cause the following MRI patterns:

1. **Periventricular hypomyelination:** Amino acid disorders such as phenylketonuria, maple syrup urine disease (MSUD), homocystinuria
2. **Diffuse demyelination:** Lowe syndrome (oculo-cerebral-renal syndrome)
3. **Agenesis of the corpus callosum:** nonketotic hyperglycinemia (NKH), pyruvate dehydrogenase complex (PDHC) deficiency, Menke's kinky hair disease, and glutaric aciduria II (GA-II)
4. **Migrational disorders:** NKH, PDHC, GA-I, GA-II, peroxisomal diseases (Zellweger), mevalonic aciduria (progressive cerebellar atrophy)
5. **Brain edema:** NKH, MSUD, urea cycle disorders, galactosemia, and pyruvate carboxylase deficiency
6. **Cystic changes:** Hurler disease (dilated perineuronal spaces filled with mucopolysaccharide gargoyle cells) and Lowe syndrome

Pelizaeus-Merzbacher Disease and Hereditary Spastic Paraparesis 2

Pelizaeus-Merzbacher disease (PMD), due to **mutations in the *PLP1* gene,** is the prototypic hypomyelinating disorder. The transmembrane PLP1 protein constitutes about 50% of the CNS myelin protein mass. Extra copies of *PLP1* (duplications, triplications, etc., 60%–70% of PMD cases) result in increased PLP1 expression and greater severity. Point mutations (missense or frame shift, 20%) results in mild or severe phenotype depending on whether the endoplasmic reticulum retains only PLP1 or PLP1 *and* DM20, respectively.

Classical PMD is recognized by the development of rotatory, vertical, or horizontal **nystagmus** within the first 2 months of life, followed by **optic atrophy,** axial-predominant hypotonia, and developmental delay. Spastic para- or quadriparesis and ataxia eventually occur. The nystagmus may improve in some. Any spastic-ataxic ambulation is eventually lost. Patients usually survive into adulthood, often into the fourth and fifth decades or even longer.

Connatal PMD children (most severe) have neonatal hypotonia resembling spinal muscular atrophy, nystagmus, **stridor,** and seizures. The stridor can be severe enough to prompt emergent intubation and tracheostomy placement, although breathing is usually possible otherwise. The severe hypotonia is followed by spastic quadriplegia and scoliosis. This form of PMD is usually fatal during childhood, but with comprehensive care, survival can be extended into the second or third decade.

Hereditary spastic paraparesis 2 (X-linked HSP, SPG2) is a relatively milder syndrome consisting of delayed motor milestones and spastic paraparesis. Nystagmus may occur during infancy. Patients with null *PLP1* mutations (complete lack of PLP1) have childhood-onset spastic paraparesis but without nystagmus and milder developmental delay. However, they tend to progress more rapidly during late adolescence or early adulthood. The MRI abnormalities are milder. Survival into the fifth or sixth decade is typical.

The normal, full-term newborn brain is largely unmyelinated, except for some brainstem tracts, such as the medial longitudinal fasciculus and the medial and lateral lemnisci, and the posterior limb of the internal capsule. The bulk of brain myelination occurs in the first year of life and is largely complete by about 2–2.5 years of age. MRI normally shows progressive hyperintensity in the T1W and hypointensity in T2W signal in the white matter relative to the gray matter. The recognition of PMD is easier after about 18 months of age, when the T2W and T1W signals approach those of a normal adult brain. **The MRI of a child with classical PMD remains immature accounting for age.** Myelin islands or **tigroid myelination** may be present. If the MRI is done at an earlier stage, it may be possible to recognize the failure of maturation of the posterior limbs of the internal capsule and the superior and middle cerebellar peduncles.

Primary Gray Matter Disorders

		Deficiency	Features (pathology, MRI)
Neuronal Ceroid Lipofuscinosis	Cortical involvement	No enzyme defect CLN1: Chr. 1 (inf) CLN2: Chr. 11 CLN3: Chr. 16 (juv)	Granular (1), curvilinear (2), or fingerprint (3) osmiophilic bodies. CLN1: ↑T2 signal in WM and ↓ in striatum/thalami. Juvenile: No WM disease
Gangliosidosis GM$_2$ (Tay-Sachs disease)		**Hexosaminidase A** Chr 15 (α subunit) Chr 5 (β subunit)	**Enlargement of the caudate, hyperdense thalami** on HCT, high signal in caudate and putamen on T2W MRI; severe cortical atrophy in later stages
Mucolipidoses		Accumulation of lipids and muco-polysaccharide	**Thin cortex** with nonspecific white matter changes in I-cell disease, fucosidosis, and mannosidosis
Alpers disease	Micro-cephalic	Respiratory chain enzyme deficiency (**POLG1** mutations)	**Occipital cortex and thalamic lesions** in refractory epileptic encephalopathy and liver insufficiency (visual symptoms in adolescent onset)
Menkes' kinky hair disease		Defective gene coding for **ATP-7A** (copper transporter)	Growth retardation, brittle hair, and cerebral and cerebellar degeneration; thin corpus callosum and tortuous cerebral arteries are main MRI findings
Mucopolysaccharidoses	Macro-	I: α-L-iduronidase (Hurler)	I: Prominent Virchow-Robin spaces, macrocephaly; III: cortical atrophy; IV: Atlantoaxial subluxation

Prominent Basal Ganglia Involvement

Globus Pallidus	Thalamus	Caudate	Putamen
Hallevorden-Spatz Canavan disease Kearns-Sayre Maple syrup urine Wilson's disease	Krabbe disease MLD Alpers disease GM$_2$ gangliosidosis Wilson's disease	Biotinidase def. Glutaric aciduria I Glutaric aciduria II GM$_2$ gangliosidos Huntington Wilson's disease	Leigh syndrome Glutaric aciduria I **Subthalamic Nucleus** Cytochrome C oxidase def.

Calcifications on the basal ganglia are seen in mitochondrial diseases (MELAS, MERRF, KS), post-inflammatory disorders (**TORCH,** cysticercosis, TB, congenital HIV), **Fahr disease, Cockayne syndrome, neurofibromatosis,** biotinidase deficiency, methemoglobinopathy, **Krabbe, GM$_2$ gangliosidosis,** and **Aicardi-Goutiéres syndrome** (microcephaly, chronic CSF lymphocytosis, generalized dystonia with truncal hypotonia, and chilblain lesions in the setting of mental retardation, often misdiagnosed as cerebral palsy).

Symmetrical Bilateral Signal Abnormalities within the Basal Ganglia

1. **CT hypodensity, T1W MRI hypo-, T2W MRI hyperintensities:**

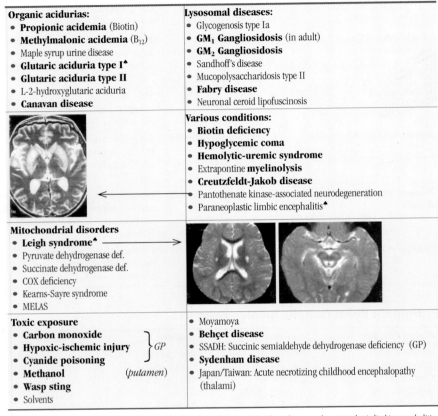

Organic acidurias:	Lysosomal diseases:
• **Propionic acidemia** (Biotin) • **Methylmalonic acidemia** (B_{12}) • Maple syrup urine disease • **Glutaric aciduria type I**[▲] • **Glutaric aciduria type II** • L-2-hydroxyglutaric aciduria • **Canavan disease**	• Glycogenosis type Ia • **GM₁ Gangliosidosis** (in adult) • **GM₂ Gangliosidosis** • Sandhoff's disease • Mucopolysaccharidosis type II • **Fabry disease** • Neuronal ceroid lipofuscinosis

Various conditions:
• **Biotin deficiency** • **Hypoglycemic coma** • **Hemolytic-uremic syndrome** • Extrapontine **myelinolysis** • **Creutzfeldt-Jakob disease** • Pantothenate kinase-associated neurodegeneration • Paraneoplastic limbic encephalitis[▲]

Mitochondrial disorders
• **Leigh syndrome**[▲] • Pyruvate dehydrogenase def. • Succinate dehydrogenase def. • COX deficiency • Kearns-Sayre syndrome • MELAS

Toxic exposure	
• **Carbon monoxide** • **Hypoxic-ischemic injury** ⎫ *GP* • **Cyanide poisoning** ⎭ • **Methanol** *(putamen)* • **Wasp sting** • Solvents	• Moyamoya • **Behçet disease** • SSADH: Succinic semialdehyde dehydrogenase deficiency (GP) • **Sydenham disease** • Japan/Taiwan: Acute necrotizing childhood encephalopathy (thalami)

[▲]Exclusive putaminal involvement may be caused by glutaric aciduria type I, Leigh syndrome, and paraneoplastic limbic encephalitis caused by CRMP-5 neuronal antibody.

2. **Bilateral T1W MRI BG hyperintensities:** Wilson disease, acquired hepatolenticular degeneration, long-term TPN (probably caused by manganese toxicity), neurofibromatosis, and calcification; **unilateral BG hyperintensity on T1W MRI** is largely an imaging domain of nonketotic hyperglycemia (causing hemiballism-hemichorea)

3. **CT hyperdensity, T2W MRI hypointensities** (besides normal aging-induced iron deposition): NBAI-1 (GP), Krabbe, PMD, Canavan, MLD (thalami), and MSA (with hyperintense lateral rim)

Angelman Syndrome

Angelman syndrome (AS) is the prototypical neurogenetic disorder involving epilepsy and severe developmental delay. It consists of **microbrachycephaly,** severe mental retardation with **absence of speech,** tremulous or myoclonic movements, ataxic gait without cerebellar features, and an unusually happy disposition (*happy-puppet syndrome*) often with inappropriate bursts of laughter hyperactivity, and **hand-flapping movements.** These patients have multiple-type seizures before the age of 3 years, with a minority developing hypsarrhythmia and Lennox-Gastaut syndrome. The EEG may be normal or demonstrate characteristic trains of high-voltage 4–6 Hz activity. About 20%–50% of patients have additional features, such as strabismus, tongue protrusion, prominent mandible, wide mouth, flexed arms on walking, and **"fascination with water."**

The five genetic mechanisms potentially causing Angelman syndrome are:
1. **Maternal deletion of the chromosomal region 15q11-q13** (about 75%); paternal deletion of 15q leads to Prader-Willi syndrome (infantile hypotonia, mild to moderate mental retardation, hyperphagia with subsequent obesity, hypogonadism, short stature, and mild facial dysmorphism)
2. **Uniparental disomy** (UPD) (3%); both 15q come from the father
3. **Imprinting center defect** (5%)
4. **UBE3A mutations** (8%–11%); UBE3A is an ubiquitin ligase gene whose protein product, E6-AP, transfers small ubiquitin molecules to their degradation sites
5. **AS phenotype with negative genetic testing** (20%)

Genetic evaluation includes **methylation** (confirms AS without ascertaining whether it is due to deletion, uniparental disomy, or imprinting defect), **FISH** (which detects microdeletions), and **RFLP** (restriction fragment length polymorphism, which evaluates the contribution of each parent to chromosome 15). In methylation positive-FISH negative patients, RFLP will distinguish between UPD and imprinting defect (negative RFLP). In a suspected AS patient, normal methylation should prompt the direct **UBE3A mutation** search. Milder phenotype but increased risk of recurrence occurs in those with imprinting center defects and UBE3A mutations. Gene-negative AS-like conditions include:
- Single gene disorders: **Rett syndrome** is the most common mimicker early on as hypotonia, seizures, awkward gait, and mild microcephaly are features of RS girls between 1 and 3 years of age. Other AS-like disorders include methylene tetrahydrofolate reductase deficiency (MTHFR), X-linked alpha-thalassemia/mental retardation syndrome (ATR-X), and Gurrieri syndrome (AR inheritance with iliac hypoplasia and tall vertebral bodies)
- Chromosome disorders: **22q13.3 terminal deletion** (severe speech delay and mental retardation without major malformations and less prevalent epilepsy), 15q11-q13 duplication instead of deletion (autistic features may be present), 2q22-q23 deletion (may have Hirschsprung disease and/or callosal agenesis), and other deletions (17q23.2, 4q12, and 4p15.2)

Neurocutaneous Syndromes (Phakomatoses)

Neurofibromatosis (NF, Von Recklinghausen Disease)

> Genes: • **NF1** ("peripheral") → **17q** → *neurofibromin*   1:3,000
> • **NF2** ("central") → **22q** → *merlin/schwannomin* 1:50,000

NF is the most common neurocutaneous disorder. Spontaneous mutations cause half of all NF1 cases. The pathogenesis involves excessive proliferation of neural crest derivatives. In a small minority of cases, tumors may become sarcomas peripherally and astrocytomas or glioblastomas centrally.

NF1 diagnosis requires two or more of the following: **six café-au-lait** (>5 mm in prepuber; >15 mm in postpuber age), axillary or inguinal freckling, **optic glioma** (astrocytoma), **two or more Lisch nodules** (hamartoma of the iris), two or more cutaneous **neurofibromas,** or one plexiform neurofibroma, a first-degree relative with NF1, **sphenoid dysplasia** ("pulsating exophthalmos"), and cortical bone thinning. **Moyamoya** syndrome is common. **Hypertension is secondary to renal artery stenosis or pheochromocytoma.** Neurofibromas may resemble multiple symmetrical lipomatosis with axonal polyneuropathy (Launois-Beusaude disease).

NF2 diagnosis is made with either of the following combinations: **bilateral VIII nerve schwannoma,** *or* first degree relative with NF2 *and* unilateral VIII CN, *or* first-degree relative with NF2 *and* two of the following: neurofibroma, meningioma, schwannoma, glioma, or **posterior subcapsular cataracts.**

Tuberous Sclerosis Complex

> Genes: • **TSC1** → **9p** → *Hamartin*, more prominent in familial cases
> • **TSC2** → **16p** → *Tuberin*, more severe disease

Referred to as tuberous sclerosis complex (TSC), this autosomal dominant disorder, with a prevalence of 1 in 6,000–9,000, is the second most common neurocutaneous disorder. The Vogt's clinical triad of seizures, mental retardation, and adenoma sebaceum manifest in less than one-third of patients. **Renal malignancies (renal cell, malignant angiomyolipoma) and glioblastoma multiforme** may rarely occur in TSC, especially in those with TSC2 mutations.

Major features include **facial angiofibromas** (adenoma sebaceum), periungual fibroma, **ash-leaf spots** (hypomelanotic macules), Shagreen patch, multiple retinal hamartomas, cortical tuber, subependymal giant cell astrocytoma (SEGA, usually in the foramen of Monro, often causing obstructive hydrocephalus), and renal angiomyolipoma. **Minor features** include dental enamel pits, bone cysts, hamartomatous rectal polyps, multiple renal cysts, and nonrenal hamartomas. Typical neuropathological lesions include **subependymal nodules, cortical hamartomas** (cortical tubers), focal **cortical hypoplasia,** and **heterotopic gray matter.** *Hamartin* and *Tuberin* have tumor suppressor activity.

Hypomelanosis of Ito or Incontinentia Pigmenti Achromianses

This third most common neurocutaneous syndrome (after NF1 and TSC) is a clinical diagnosis that rests on the recognition of **hypopigmented whorls or streaks** on at least two body parts, which appear at birth or shortly thereafter but tend to normalize with age. **Seizures** (West syndrome), mental retardation, and musculoskeletal malformations are common. Ophthalmologic findings include **strabismus, optic atrophy, micro-ophthalmia,** eyelid ptosis, and heterochromia iridis. Facial dysmorphic features, including microcephaly, may be present.

Incontinentia Pigmenti (Bloch-Sulzberger Syndrome)

IP is distinguished from hypomelanosis of Ito by the *evolution* of the skin lesions into three stages: **inflammatory vesicular rash** on flexor surfaces of the limbs and lateral trunk at birth, verrucous and **hyperpigmented** ("marble cake") a few months later, and **hypopigmented** finally. The neurologic and ophthalmologic features are largely those of hypomelanosis of Ito. It has also been associated with a **spinal muscular atrophy-like syndrome** and **recurrent encephalomyelitis.** In its X-dominant form (Xp11), incontinentia pigmenti is lethal in homozygous males. There is a common locus in Xp11 between incontinentia pigmenti and hypomelanosis of Ito. Neuropathology may show cerebral atrophy with microgyria.

Hereditary Hemorrhagic Telangiectasia (Osler-Weber-Rendu Disease)

This autosomal dominant disorder is characterized by enlarging telangiectasias of the retinal, nasal, and conjunctival mucosa. The neurologic features are headache, dizziness, seizures, and **ICH or SAH from AVM** more often than aneurysms. Cerebral abscess and septic embolic meningitis may occur. Dental and surgical procedures require **antibiotic prophylaxis** in this population.

Sturge-Weber Syndrome (SWS)

SWS is a sporadic disorder consisting of facial angiomas **(port-wine nevus)** associated with **leptomeningeal** and **brain angiomas,** usually ipsilateral to the facial lesion. Seizures, mental retardation, glaucoma, contralateral hemiparesis, hemiatrophy, and hemianopsia are the common clinical findings. "Trolley track" or *tramline* gyral calcification is the hallmark CT abnormality.

Chédiak-Higashi Syndrome (CHS)

This disorder (**CHS1** mutation; **1q**), which causes areas of depigmentation resembling giant fingerprints **(oculocutaneous albinism),** is associated with **recurrent infections** (immunologic defects), **bleeding diathesis,** and progressive neurologic dysfunction (seizures, mental retardation, **peripheral neuropathy,** and **dysautonomia**). A **spinocerebellar** form has been described.

Von Hippel-Lindau syndrome, ataxia-telangiectasia, and **Fabry disease** are discussed under *Brain Tumors, Ataxia,* and *Neuropharmacology* sections, respectively. **Klippel-Trenaunay-Weber syndrome** (port-wine stain, varicose veins, and bony and soft tissue hypertrophy suggesting SWS) rarely causes a neurologic disorder but may be associated with spinal hemangiomas.

2 Stroke, Migraine, and Epilepsy

These three groups of disorders share tantalizingly common pathogenic mechanisms, even long before migraine was considered a vasospastic disorder with "aural" constriction and "algia" dilation. **Chromosome 19** became the ultimate common denominator when its *Notch3*[1] and *CACNL1A4*[2] genes were found responsible for cerebral autosomal dominant arteriopathy with subcortical **infarcts** and leukoencephalopathy (CADASIL) and familial hemiplegic **migraine** (FHM), respectively. Interestingly, the *CACNL1A4* mutation in the P/Q type calcium channel was found in the recessive tottering mice,[3] the animal model for human absence and motor **seizures,** as well as mild ataxia.

Migraine and epilepsy may have the same "positive phenomena" that "march" at the pace of the cortical spreading depression (CSD), the result of oligemia and electrical changes, which reciprocally appear to activate each other. Migraine, then, follows epilepsy as an electrical disease in which excessive neuronal activation is mediated in part by serotonergic "pacemaker" raphe nuclei cells.

Migraine and stroke may share a reciprocal causal relationship by also leading to each other. Although migraine has established itself as a risk factor for cerebral infarction, at least in young women, the classic textbook, *Wolff's Headache,* highlights the directional vagaries by stating that ischemia-induced migraine might even be more frequent than migraine-induced ischemia. **Migrainous infarctions** are the rare outcome of auras that overstay their welcome with severe hypoperfusion, especially in the territory of the posterior cerebral artery. If this example is followed partially (i.e., overstay is not permanent), before the third decade of life, **FHM** is a suspect. These migraines with hemiparesis, aphasia, hemianopsia, and sometimes coma, leave no trail of evidence on their way out, which is much unlike the way **CADASIL** declares itself. Once migraine-with-aura attacks begin to suggest TIAs, strokes, and dementia, a testimonial of widespread white matter abnormalities would have been secretly collecting for many years, as unveiled by T2W sequences. The pathogenic highly stereotyped missense mutation in *Notch3* allows for reliable diagnosis in about 75% of subjects. Other conditions linking migraine (usually with aura) and ischemic strokes are thrombocytopenia, essential thrombocythemia, systemic lupus erythematosus, antiphospholipid antibody syndrome, and mitochondrial cytopathies (especially mitochondrial encephalopathy, lactic acidosis, and strokelike episodes, or **MELAS,** which result from a point mitochondrial DNA mutation in the tRNA *Leu* gene). Finally, a polymorphism in the methylenetetradohydrofolate reductase gene (*C677T*) is associated with moderately elevated homocysteine, which in turn increases the risk of stroke. The same polymorphism is overexpressed in migraine-with-aura patients.

---

[1] Joutel A et al. Notch3 mutations in CADASIL, a hereditary adult-onset condition causing stroke and dementia. *Nature* 1996; 383(6602):707–710.
[2] Ophoff RA et al. Familial hemiplegic migraine and episodic ataxia type-2 are caused by mutations in the Ca2+ channel gene CACNL1A4. *Cell* 1996; 87(3):543–552. [3] Doyle J et al. Mutations in the Cacnl1a4 calcium channel gene are associated with seizures, cerebellar degeneration, and ataxia in tottering and leaner mutant mice. *Mamm Genome* 1997; 8(2):113–120.

Stroke

Stroke applies to the sudden onset of deficits localized to the distribution of an arterial or venous territory, which either resolve within minutes to hours (TIA) or persist (completed stroke). It may be caused by atherothromboembolism, cardiogenic embolism, small-vessel ischemic disease, or a combination of these.

Independent risk factors for stroke include advanced age, prior TIA, atrial fibrillation, chronic hypertension (systolic > diastolic), poor left ventricular function, diabetes mellitus, coronary artery disease, mitral regurgitation, hypercholesterolemia and hyperhomocysteinemia. **Hyperthermia, hyperglycemia,** and **diastolic hypotension** threaten full functional recovery. *Early* **recurrence of stroke** is around 2% within the first 14 days. Most infarcts are visible on CT within 48 hours after symptom onset, become isodense from days 10–21, and achieve CSF-like density by 3 months.

- **Lacunar syndrome** presents as a (1) **pure motor stroke** from an internal capsule, corona radiata, or basis pontis lacune, with hemiparesis or plegia involving the face, arm, and to a lesser extent the leg, accompanied by dysarthria; (2) **pure sensory stroke** due to a thalamic ventroposterolateral nucleus lacune, with unilateral hemisensory deficits involving the face, arm, trunk, and leg; (3) **clumsy hand-dysarthria syndrome** from a basis pontis or genu of the internal capsule lacune, causing supranuclear facial weakness, tongue deviation, dysphagia, dysarthria, and impaired hand fine motor control; or (4) **ataxic hemiparesis** from a capsular, thalamocapsular or pontine lacunae, with ipsilateral ataxia and crural paresis. Lacunes are strongly related to age and hypertension but not to thrombogenesis.

- **Cardioembolic syndrome** results in deficits from any vascular territory, especially due to atrial fibrillation, the most prevalent dysrhythmia, which carries at least a 5-fold increased risk of ischemic stroke in nonvalvular and 17-fold in valvular types.

- **Intracerebral hemorrhage (ICH)** is caused by hypertension, arteriovenous malformations (AVM), and saccular aneurysms. Lobar hematomas in older patients are often caused by cerebral amyloid angiopathy (CAA).

- **Subarachnoid hemorrhage (SAH)** is due to ruptured intracranial aneurysms in most spontaneous (nontraumatic) cases. Less common causes include nonaneurysmal perimesencephalic SAH, bleeding diatheses, CAA, primary or metastatic tumors, vasculitis, intracranial dissections, cerebral venous thrombosis, bacterial meningitis, spinal cord vascular malformations, and spinal cord tumors.

- **Cerebral venous sinus thrombosis (CVST)** presents more gradually than arterial strokes, with disorders ranging from idiopathic intracranial hypertension (IIH) to lobar hematoma or cortical hemorrhage. CVST usually occurs during pregnancy or puerperium and is suspected in someone with seizures and family history of venous thromboembolism or thrombophilia.

Stroke of the Young

Carotid artery dissection causes neck pain and Horner syndrome and is suspected in **Marfan syndrome, pseudoxanthoma** elasticum, fibromuscular dysplasia, **Ehlers-Danlos IV**, α-**1-antitrypsin deficiency**, and Menkes disease.

Hemiplegic migraine: recurrent familial episodes associated with fever, confusion or coma. **MELAS** and **CADASIL** may be associated. **Migrainous infarction** may follow after a migraine-with-aura attack.

Antiphospholipid antibody syndrome: recurrent venous and arterial thrombosis, thrombocytopenia, and recurrent miscarriages in younger women. **Anticardiolipin antibody** is the commonest antibody but its presence alone does not convey a higher risk of recurrence unless there is active SLE, a positive **lupus anticoagulant**, and evidence of recurrent thrombotic events

Primary angiitis of the CNS: angiography/MRA may show beading and confirmation with brain biopsy may be needed. Intensive immunosuppression with **cyclophosphamide** is required for adequate control.

Workup:
- Sickle cells
- FVL mutation, APC resistance, prothrombin 20210A gene mutation, homocysteine, factor VIII, lupus anticoagulant
- Protein C, S, antithrombin, anticardiolipin antibody
- Syphilis
- Lactate
- Drug screen
- EKG, two-dimensional echo
- Angiography

Moyamoya ("puff of smoke") is a progressive stenosis of the arteries of the circle of Willis, which may be secondary to Down syndrome, **sickle cell anemia**, neurofibromatosis type 1. **Revascularization** may be indicated.

Takayasu arteritis (aortitis of granulomatous origin) leads to occlusion of the origin of the great vessels, diagnosed by **angiography** in someone with pronounced **asymmetry of BP** readings between upper and lower limbs. **Corticosteroids** prevent its progression.

Patent foramen ovale may be a coincidental finding in up to 40% of stroke patients but **paradoxical embolism** may occur when there is associated prior DVT, pulmonary embolism, or pulmonary hypertension.

Thrombophilia (discussion later): tendency to thrombosis associated with deficiency in any natural anticoagulant factor (antithrombin [AT], protein C, protein S, heparin cofactor 2, and FVL mutation). **FVL mutation (activated protein C resistance) is the commonest abnormality** associated with cerebral **venous** thrombosis. AT and proteins C and S are depressed (and factor VIII is increased) after stroke and should be measured at least 3 months after the acute event. Warfarin also lowers the concentrations of proteins C and S. **Hyperhomocysteinemia** alone or in combination with FVL increases the risk of venous thrombosis.

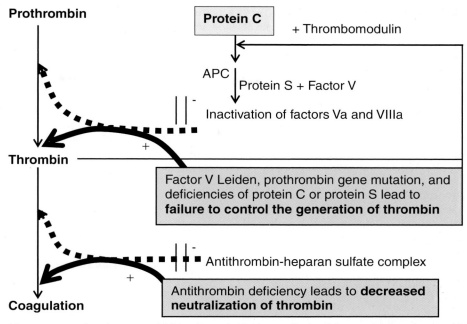

Measurement of resistance to APC in plasma is highly specific for FVL mutation but also sensitive for the presence of lupus anticoagulant, increased factor VIII levels, pregnancy, and the use of oral anticoagulant therapy.

Venous thrombosis results more often from homozygosity for FVL or the G20210A prothrombin gene mutation. Heterozygotes have lesser predisposition to thrombosis. **Hyperhomocysteinemia** can be caused by vitamins B_{12}, B_6, and folate deficiencies, renal failure, hypothyroidism, increasing age, menopause, smoking, psoriasis, and genetic disorders affecting the homocysteine pathway (MTHFR gene mutation and classic homocystinuria due to cystathionine β-synthase deficiency)

Lifelong anticoagulation needed for:
    Recurrent thrombosis
    CVT due to any thrombophilia
    Multiple thrombophilias
    FVL homozygous mutation
    Antithrombin deficiency
    Antiphospholipid antibodies

Drugs causing high homocysteine:
- Methotrexate
- Phenytoin and carbamazepine
- Nitrous oxide
- Lipid-lowering agents colestipol, cholestyramine, niacin, and fibrates
- Methylxanthines
- Levodopa

Arterial and venous thrombosis can only be caused by hyperhomocysteinemia and antiphospholipid antibody syndrome. Prophylaxis is initiated during high-risk situations (surgery, trauma, immobilization) and involves using unfractionated or low-molecular-weight heparin, avoidance of hormone replacement therapy, and maintenance of normal homocysteine level (vitamins B_{12}, B_6, and folate).

Anticoagulation: Warfarin (INR 2.0–3.0) was shown to be better than aspirin in the secondary prevention of recurrent stroke and thromboembolism in **patients with atrial fibrillation** (AF) of high risk (CHF, previous embolism, SBP >160, woman older than 75 years), according to the **Stroke Prevention in Atrial Fibrillation III study (1996).** Anticoagulation reduces the annual stroke risk of patients with AF from 4.5% to 1.4%. The **Warfarin-Aspirin Recurrent Stroke Study (2001)** showed no advantage of warfarin (INR 1.4–2.8) over aspirin for the prevention of recurrent **noncardioembolic** ischemic stroke or death. In this population, greater INR targets (3.0–4.5) are to be avoided to prevent hemorrhagic complications. Other patients that may still benefit from the use of warfarin (level 3 evidence) include those with antiphospholipid antibodies (INR >3.0) and aortic atheroma. **Low-molecular-weight heparinoids** do not offer significant benefit and are not used routinely in stroke management.

Thrombolysis: Intravenous recombinant tissue plasminogen activator **(rt-PA)** at a dose of **0.9 mg/kg (maximum 90 mg)** given over 1 hour for use within 3 hours from ischemic stroke onset was approved following the NINDS rt-PA study findings of excellent outcome achieved in 34% of patients at 3 months from infusion. Ten percent of the total dose is given as an initial bolus, and the rest of the dose is infused over 60 minutes. The BP must be **<185/110** and should be kept **<180/105 during the infusion** and for the next 24 hours. Newer data suggest that the window for use of IV tPA may be extended to 4.5 hours. The risk of symptomatic intracerebral hemorrhage within 36 hours of IV rt-PA infusion is 6%, half of which may be fatal. Hyperglycemia is associated with ICH following rt-PA. The mortality rate at 3 months after stroke is the same in those who receive rt-PA versus those who do not. New data (ECASS III) suggest that selected patients with acute ischemic stroke with symptom onset from 3 to 4.5 hours can be safely treated with intravenous thrombolytic therapy.

SELECTIVE STUDIES OF THROMBOLYSIS IN ACUTE ISCHEMIC STROKE

Study	Year	Comments	Odds ratio
NINDS	1995	Pivotal trial: most of the data supporting rt-PA	1.82
ECASS I	1995	rt-PA 1.1 mg/kg within 6 h: ↑ mortality	1.34
ECASS II	1998	rt-PA 0.9 mg/kg within 6 h: marginal	1.11
ATLANTIS	1999	rt-PA 0.9 mg/kg between 3 and 6 h: negative	1.05
PROACT II	1999	Potential benefit of intra-arterial thrombolysis with **rpro-UK*** within 6 h from MCA stroke.	
ECASS III	2008	rt-PA yields favorable outcome (modified Rankin scale of 0 to 1 at 3 months) when given between 3 and 4.5 h	1.28

NINDS: National Institute of Neurological Disorders and Stroke; ECASS: European Cooperative Acute Stroke Study; **ATLANTIS**: Alteplase Thrombolysis for Acute Noninterventional Therapy for Ischemic Stroke; PROACT: Prolyse in Acute Cerebral Thromboembolism Trial.
*Prolyse (rpro-UK): recombinant prourokinase.

The intra-arterial delivery of thrombolytics has several potential advantages including direct visualization and manipulation of the thrombus, delivery of lower effective dose of drugs (rarely over 20 mg of rt-PA) at slightly **longer time windows,** and use of angioplasty and stenting or mechanical devices.

Heparin-induced thrombocytopenia type 2 (risk <1%) may occur **3–15** days after initiation of heparin, causing potentially fatal **arterial and venous thrombosis** by "white clots" (platelet-rich thrombi and immune complex with platelet factor 4 **[PF4]**). **LMW heparins or heparinoids** have antifactor Xa activity and low tendency to induce thrombocytopenia compared with unfractionated heparin.

Emergency Treatment of Ischemic Stroke

Blood pressure control to ensure that systolic blood pressure (SBP) <185 mm Hg and diastolic blood pressure (DBP) <105 mm Hg, in which case antihypertensive therapy is not indicated

- If DBP >140 mm Hg on two readings 5 minutes apart, start continuous IV infusion of sodium nitroprusside (0.25–0.5 μg/kg/min). These patients are *not* candidates for rt-PA therapy
- If SBP >220 mm Hg or DBP is 120–140 mm Hg or mean arterial pressure >130 mm Hg on two readings 15 minutes apart, give:
  - **Labetalol** 10 mg IV over 1–2 minutes, repeating every 10–20 minutes if necessary for a maximum cumulative dose of 300 mg; or
  - **Enalapril** 0.625–1.25 mg IV over 5 minutes, repeating every 6 hours or as needed (useful in cardiac failure patients); or
  - **Esmolol** IV at 50 μg/kg/min, increasing by 50 μg/kg/min every 5 minutes if needed.

Thrombolysis may not be prudent if three antihypertensive doses have been given.

RULE OUT EXCLUSION CRITERIA

Potential Mimickers	Hemorrhagic Conditions
Glucose <50 mg/dL (<2.8 mmol/L), seizure at stroke onset (if residual impairments are postictal), and rapidly improving symptoms (~TIA)	Intracranial hemorrhage or subarachnoid hemorrhage, Previous intracranial bleed, stroke, or head trauma within last 3 months, low platelets, high PT, recent lumbar puncture or arterial puncture at a noncompressible site

Hypodensity on initial CT and severe stroke (NIH score >22) may predict ICH but these patients still benefited in the overall analysis of the NINDS trial.

Administration of rt-PA should occur within 3 hours from stroke onset, with a dose of 0.9 mg/kg (maximum 90 mg), infused over 1 hour with 10% of the total dose administered in a bolus given over 1 minute. Neurologic status is monitored every 15 minutes for 2 hours, every 30 minutes for the next 6 hours, and hourly thereafter up to 24 hours. If ICH is suspected (neurologic deterioration, new headache, acute hypertension, nausea, vomiting), discontinue rt-PA infusion, obtain STAT head CT scan and draw blood for PT, PTT, platelets, and fibrinogen. Prepare 6–8 units of cryoprecipitate containing factor VIII and 6–8 units of platelets if hemorrhage is confirmed. A neurosurgeon may need to be consulted for the potential need for hematoma evacuation. Consider a second CT scan to assess for change in size. No antiplatelet agent, heparin, heparinoids, or warfarin should be given within 24 hours of symptom onset.

Additional measures include the prevention of complications from cerebral edema (hyperventilation aiming at Pco_2 of 30–35 mm Hg and mannitol 20% solution 1 g/kg bolus over 30 minutes followed by 0.25 g/kg q4–6h), dehydration, aspiration pneumonia (speech therapy, modified barium fluoroscopy), deep vein thrombosis (SC unfractionated heparin 5,000 U twice daily or SC enoxaparin 40 mg daily), fever, hyperglycemia, infection, contractures, decubitus ulcers, and depression.

Antiplatelet Drugs

Antiplatelet agents such as aspirin, aspirin and extended release dipyridamole, or clopidogrel may be used to prevent stroke recurrence for patients with non-cardioembolic ischemic stroke.

- **Aspirin,** a selective **cyclo-oxygenase** inhibitor, at low doses (50–325 mg), prevents early recurrence and reduces disability and death at 3–6 months after a stroke with a small risk of increased intracranial hemorrhage. Aspirin remains the drug of choice for secondary stroke prophylaxis.
- **The combination of aspirin 25 mg plus extended release dipyridamole 200 mg twice daily** increases the benefit of monotherapy with aspirin, although perhaps only modestly. The **phosphodiesterase inhibitor dipyridamole potentiates the antiadhesive effect of adenosine,** resulting in decreased platelet adhesion and aggregation. **Headaches** are a potential side effect.
- **Clopidogrel (Plavix)** (75 mg daily), **an adenosine diphosphate antagonist** like ticlopidine, can be initiated in patients allergic to aspirin. Clopidogrel may cause polyarticular arthritis and thrombotic thrombocytopenic purpura (TTP, also caused by ticlopidine, the drug clopidogrel replaced), the latter within 14 days after initiation of therapy.

EARLY MAJOR ANTIPLATELET CLINICAL TRIALS

IST	1997	ASA given within 48 hours of stroke onset improved outcome (13 fewer dead or disabled per 1,000 treated)
CAST	1997	
CAPRIE	1996	Clopidogrel better than ASA in reducing vascular events
ESPS-2	1996	Combination of aspirin plus extended release dipyridamole twice as better as aspirin given alone
MAST-I	1995	ASA did not reduce 10-day mortality or 6-month disability

ASA, aspirin; **IST**: International Stroke Trial; **CAST**: Chinese Acute Stroke Trial; **CAPRIE:** Clopidogrel versus Aspirin in Patients at Risk for Ischemic Events; **ESPS**: European Stroke Prevention Study; **MAST-I:** Multicenter Acute Stroke Trial-Italy.

- **GPIIb/IIIa receptor antagonists** such as abciximab, eptifibatide, and tirofiban block the activation of the specific platelet-aggregating membrane glycoprotein receptor GPIIb/IIIa. Despite their short-term efficacy, long-term use increases mortality by a partial agonist effect.
- **Direct thrombin inhibitors** show great promise as substitutes for warfarin for the prevention of stroke in patients with atrial fibrillation. **Dabigatran** has been recently approved in the United States. It has similar efficacy to warfarin but does not require monitoring of prothrombin time. Dabigatran 110 mg was non-inferior to warfarin for stroke or systemic embolization, while 150 mg was more effective than warfarin or dabigatran 110 mg. Major bleeding occurred significantly less often with dabigatran 110 mg than warfarin; dabigatran 150 mg showed similar bleeding to warfarin (RE-LY, 2009).
- **Combination therapy with aspirin and clopidogrel** does not provide significant additive benefits compared to the use of clopidogrel alone for secondary stroke prophylaxis. The risk of major bleeding outweighs any benefits at 18 months (MATCH, 2004).
- **Aspirin plus dipyridamole and clopidogrel** are similar in reducing the risk of recurrent stroke at 2.5 years or to prevent MI or vascular death in secondary prophylaxis (PRoFESS, 2008). The risks of hemorrhagic events and headache are higher with aspirin-dipyridamole. In addition, this drug has not been proven effective for the treatment of atherothrombotic disease in other vascular beds (such as coronary artery disease).

HMG-CoA reductase inhibitors ("statins") pravastatin and simvastatin and the fibrate **gemfibrozil** reduce the risk of stroke. Cholesterol reduction not only lowers the risk of stroke, myocardial infarction, and death from vascular causes but also the need for vascular surgical procedures in patients with previous vascular diseases.

ANTIDISLIPIDEMIC AGENTS, INDICATIONS, AND DOSAGES

Classes of Agents	Classic Indications	Agents and Dosage Range
HMG-CoA Reductase inhibitor (**statins**): inhibit rate-limiting enzyme in cholesterol synthesis	**High LDL**, familial **hypercholesterolemia**, diabetes or renal failure-related hyperlipidemia	Lovastatin 40–80 mg/day **Pravastatin** 40–80• mg/day **Simvastatin** 20–80• mg/day Fluvastatin 40–80 mg/day Atorvastatin 10–80 mg/day Rosuvastatin 5–80 mg/day
Bile acid-binding sequestrants (**resins**): shifts cholesterol into bile acid	**Hypercholesterolemia** without high triglycerides (triglycerides <300 mg/dL)	Cholestyramine 4–24 g bid Colestipol 5–30 g bid Colesevelam 1,250 bid-tid
Nicotinic acid (**niacin**): reduce use of FFA for synthesis of TG and VLDL	**Low HDL**, familial **hypercholesterolemia** or combined **hyperlipidemia** in combination with statins	Niacin 100–4000 mg/day Niacin ER 500–2000 mg/day Niacin SR 500–2000 mg/day
Fibric-acid derivatives (**fibrates**): activates FA uptake and LPL-induced VLDL catab.	Hypertriglyceridemia **Low HDL *and* LDL** in patients with CAD	**Gemfibrozil** 300–600 bid• Fenofibrate 67–200 mg/day Clofibrate (no longer used: high mortality, cholelithiasis)

LDL, low-density lipoprotein; FFA, free fatty acid; TG, triglyceride; VLDL, very-low-density lipoprotein; FA, fatty acid; LPL, lipoprotein lipase; HDL, high-density lipoprotein.

• Secondary prevention of stroke was proven in the Scandinavian Simvastatin Survival Study (4S, 1994), the Cholesterol and Recurrent Events (CARE, 1996), and the Long-term Intervention with Pravastatin in Ischemic Disease (LIPID, 1998). Myositis is common in patients taking statins with gemfibrozil, niacin, or erythromycin, and in patients with renal insufficiency.

Blood pressure, stroke, and vascular mortality have a log-linear relationship, with the risk of stroke and vascular mortality falling with lower BP, with no cutoff established. The prospective Perindopril Protection Against Recurrent Stroke Study (**PROGRESS,** 2001) showed that BP reduction, even in those considered normotensive (<140/90 was present in 50% of this cohort), by 9/4 mm Hg on average resulted in a 28% risk reduction of major stroke (one stroke could be prevented among every 14 patients treated for 5 years). This study was also important because it supported the hypothesis that **diuretics,** in addition to their antihypertensive action, may confer a **neuroprotective effect.** There are no guidelines regarding how soon to start antihypertensive therapy but 1 month after the acute event is the prevailing recommendation. If ACE inhibitors are not tolerated (because of cough, for example), BP reduction with other agents (such as calcium antagonists or β-blockers) is likely to reduce the risk of stroke, although the evidence comes from studies in primary stroke prevention.

Although **hyperhomocysteinemia** is believed to be an independent risk factor for stroke, the Vitamin Intervention for Stroke Prevention (VISP, 2004) study failed to demonstrate the benefit of using a combination of folic acid, pyridoxine (vitamin B6), and cobalamin (vitamin B_{12}) in reducing stroke recurrence.

Carotid Endarterectomy (CEA)

The severity of carotid stenosis is the best predictor of stroke recurrence. There is an annual stroke rate of 18% in patients using antiplatelets with a history of TIA or strokes and a 70%–99% stenosis (WASID, Warfarin vs. Aspirin for Symptomatic Intracranial Disease study, 2006). CEA offers the greatest risk reduction in recurrent ipsilateral ischemic stroke for those with **symptomatic carotid stenosis >70%**, (**NASCET,** North American Symptomatic Carotid Endarterectomy, 1991; **ECST,** European Carotid Surgery Trials, 1998). The greatest gain occurs in men, the elderly, and those with hemispheric rather than retinal symptoms. Only six patients needed to be treated to prevent one stroke in 2 years. For symptomatic stenosis of 50%–69% (lower stroke risk) and perioperative risk of 6%, the number needed to treat to prevent one stroke was 15 (NASCET). The procedure's benefit is greatest if performed within the first 2 weeks from the ischemic event, greatly reduced by 12 weeks in those with at least 70% stenosis, and absent in those with 50%–69% stenosis.

In **asymptomatic carotid atherosclerosis of 60%–99%,** the absolute risk reduction for major stroke ranges between 5.4% and 5.9% at 5 years, according to reports from the Asymptomatic Carotid Surgery Trial (**ACST,** 2004) and the Asymptomatic Carotid Atherosclerosis Study (**ACAS,** 1995), respectively. This modest benefit favoring CEA assumes that operative complications are below 3%. Unlike trials in symptomatic patients, the benefit was not dependent on the severity of the stenosis (which may be the result of ascertainment bias, as the stenosis was determined by ultrasound rather than angiography). Asymptomatic patients face only a 2% annual stroke rate, which falls below 1% after successful CEA. Hence, the number needed to treat to prevent one stroke was found to be at least 67. Although it has not been established that asymptomatic individuals at highest risk are those with the greatest severity of stenosis, the American Heart Association has published the following **guidelines for asymptomatic stenosis:**
- **For patients with a surgical risk <3%** and life expectancy of at least 5 years, ipsilateral CEA is considered "proven indication" for asymptomatic stenotic lesions ≥60% regardless of contralateral artery status
- **When the surgical risk is between 3% and 5%,** ipsilateral CEA for stenosis ≥75% in the presence of contralateral ICA stenosis ranging from 75% to total occlusion is "acceptable but not proven."

Extracranial carotid angioplasty with stenting (CAS) is a less invasive alternative to CEA. The periprocedure risks in symptomatic patients who had CAS (~10%) were as high as (**CAVATAS,** 2001), or higher than (**EVA-3S,** 2006), CEA with similar benefits (average annual risk of ipsilateral stroke was ≤1% despite a significantly higher risk of restenosis in CAS [~11%] vs. CEA [~5%]; **SPACE,** 2008). The Carotid Revascularization Endarterectomy versus Stenting Trial (**CREST,** 2010) showed no significant difference in the composite of any stroke, myocardial infarction, or death between symptomatic and asymptomatic patients receiving carotid artery stenting or carotid endarterectomy.

Transient Ischemic Attack (TIA)

TIAs are short-lived episodes of neurologic deficit attributed to focal cerebral or retinal ischemia of sudden onset and offset. Symptoms and signs usually last <1 hour, and in **90% of cases last <10 minutes.** Using the formal 24-hour time cutoff, up to 50% of patients have evidence of acute infarction by DWI. The incidence of TIA reaches 500,000 cases per year. **The 90-day risk of stroke after a TIA is about 10%,** with half occurring within 2 days. As such, TIAs are considered medical emergencies. If a nonretinal TIA is attributable to a 70% to 99% stenosis of the ICA, the 90-day risk exceeds 25% (retinal TIAs carry half the risk of nonretinal events). The **ABCD2 score** is useful for stroke risk stratification in patients with TIAs: **A**ge ≥60 years = 1 point; **B**lood pressure ≥140/90 mm Hg = 1 point; **C**linical unilateral weakness = 2 points; speech-only impairment = 1 point; **D**uration ≥60 minutes = 2 points, < 60 minutes = 1 point; **D**iabetes = 1 point. ABCD2 score ≥4 indicate a moderate to high stroke risk (Johnston SC et al. *Lancet* 2007; 369:283–292).

> The following conditions may cause symptoms or signs suggestive of TIA: migraine, vestibulopathy, **postictal paralysis**, arterial dissection, **transient global amnesia**, subdural hematoma, **vasovagal syncope**, **hypoglycemia**, thrombocythemia, severe **orthostatic hypotension**, cervical disc disease, **cerebral venous thrombosis**, temporal arteritis, and conversion disorder.

Evaluation of TIAs aims at localizing the affected vessel and ruling out metabolic and hematologic causes of neurologic symptoms (hypoglycemia, hyponatremia, thrombocytosis). An elevated ESR may suggest temporal arteritis or infective endocarditis. EKG rules out atrial fibrillation or a myocardial infarction. Carotid stenosis should be explored by Doppler ultrasonography, magnetic resonance angiography, or computed tomography angiography (CTA). MRA and CTA have replaced catheter angiography for many patients.

Aspirin (75–1300 mg) provides a relative risk reduction of 22% for stroke and cardiovascular events after a TIA or stroke. The benefit is smaller (~10%) during acute stroke partly because of the risk of intracranial hemorrhage. Clopidogrel and extended-release dipyridamole/acetylsalicylic acid are alternatives in patients who cannot tolerate aspirin or who were taking aspirin at the time of the event. For patients with atrial fibrillation, **anticoagulation** with warfarin is compulsory. Given the high short-term risk of stroke after a TIA, treatment with unfractionated or low-molecular weight heparin is justified. For symptomatic patients with 70% to 99% stenosis, the absolute risk reduction with carotid endarterectomy based on a 5-year risk of stroke is 15.65 (number needed to treat [NNT] = 6). For symptomatic patients with 50% to 69% stenosis, the absolute risk reduction is 7.8% (NNT = 13). **Statins** may have a protective value beyond that provided by the correction of lipid profiles. **Antihypertensive drugs** also reduce the long-term risk of stroke (relative risk reduction, 25%-30%) after TIA or stroke even among those without hypertension. The BP target is <140/90 mm Hg in nondiabetics and <130/80 mm Hg in diabetics.

Subarachnoid Hemorrhage (SAH)

Nontraumatic SAH is a medical emergency most commonly caused by **ruptured cerebral aneurysms.** Saccular or berry aneurysms are the most common. There is a 51% mortality or significant morbidity after aneurysm bleeds. Aneurysm rebleeding is greatest in the first 24 hours (2.6%–4%). A **sentinel headache** or warning leak may be the event preceding a major hemorrhage in 40% of the patients. The classic presentation consists of abrupt onset of the worst headache of one's life followed by altered consciousness, meningismus, photophobia, nausea, and vomiting. They are all **poorly localizing findings,** except for:

- **Complete oculomotor palsy** is often due to **posterior communicating artery** (PcomA) or basilar apex artery aneurysm
- **Crural-predominant hemiparesis** results from **anterior communicating artery** (AcomA) aneurysm
- **Carotid-cavernous fistula** occurs with **intracavernous ICA** aneurysm

A noncontrast head CT shows blood filling the skull base cisterns until 6–10 days from the bleed (MRI yields delayed identification but blood changes persist longer than 30 days). **Lumbar puncture** is the next step if the HCT is normal. LP may be negative if done within 6 hours (up to 12 hours) from onset of symptoms.

> **Xanthochromia** is always present by 12 hours, peaks at 1 week, and remains visible for an average of 2 weeks. A traumatic tap is not reliably excluded by reduced red cell counts of the fourth CSF tube. **CSF spectrophotometry** is more reliable than the naked eye in the detection of xanthochromia.

- **Four-vessel cerebral angiography or CTA** confirms the presence and location of the aneurysm; additional ones may coexist in 10%–15% of patients. Aneurysms <10 mm in diameter have a rupture risk of 0.05% per year.
- **Brain MRI** ascertains angiographically occult AVMs, cavernous malformations, external carotid circulation aneurysm, and dural AVMs

Preoperative management is based on correction of any underlying physiologic derangements, discontinuation of antithrombotics, deep vein thrombosis (DVT) prophylaxis, and the use of **nimodipine** 60 mg POr or NG every 4 hours for 21 days. The use of antiepileptic drugs for seizure prophylaxis and glucocorticoid is controversial. **Cerebral vasospasm with delayed cerebral ischemia** is the major cause of late neurologic deficits and correlates with the amount of blood collected in the basal cisterns. It typically occurs 3 days, and peaks between 7 and 8 days, after SAH. In the presence of hydrocephalus, **ventriculostomy** helps maintain the cerebral perfusion pressure (CPP) >60 torr and ICP <20 torr (other measures to decrease ICP are hyperventilation, elevation of the head of the bed, and hyperosmolar agents). **Surgical treatment** consists of **aneurysm clipping or coiling** (for Hunt-Hess scale 1–2). **Postoperative management** is intended to treat ischemic deficits due to vasospasm with avoidance of hypovolemia and the "3 H approach": **h**ypertension, **h**ypervolemia, and **h**emodilution.

Intracerebral Hemorrhage

ICH accounts for 10% of all strokes and is associated with ~60% mortality within the first year. **Hypertension** is the most common cause and accounts for the higher incidence of ICH among blacks (50 per 100,000), twice that of whites. **Excessive alcohol use** increases the risk by impairing coagulation. The most common sites of ICH are the putamen (lenticulostriate branches of the MCA), thalamus (thalamogeniculate branches of the PCA), cerebral lobes (penetrating cortical branches of the major brain vessels), pons (paramedian branches of the basilar artery), and the dentate nucleus region of the cerebellar hemisphere (branches of the superior cerebellar artery). **CAA,** presenting as **lobar hemorrhages** in the elderly, is caused by the deposition of β-amyloid protein (mostly in Apolipoprotein allele E2 carriers) or fracture of the amyloid-laden vessel wall in cortical and leptomeningeal *small and medium*-sized arteries. Hereditary CAA is caused by mutations in various genes, including APP, cystatin C, gelsolin, and transthyretin.

Primary ICH (~80%)		Secondary ICH (~20%)	
Spontaneous rupture of small vessels	Annual risk of recurrence	Associated with vasculopathies, tumors, or coagulopathies	Annual risk of recurrence
Hypertension	2%	**Arteriovenous malformations**	18%
Amyloid angiopathy	10.5%	**Intracranial aneurysms**	50%–3%*
Vasculitis	Variable	**Cavernous malformations**	4.5%
Hemorrhagic infarct	Variable	**Developmental venous anomalies**	0.15%
		Dural venous thrombosis	10%–1%♣
		Coagulopathies	Variable

*The risk of recurrent (usually *subarachnoid*) hemorrhage from a saccular aneurysm is 50% within the first 6 months, decreasing to 3% per year thereafter. Surgical clipping or placement of endovascular coils significantly reduces the risk.
♣ The risk of recurrent dural venous sinus thrombosis is 10% within the first year and <1% thereafter.

Neurologic deterioration is primarily due to hematoma expansion within the first 3 hours, but also to worsening cerebral edema 24–48 hours after the onset of hemorrhage. Poor predictive factors (leading to a mortality rate of 90% at 1 month) are a **low Glasgow coma score** (<9), **large volume of hematoma** (>60 mL), and presence of **intraventricular blood** on initial CT scan.

> The **volume of the hematoma** can be empirically measured by: **A × B × C / 2,**
> where: **A** = greatest diameter of hemorrhage; **B** = diameter perpendicular to A;
> and **C** = number of slices showing hematoma multiplied by the slice thickness.

MRA and/or CTA are useful tools in detecting underlying structural abnormalities. Conventional angiography may be needed for selected individuals who have no obvious cause for their hemorrhage. Surgical removal of supratentorial intracerebral hemorrhage remains unproven in the majority of patients. Large volume, superficial lobar hemorrhages with neurologic deterioration often require surgery. Surgery is indicated in most instances of cerebellar hemorrhages in an effort to prevent brainstem compression.

Increased Intracranial Pressure (ICP)

Any process displacing the rigid cranial volume (a volume of about 1,500 cm^3) increases the pressure in the intracranial compartment, which causes anatomical displacement on the parenchyma, impairs cerebral blood flow, and causes ischemia, neuronal death, and/or blood–brain barrier disruption with brain **edema:**

- **Vasogenic edema** is caused by neoplasm and infections, accumulating *extracellular* water from primary cerebral vasculature damage. This variant of brain edema responds to corticosteroids.
- **Cytotoxic edema** caused by hypoxia and ischemia that occurs in head injury and stroke, consists of accumulation of *intracellular* water from primary neuronal dysfunction.
- **Ischemic edema** is initially cytotoxic and later vasogenic, reaches its peak ~72–120 hours after stroke, and does not respond to corticosteroids.

> **Imaging distinction**: Hyperintensity on DWI and reduced ADC strongly suggest cytotoxic edema (ischemia), whereas hypointensity on DWI with bright ADC signal points toward vasogenic edema (infection, neoplasm).
>
> DWI = diffusion-weighted MRI sequence; ADC = apparent diffusion coefficient sequence

Monitoring of ICP is standard of care in high-risk and comatose patients. Conventionally, 20 mm Hg (normal ICP = 0–10 mm Hg) is the threshold beyond which CPP may fall and lead to ischemia. CPP is obtained as MAP − ICP (where MAP is the mean arterial pressure).

Treatment of increased ICP may require removal of tumor or hematoma; CSF drainage, fluid restriction, correction of hyperglycemia, and head elevation.

- **Mannitol 20%** in acutely increased ICP is administered as 1 g/kg bolus infusion over 30 minutes followed by 0.25–0.5 g/kg every 4–6 hours thereafter for only a brief period to avoid rebound or paradoxical increased ICP. The serum osmolarity is allowed to increase to 315–320 mOsm/L.
- **Hypertonic saline** solutions may decrease elevated ICP in stroke patients who are refractory to mannitol administration.
- **Cautious hyperventilation** (Paco$_2$ = 33 ± 2 mm Hg) leads to vasoconstriction and subsequent reduction in blood volume in the "vascular subdivision of the intracranial compartment," reducing ICP. Aggressive hyperventilation (Paco$_2$ = 25 mm Hg) may reduce CPP, cause secondary ischemia, and worsen neurologic outcome.
- **Barbiturates** decrease cerebral metabolism and may inhibit free radical-mediated lipid peroxidation. **High-dose pentobarbital** (10 mg/kg over 30 minutes, followed by 1–1.5 mg/kg/h, keeping levels at ~3 mg/dL), *when other measures have failed* reduces ICP but may cause hypotension.
- **Moderate hypothermia** (33°C–36°C for 24–48 hours) for intractable cases may improve neurologic outcome.
- In selective patients with malignant cerebral edema associated with hemispheric infarction, hemicraniectomy and durotomy may be indicated.

Patent Foramen Ovale (PFO)

About **30% of the population** has a patent interatrial channel that normally closes soon after birth when pressure in the left atrium exceeds that in the right. A PFO provides a way through which **right-to-left shunting** takes place. Most people with a PFO remain asymptomatic throughout life. PFO is associated with cryptogenic strokes in patients younger than 55 years, but the causal link has not been confirmed. Stroke presumably results from **paradoxical embolism** of thrombotic material from the venous into the arterial circulation. Intracardiac thrombosis or arrhythmias have not been proven mechanisms of stroke. The size of the foramen ranges from 1 to 19 mm (mean, 4.9 mm).

Because PFO is also common in individuals without stroke and may coexist by chance alone in a subset of young adults with stroke, the following conditions are believed to increase the risk of stroke:
- **Coexistence with atrial septal aneurysms,** lesions characterized by redundant hypermobile septal tissue causing turbulent flow, and present in combination with PFO in about 20% of cases.
- **Large opening of the PFO** correlates with a more severe right-to-left shunting at rest.

PFO of any opening size, by itself, does not predict recurrent cerebrovascular events.

Diagnosis of PFO is established through the following tests:
- **Transesophageal echocardiography with intravenous injection of microbubble contrast agents** is more sensitive than the transthoracic approach. Right-to-left shunt is indicated by the passage of microbubbles into the left atrium within three cardiac cycles after opacification of the right atrium. Testing is performed at rest and during Valsalva maneuvers.
- **Transcranial Doppler (TCD)** of the middle cerebral artery is highly sensitive and specific to detect arterial bubbles compared with TOE. Although TCD may avoid the need for transesophageal echocardiography, it does not provide any information about other potentially important cardiac embolic sources.
- **Documentation of deep venous thrombosis or pulmonary embolism** is critical if the diagnosis of paradoxical embolism is entertained, although when there is evidence for simultaneous pulmonary and systemic embolism, paradoxical embolism is not necessarily confirmed (venous thrombosis may be result rather than the cause of stroke).

Therapeutic options for PFO include antiplatelet drugs, oral anticoagulants, transcatheter closure of the foramen, and open-heart surgery. There are no data to support the relative superiority of any one of these strategies. The long-term risks and benefits of PFO closure are not known. Results of the CLOSURE I Trial (2009) failed to demonstrate superiority of PFO closure with STARFlex plus medical therapy over medical therapy alone.

Neurovascular Syndromes

Middle cerebral artery (MCA) syndromes:

- Stem occlusion causes contralateral hemiplegia, conjugate eye deviation toward the side of the infarct, hemianesthesia, and homonymous hemianopsia. **Global aphasia** lateralizes the lesion to the dominant hemisphere whereas **hemineglect** lateralizes the lesion to the nondominant hemisphere.

- **Upper division MCA strokes** are recognized by a gradient of face and arm greater than leg involvement and a greater tendency for aphasia of the Broca rather than Wernicke type (**lower division MCA strokes**).

- **Lenticulostriate branches** may cause a lacunar infarction within the internal capsule expressed as a pure motor hemiparesis.

Amaurosis fugax and Horner syndrome (from oculosympathetic damage) are the only features that indicate a lesion proximal to the MCA, at the carotid level.

Anterior cerebral artery (ACA) syndrome produces a gradient of hemiparesis that affects the legs more than the arms, as well as abulia, **akinetic mutism,** sphincter incontinence, **transcortical motor aphasia** (dominant hemisphere), position greater than vibration sensory loss in the legs, and paratonia. An anterior disconnection syndrome (left arm apraxia) may be present.

Anterior choroidal artery syndrome is characterized by the clinical triad of hemiparesis (posterior limb of the internal capsule), hemihypesthesia (posteroventrolateral thalamus), and hemianopsia sparing the horizontal meridian (lateral geniculate body).

Posterior inferior cerebellar artery syndrome, also resulting from vertebral artery occlusion or dissection, leads to the Wallenberg or **dorsolateral medullary** syndrome. Its onset may be preceded by **neck pain** hours, days, or months in advance. The constellation of deficits include vertigo, **nystagmus, Horner syndrome,** dysphagia, dysarthria, diplopia, and ipsilateral facial hypesthesia to pain and temperature (trigeminal nucleus) with contralateral arm and leg hypesthesia to the same sensory modalities (lateral spinothalamic tract).

Anterior inferior cerebellar artery (AICA) syndrome, or ventral cerebellar syndrome, is distinguished by the presence of Horner syndrome, ipsilateral facial and corneal hypesthesia to pain and temperature (trigeminal spinal nucleus and tract), and **ipsilateral deafness** and facial paralysis from lateral pontomedullary tegmentum involvement.

Superior cerebellar artery (SCA) syndrome, or dorsal cerebellar syndrome, is recognized by the presence of a **cerebellar outflow tremor** (Holmes tremor) in addition to Horner syndrome, nystagmus, and ipsilateral ataxia. A fourth nerve palsy may be seen contralaterally.

Middle cerebral artery (MCA) syndromes of the midbrain:

- **Weber syndrome (cerebral peduncle;** PCA penetrators): fascicular CN III and contralateral pyramidal deficit of the face, arm, and leg
- **Benedikt syndrome (ventral mesencephalic tegmentum):** ipsilateral CN III and contralateral cerebellar outflow tremor, hemiathetosis, and chorea from red nucleus and brachium conjunctivum involvement
- **Claude syndrome (dorsal mesencephalic tegmentum):** ipsilateral CN III and cerebellar deficits from dorsal red nucleus involvement
- **Parinaud syndrome (mesencephalic tectum):** supranuclear vertical gaze palsy, light-near dissociation, convergence-retraction nystagmus, skew deviation, and lid retraction (Collier sign)
- **Top-of-the-basilar syndrome:** midbrain, thalamus, and temporal and occipital lobes from thromboembolic disease of the rostral basilar artery
  - **Behavioral abnormalities:** peduncular hallucinosis, somnolence
  - **Ocular findings:** full Parinaud syndrome plus visual field deficits such as hemianopsia, cortical blindness, and Balint syndrome

Midline vertebrobasilar syndromes of the pons

- **Medial inferior pontine syndrome** (paramedian basilar penetrators): Ipsilateral paralysis of conjugate gaze to the side of the lesion and ataxia with contralateral hemiparesis and hemihypesthesia
- **Medial midpontine syndrome:** as in previous list plus ipsilateral limb ataxia
- **Bilateral ventral pontine syndrome (Locked-in syndrome):** impairment of horizontal eye movements and quadriplegia with intact wakefulness, blinking, and vertical gaze movements (intact supranuclear pathways).

Midline and lateral medullary syndromes

- **Lateral medullary syndrome (Wallenberg syndrome):** ipsilateral Horner syndrome, facial analgesia and thermoanesthesia, dysphagia, dysphonia, and cerebellar ataxia with contralateral hemihypesthesia due to vertebral artery and, less commonly, PICA occlusion
- **Medial medullary syndrome:** ipsilateral CN XII and contralateral hemiparesis-hemihypesthesia from distal vertebral artery steno-occlusive disease or atheromatous disease of penetrating branches of the anterior spinal artery

Posterior cerebral artery (PCA) syndrome: Any combination of contralateral homonymous hemianopsia or quadrantanopsia with macular sparing, visual field neglect (nondominant lesion), visual and color agnosias, prosopagnosia, alexia without agraphia, transcortical sensory aphasia, and Dejerine-Roussy syndrome (thalamic pain, vasomotor disturbances, and choreoathetosis or hemiballism).

Spinal artery (SA) syndromes: Anterior: paraplegia, thermoanesthesia, and analgesia below the level of the lesion with preservation of proprioception, commonly occurring in the border zone segments between **T1 and T4** and **L1; Posterior:** loss of proprioception and vibration below the lesion.

Thalamic Syndromes

Except for olfaction, most sensory modalities are somatotopically organized in the thalamus, from which projections are sent to the cortex. Only very fine discriminative sensory functions such as stereognosis, graphesthesia, two-point discrimination, and precise tactile localization require the cortex.

The **internal medullary lamina** divides the thalamus into the anterior, medial, and lateral nuclear groups. The **centromedian nucleus,** within the intralaminar nuclei of the internal medullary lamina, is the rostral extension of the brainstem reticular formation (arousal). The **anterior nucleus,** which lies between the Y-shaped arms of the internal medullary lamina, connects with the mamillary bodies and the cingulate gyrus (limbic system). The **dorsomedial nucleus** (cognition, affect, memory), is a target in Wernicke encephalopathy, as are the mamillary bodies. **The ventral posterior lateral (VPL) and ventral posterior medial (VPM) nuclei** are the major sensory relay nuclei for body (VPL) and face (VPM). They relay lemniscal (light touch, pressure, vibration, and position) and spinothalamic (pain and temperature) sensation to the somesthetic cortex (Brodmann areas 1–3). Strokes affecting them may produce the syndrome of thalamic pain. **The ventrolateral nucleus** receives input from the globus pallidus and cerebellum and projects to the motor and premotor cortices.

Four specific stroke syndromes according are recognized:
- **Anterior infarcts** (occlusion of tuberothalamic or polar artery, arising from the posterior communicating artery or paramedian or thalamoperforating arteries) consist of perseverations, apathy, and amnesia
- **Paramedian infarcts** (occlusion of thalamoperforating arteries which originate from the first [P1] segment of the PCA) may lead to cyclical psychosis, manic delirium, personality changes, amnesia, vertical gaze paresis, and "thalamic dementia" in extensive lesions
- **Inferolateral infarcts** (occlusion of thalamogeniculate arteries, from the second [P2] segment of the PCA) may lead to hypesthesia and ataxia

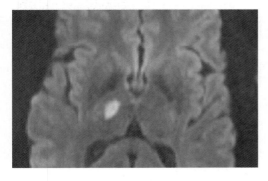

53-year-old man with acute onset of isolated, painless, left hemiataxia. Brain MRI shows restricted diffusion in the right thalamus. Acute isolated hemiataxia, most often due to infratentorial (cerebellar) stroke, may occur with supratentorial (thalamic) lesions or damage to cerebellar pathways (dentatorubrothalamocortical or corticopontocerebellar).

- **Posterior infarcts** (occlusion of medial and lateral branches of the posterior choroidal artery, which originates from the P2 segment of PCA) consists of hypesthesia, homonymous horizontal sectoranopsia (due to involvement of the lateral geniculate body), neglect and aphasia.

Stroke patterns (A)

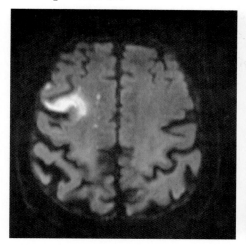 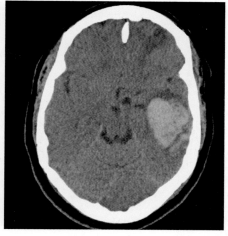

Diffusion-weighted (DW) MRI shows restricted diffusion on the anterior right frontal region consistent with an acute infarct in the superior division of the right MCA.

CT head without contrast shows a large parenchymal hemorrhage centered in the left temporal lobe measuring ~4.7 × 3.2 cm extending into the parietal region. There is slight rightward shift

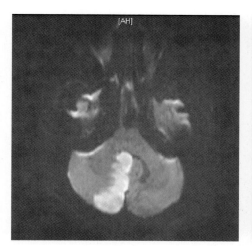 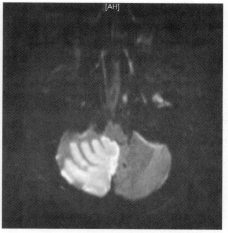

Diffusion-weighted MRI shows restricted diffusion on the distribution of the posterior inferior cerebellar artery consistent with an acute infarct.

Stroke patterns (B)

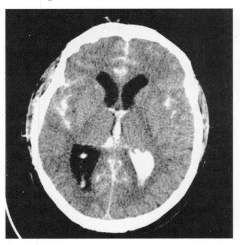 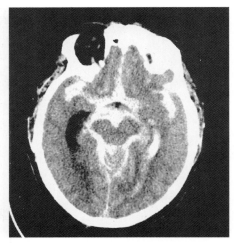

Noncontrast CT of the head shows extensive amount of subarachnoid hemorrhage. There is also large amount of intraventricular hemorrhage that extended caudally to the upper cervical spinal canal. The patient was found to have a ruptured left posterior communicating artery aneurysm.

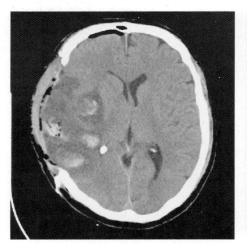 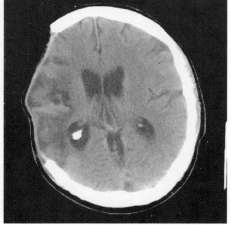

CT head without contrast. Left: status post right frontal parietal craniectomy with decompression of hemorrhagic right MCA territory infarction in a patient with cervical right ICA occlusion; Right (6 weeks later): resolution of previously seen mass effect and edema in the right MCA territory infarct with no evidence of new ischemic change or hemorrhage.

Stroke patterns (C)

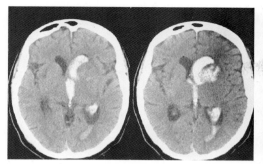

CT head without contrast shows an acute hemorrhage in the left caudate nucleus dissecting into the ventricles

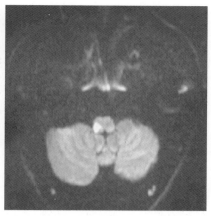

Diffusion-weighted (DW) MRI shows a focal area of restricted diffusion in the right posterolateral medulla (Wallenberg syndrome)

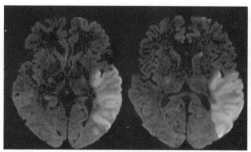

DW MRI shows signal changes with an acute infarction of the left temporal lobe in a patient with Wernicke aphasia.

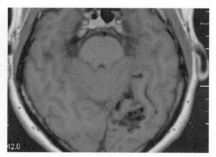

Axial T1W of a left PCA arteriovenous malformation.

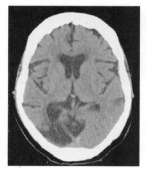

CT head without contrast shows remote right PCA distribution infarct.

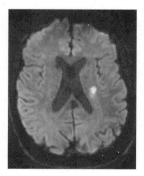

DW MRI shows an acute lacunar infarction in the left periventricular white matter and posterior limb of the internal capsule.

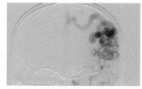
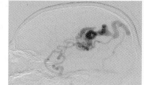

Cerebral angiogram of a large left parietal AVM from a 51-year-old man with partial complex seizures.

Stroke patterns (D)

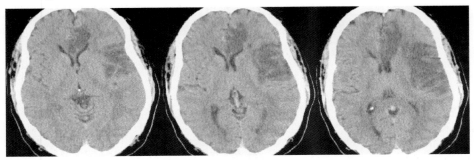

CT brain scan demonstrates hypodensity with loss of gray-white matter differentiation involving the left frontal and parietal lobes compatible with infarcts involving the left anterior and middle cerebral artery territories.

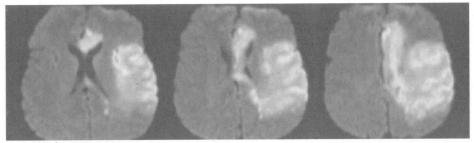

DW MRI shows restricted diffusion involving the left anterior and middle cerebral artery territories with mild effacement of the sulci of the sulci overlying the left frontal and anterior parietal lobes.

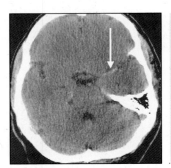

The "hyperdense" MCA sign applies to the increased attenuation of the proximal MCA on head CT (arrow), often associated with thrombosis of the M1 segment.

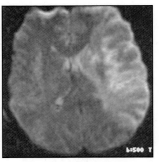

Early CT signs of ischemic stroke include: (1) hyperdense vessel, (2) loss of insular ribbon, (3) obscuration of the lenticular nucleus, (4) loss of gray-white matter differentiation, and (5) sulcal effacement, and (6) focal hypoattenuation

CT (left) shows a hyperdense MCA, an early CT diagnostic feature of an acute ischemic stroke. DW MRI (right; same patient) demonstrates restricted diffusion on the superficial and deep left MCA territory. This patient subsequently developed brain edema and herniation consistent with a **malignant left MCA infarction**. The underlying mechanism of malignant MCA infarction is either a carotid terminus occlusion or a proximal MCA occlusion.

Hemorrhagic neuroimaging patterns

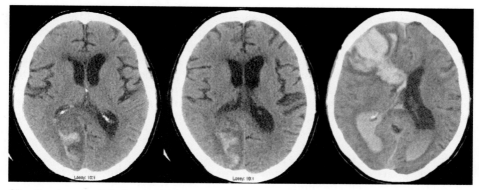

CT without contrast: Left and middle: hemorrhagic conversion of a PCA stroke. Right: intraparenchymal hemorrhage with surrounding edema, midline shift, and intraventricular extension with hydrocephalus in an 84-year-old man with a prior right temporal lobar hematoma suspected to have cerebral amyloid angiopathy.

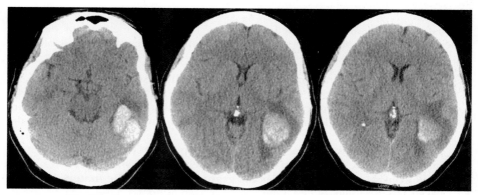

CT without contrast: hemorrhagic conversion of metastatic breast cancer.

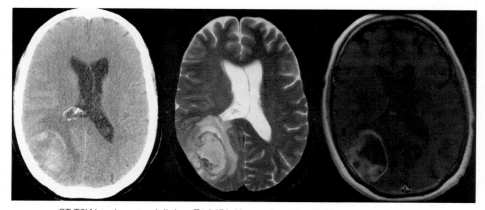

CT, T2W and postgadolinium T1 MRI: Hemorrhage in glioblastoma multiforme.

CADASIL

CADASIL is an inherited autosomal dominant condition characterized by **migraine** (most frequently migraine with aura), **recurrent ischemic strokes, and frontal-predominant dementia.** Classically, migraine occurs in the third to fourth decades, strokes in the fourth and fifth, dementia in the sixth and seventh, and death usually in the seventh decade. Psychiatric disturbances and epileptic seizures are part of the phenotypic spectrum. CADASIL is considered the most frequent cause of stroke of genetic origin. Although the clinical features are **confined to the CNS,** the pathology involves **systemic arterioles,** allowing "peripheral" tissue to be used for diagnostic purposes.

Point mutations in the *Notch3* gene cause CADASIL. This gene codes for a transmembrane protein that participates in an **intercellular signaling pathway** essential for controlling cell fate during development. Thus far, all mutations reported in CADASIL occur in the extracellular portion of the protein, in the first 23 of its 33 exons. Because **60%–70% of mutations cluster in exons 3 and 4,** a limited screen can be achieved by examining these exons alone. However, about 14% of sporadic patients with MRI suggestive of CADASIL but apparently negative family history carry the *Notch3* gene mutation in exons 10, 11, and 19.

Because of difficulties with genetic screening, the current methods of diagnosis depend on the ***combination*** of suggestive brain MRI features and, if available, specific skin biopsy findings.

- **Brain MRI** demonstrates **confluent regions of high signal** on T2W and FLAIR sequences in the periventricular and deep white matter (with U-fiber involvement), **anterior temporal pole, external capsule, basal ganglia,** and brainstem. Hemosiderin deposits due to microbleeds have been described in the thalamus.
- **Skin biopsy** shows PAS-positive granular deposits adjacent to the basement membrane of the smooth muscle cells of arterioles, which, on electron microscopy, consists of the pathognomonic **granular osmiophilic material** (GOM). Given the variability of GOM deposition in skin arterioles, false-negative results are possible. Immunostaining the tissue specimen with a *Notch3* monoclonal antibody increases the sensitivity.

Patients with an autosomal dominant pattern of transmission of headache, stroke, and/or dementia, especially when the MRI findings are suggestive of leukoaraiosis, can be directly tested for *Notch3* mutation status without first undergoing **skin biopsy with electron microscopy.** Other small-vessel vasculopathies that need consideration in the differential include other hereditary vasculopathies (Fabry disease, homocystinuria), arteriosclerosis (often associated with smoking, hyperlipidemia, and hypertension), vasculitis, and cerebral amyloid angiopathy.

Classic Brain MRI Findings of CADASIL

The axial brain MRI shown here of a *Notch3*-positive patient, admitted for recurrent headaches, demonstrated confluent white matter abnormal signal on FLAIR (left column) and T2W (right column) sequences in, among others, two classic regions: (1) the anterior temporal pole (upper row; rarely affected in other leukoencephalopathies) and (2) the external capsule (lower row). Basal ganglia and pons are often affected. Cystic infarcts or enlarged perivascular spaces are also common.

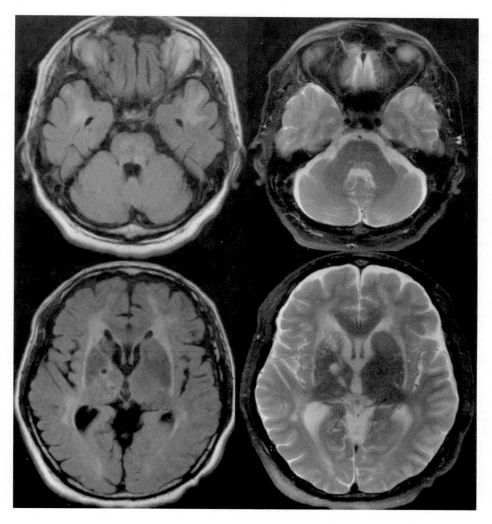

Important Stroke Mimickers

Migraine

Focal symptoms *march* from visual (fortification spectra) to sensory (perioral or arm tingling) to mild dysphasia. History of headache or typical fortification spectra is important when the aura is not followed by headache (see next section).

Late-life migraine accompaniments (migraine equivalent of middle age) These accompaniments refer to such deficits as scintillating scotomas, numbness, aphasia, dysarthria, and focal weakness that occur for the first time after the age of 45 years in the form of **acephalgic migraine** (headache does occur in 50%). The episode lasts between 15 and 25 minutes (90% of TIAs last <15 minutes). History of recurrent headache is present in 65% of cases. The critical **visual accompaniments** (hemianopsia, diplopia, blindness, and blurred vision besides scotoma) "build up" gradually, the paresthesias "march" as in classic migraine, and the progression of one accompaniment to another rules out cerebrovascular disease. Remarkably focal and brief numbness (tip of tongue, half of digit, one toe or finger) is a relatively common observation. Vascular risk factors are absent and there are no permanent sequelae.

Transient global amnesia is a transitory deficit of anterograde memory (inability to acquire new information) of sudden onset and gradual remission, lasting a few hours (longer than most transient ischemic attacks: 4–8 hours instead of minutes). The patient repetitively asks the same questions and appears perplexed, disoriented to time, sometimes to place, **but never to family or self** (identity is always preserved). Immediate recall and the ability to perform complex activities are preserved. There are no other focal neurologic deficits. When memory returns, the patient retains a memory gap for the span covered by the spell. It has a benign prognosis and there is a low rate of recurrence. The cause remains unsolved and ischemia, epilepsy, and migraine have been largely excluded, whereas behavioral disorders (phobic personality traits) are believed to be at least contributory.

Intravascular Lymphomatosis (Malignant Angioendotheliomatosis)

This rare angiotropic large-cell lymphoma presents in the sixth decade of life with widespread vascular occlusion of **small vessels** (arterioles, capillaries, and venules) and a fatal course within weeks to months. A significant proportion of patients have CNS involvement from **multiple infarcts and hemorrhage** causing encephalopathy, seizures, myelopathy, and peripheral and cranial neuropathies. Because of the sparing of the hematopoietic system, peripheral blood or bone marrow analysis is unrevealing and only biopsy or autopsy offers definitive confirmation: distention and plugging of small vessels by **neoplastic mononuclear cells** (mostly of B-cell lineage). This condition has been confused with **Creutzfeldt-Jakob disease** (when myoclonus is present), and **primary angiitis of the CNS.**

VASCULITIDES

Vessel Size	Disease Entity	Neurologic Dysfunction
Large	**Giant cell arteritis** (see Neuroophthalmology)	**Polymyalgia rheumatica, temporal arteritis**
	Takayasu arteritis	Encephalopathy (young women with pulse deficits, aortitis, and aortic dissection)
Medium	**Primary CNS angiitis**	"Primary" (see separate text)
	Kawasaki disease	Aseptic meningitis (children with fever, rash, "strawberry tongue", redness of palms and soles, and conjunctivitis)
Medium and small Lungs are largely spared in polyarteritis nodosa ANCA as tested by ELISA provides two antibody patterns: *antiproteinase 3*, present with c-ANCA (specific for Wegener granulomatosis) and *antimyeloperoxidase*, present with p-ANCA (PAN)	**Polyarteritis nodosa** (PAN) *Hepatitis B surface antigen*, Hepatitis C, or HIV may be present	Mononeuritis multiplex; strokes and seizures are rare (other classic neurologic deficits are **iritis, episcleritis, and retinal hemorrhage;** systemic features include livedo reticularis, *renal insufficiency, hypertension*, abdominal pain)
	Churg-Strauss syndrome p-ANCA may be present	Mononeuritis multiplex, (painful) cranial neuropathies (AION) (lung involvement, *eosinophilia*, diffuse subcutaneous nodules and late-life asthma)
	Wegener granulomatosis c-ANCA may be present	Mononeuritis multiplex and lower cranial neuropathies (kidneys, lungs, *sinuses*, and cutaneous vasculitis)
Small Other small-vessel vasculitis are urticarial hypersensitivity vasculitis, and those associated with arthropod stings: spiders and hymenoptera (bees, hornets, fire ants), which cause mononeuropathy, radiculopathy, mononeuritis multiplex, Guillain-Barré syndrome, and myeloradiculopathy	**Henoch-Schönlein purpura** Self-limited but often relapsing	Headache, PRES, seizures, peripheral neuropathy is rare (purpura below the waist, abdominal pain, arthralgias, and kidney involvement)
	Cryoglobulinemia Sensorimotor polyneuropathy (purpura, arthralgia, nephropathy, liver disease) *Types* 1: Waldenström's macroglobulinemia, myeloma, and lymphoma 2: *Hepatitis C* and B, EBV, bacterial and parasitic infections 3: Hepatitis C, lupus, lymphoma	
	Infection (mostly associated with rash and glomerulonephritis): Hepatitis C: mixed cryoglobulinemia Bartonella henselae (cat scratch disease): encephalitis Lepromatous leprosy (erythema nodosum leprosum): painful neuritis **Connective tissue disease** (limited to a few organs) SLE: psychosis, seizures, cranial neuropathies, chorea RA: pachymeningitis (seizures, stroke), mononeuritis, myopathy Scleroderma: myopathy, cranial neuropathies Sjögren syndrome: trigeminal neuropathy, myelopathy, stroke **Malignancy**	
Any size (pseudo-vasculitis)	**Antiphospholipid syndrome,** embolic phenomena (atrial myxomas, cholesterol emboli, or infective or marantic endocarditis), and drugs (amphetamines, phenylpropanolamine, phencyclidine, ephedrine, cocaine, and heroin)	

HIV, human immunodeficiency virus; ANCA, antineutrophil cytoplasmic antibodies; ELISA, enzyme-linked immunosorbent assay; PRES, pposterior reversible encephalopathy syndrome; EBV, Epstein-Barr virus; RA, rheumatoid arthritis.

Hypocomplementemia distinguishes vasculitis associated with connective tissue diseases, such as SLE or cryoglobulinemia. A small-vessel arteritis is the pathogenesis in the mononeuropathies of *Lyme disease and AIDS*. Other causes of mononeuritis multiplex are *diabetic radiculoneuritis*, carcinomatous plexopathy, *sarcoidosis, inflammatory demyelinating polyneuropathies*, and inherited liability to pressure palsies.

Thrombotic Microangiopathies

These are **microvascular occlusive disorders** characterized by aggregation of platelets, thrombocytopenia, and mechanical injury to erythrocytes in the kidney, the brain, and/or other organs. There are two main microangiopathies:

- **Hemolytic uremic syndrome (HUS),** whereby platelet aggregation (thrombi) occludes predominantly the renal circulation, may result from such disorders as *Escherichia coli* enteric infection (mainly, O157:H7), transplantation, and drugs (quinine, mitomycin, cyclosporine, and tacrolimus).
- **TTP,** in which thrombi cause ischemia of the brain among other organs, results from the failure to degrade unusually large multimers of von Willebrand factor (vWF).

Acquired idiopathic TTP is a fulminant multisystem consumptive coagulopathy expressed with neurologic deficits occurring in the setting of **thrombocytopenia** (with high marrow megakaryocytes), **hemolytic anemia** (schistocytosis), and **renal dysfunction**. Renal failure and fever are present less commonly. Clotting studies during TTP episodes are normal. **Posterior reversible encephalopathy syndrome** (PRES) is the most common abnormality on brain MRI in severe TTP. Vasogenic edema in the basal ganglia may be characteristic of TTP-associated PRES. Although often not clear-cut, HUS is the appropriate nomenclature when severe renal failure is more prominent than neurologic abnormalities. TTP may occur in adults within a few weeks after the initiation of **ticlopidine** and, to a lesser extent, **clopidogrel** (inhibitors of platelet ADP receptors), and occasionally during **pregnancy** or early **postpartum** period.

The microvascular thrombi of TTP have platelet aggregates with **abundant vWF antigen but little or no fibrin,** no perivascular inflammation, and no endothelial cell damage (by contrast, the platelet thrombi in disseminated intravascular coagulation [DIC] contain fibrin but not vWF). Defective vWF-cleaving **metalloproteases** (called ADAMTS 13, encoded in chromosome 9q34) fail to cleave unusually large multimers of vWF into the smaller forms that do not induce the adhesion and aggregation of platelets during normal blood flow. Ticlopidine-associated TTP and other acquired variants result presumably from autoantibodies against ADAMTS 13, whereas the familial form come from mutations in the 9q34 gene of ADAMTS 13, whose plasma activity is barely detectable.

Daily plasmapheresis and infusion of platelet-poor, fresh-frozen plasma or cryosupernatant (containing active metalloprotease) are the basis for the treatment of acute acquired idiopathic TTP episodes. Plasma exchange is often not sufficient against the ADAMTS 13 autoantibodies of acquired TTP, and glucocorticoids or splenectomy may be necessary. Platelet transfusions are to be avoided in the absence of life-threatening hemorrhage as they can exacerbate microvascular thrombosis.

Disseminated Intravascular Coagulation (DIC)

Previously called **"consumptive coagulopathy"** or "defibrination syndrome," DIC is a complication of disorders such as bacterial **sepsis** with multiple organ failure, severe traumatic brain injury, and **obstetric complications** (abruptio placenta, retained dead fetus syndrome, eclampsia, or amniotic fluid embolism). Less common associations causing "low-grade" DIC are **malignancy** (lymphomas, mucin-secreting adenocarcinomas [associated with nonbacterial thrombotic endocarditis], and solid tumors such as prostate cancer), autoimmune diseases, and even prosthetic cardiovascular devices.

The "fulminant" form presents as rapidly progressive **thrombosis or hemorrhage** (excessive wound or deep tissue bleeding, with petechiae or purpura) on at least three unrelated sites, concomitantly with **fever** and **shocklike symptoms with tachycardia, tachypnea, and hypotension.** Microvascular thrombosis is often the cause of end-organ damage in the kidneys, liver, or central nervous system.

Endothelial or tissue injury triggers the formation of **tissue thromboplastin** into the systemic circulation with subsequent release of procoagulant cytokines interleukin-6 and tumor necrosis factor. The activation of the proteolytic enzymes **thrombin and plasmin** lead to both intravascular thrombosis and hemorrhage. Thrombin cleaves fibrinogen to form fibrin monomers. Plasmin degrades fibrin and activates complement.

Diagnosis of DIC rests on the clinical findings of hemorrhage or thrombosis or both, and laboratory evidence of procoagulant activation (thrombin), fibrinolytic activation (plasmin), and end-organ damage (elevated creatinine, liver function tests, or abnormally low Pao_2):

- **Thrombocytopenia** due to thrombin generation leads to high prothrombin (70%) and high partial thromboplastin times (50%)
- **Low fibrinogen** given fibrinolytic activation (which create high-fibrin thrombus) in 50% of patients
- **High fibrin and fibrin degradation products** (FDP)
- **Present D-dimer** (specific FDP) in over 90% of patients
- **Low antithrombin** (useful for therapeutic monitoring)
- **High schistocytes in blood smear** (present in 50% of fulminant DIC)

Schistocytosis with moderate to severe thrombocytopenia but normal coagulation tests raises the possibility of TTP or HUS rather than DIC.

DIC hemorrhage must be distinguished from that associated with coagulopathy due to liver failure, anticoagulant use or overuse, and qualitative and quantitative platelet abnormalities accompanying uremia or aplastic anemia, where there is no factor or platelet consumption due to extensive intravascular thrombosis.

Epilepsy

As part of the group of **paroxysmal focal neurologic deficits** (to which migraine, syncope, and transient ischemia belong), epilepsy is clinically suspected in the setting of stereotyped, "marching," predominantly "positive" attacks that may rapidly evolve into a tonic clonic convulsion and can only definitively be diagnosed by ictal electro-clinical correlation.

1. **Focal versus generalized:** primary generalized seizures tend to be **myoclonic** (or absence, clonic, tonic-clonic, atonic) and begin **before the age of 20 years.** EEG changes may be accompanied by photosensitivity.

2. **Symptomatic versus cryptogenic and idiopathic:** the etiology is either known, presumed but not established, or nonstructural polygenic, respectively. EEG may further help distinguishing them:

	Generalized/Idiopathic*	Secondary/Symptomatic
Characteristics of the EEG background	Normal or ≥3 cps	Abnormal or <3 cps
	Frontally dominant	Anywhere
	Bisynchronous	Asynchronous, asymmetric

*Most generalized epilepsies are idiopathic but some severe childhood generalized epilepsies are symptomatic. Examples of the latter are Lennox-Gastaut and West syndromes (associated with tuberous sclerosis).

Common idiopathic epilepsies are:

Generalized

- **Childhood absence epilepsy** begins between ages 3 and 10 years as brief staring spells that, if frequent, may lead to school failure. The ictal EEG is composed of **3-Hz generalized spike-and-wave pattern** triggered by hyperventilation. Remission occurs by age 30 in 75%.
- **Atypical absence seizures** begin before 5 years of age in conjunction with other generalized seizure types and mental retardation. They last longer than typical absence and have less abrupt onset or cessation.
- **Juvenile absence epilepsy** begins between ages 7 and 17 years, has a 90% tendency to occur with tonic-clonic seizures, may be associated with photosensitivity (20%), and requires lifelong treatment.
- **Juvenile myoclonic epilepsy** (7–30 years; 3%–12% of all epilepsies) consists of myoclonic jerks and tonic-clonic seizures (absences in 20%) occurring after awakening. *Interictal* EEG shows **3–5 Hz bisynchronous spike and PSW in the frontocentral regions.** Photosensitivity is seen in 33%. JME requires lifelong treatment.

Focal

- **Benign childhood epilepsy with centrotemporal spikes, aka benign rolandic epilepsy** (3–13 years, tends to remit after 3 years; 10%–15% of childhood epilepsy), more common in boys, consists of nocturnal **drooling** and hemifacial twitching. It may evolve into tonic-clonic seizures. EEG shows centrotemporal spikes and slow waves.
- **Childhood epilepsy with occipital paroxysms** exhibits headache and visual hallucinations. Occipital paroxysms (EEG) occur on eye closure. It usually remits after three seizures (young onset) or in late teens.

Generalized Frontally Dominant Slow (3.5 Hz) Spike and Wave:

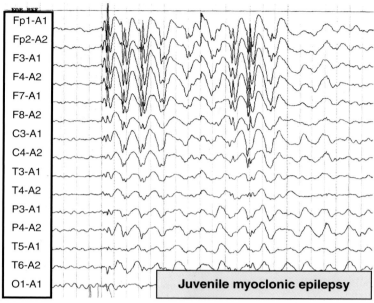

EEG tracings courtesy of Dr. Omar Markand, Indiana University.

Centrotemporal Spikes and Waves:

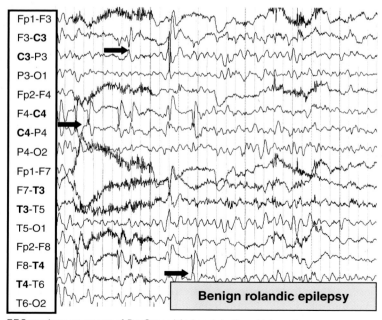

EEG tracings courtesy of Dr. Omar Markand, Indiana University.

West syndrome and Lennox-Gastaut syndrome

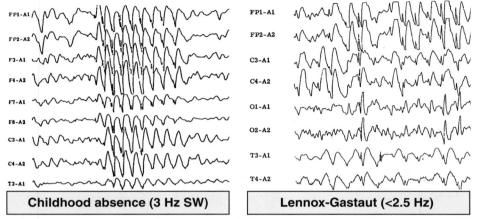

Childhood absence (3 Hz SW)	Lennox-Gastaut (<2.5 Hz)

SW = spike-wave

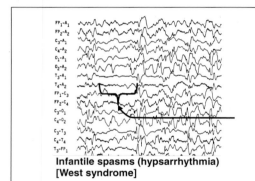

**Infantile spasms (hypsarrhythmia)
[West syndrome]**

West syndrome and Lennox-Gastaut syndrome (see "Myoclonic Encephalopathies") are considered parts of the spectrum of idiopathic or symptomatic forms of epilepsy. Classic hypsarrhythmia occurs only during NREM sleep; the ictal EEG correlate of spasms is voltage attenuation ("**electrodecremental response**"). Similarly, the hallmark of Lennox-Gastaut is its *interictal* pattern: only **beta bursts** are recorded during tonic posturing.

Febrile seizures, relatively benign, are applied to single, short, generalized motor seizures that develop with rising temperatures ("situation-related seizures," according to the ILAE) and are followed by complete recovery thereafter. Simple classic febrile seizures occur between the ages of **6 months to 5 years.**

> **Complex febrile seizures** are prolonged (>15 minutes), focal, and/or recurrent seizures with fever. The risk of later unprovoked seizure may reach nearly 50% when these three complex features are present (as opposed to the 2.4% risk in those with simple febrile seizures).

Lumbar puncture is mandatory in any patient under the age of 18 months. Prophylactic antiepileptic drugs are not indicated in simple febrile seizures but some advocate rectal diazepam when temperature rises. **The risk of recurrence** is high (50%) if the first febrile convulsion takes place before 1 year; the risk is reduced nearly by half (28%) with later onset. **Other independent predictors of seizure recurrence** are the presence of developmental delay, a short interval from fever onset to seizure, and a positive family history of febrile seizures.

ANTIEPILEPTIC AGENTS

Absorption (%)		Protein Binding (%)	Renal Metabolism (%)	Liver Metabolism	T½ VD (L/Kg)	Interaction(s)
PHT	Erratic	**90**	5	CYP 2C9 CYP 2C19	22 h 0.6	↓**CBZ, LTG**, TGB, TPM, BCP, warfarin
PB	>90	50	25	CYP 2C9 Glucuronidation	100 0.6	↓**CBZ, LTG**, TGB, TPM, BCP, VPA, PHT, Haloperidol, TCA, warfarin, steroids.
PRM	High	20	20	40%, PEMA 5% to PB	8 h 0.6	
CBZ	80	**75**	2	CYP 3A4; act met: epx	20 h 1–2	↓**VPA, LTG**, TGB, TPM, BCP, theoph.
VPA	100	**90**	2	**GT** (glucuronidation)	15 h 0.2	↑**CBZ epx, LTG**, FBM, PHT, PB
ESM	100	0	15	CYP 3A4	50 h 0.7	None
FBM	>90	25	50	CYP 3A4	20 h 0.8	↓**CBZ**, BCP; ↑**PHT**, ↑**VPA, CBZ epx**
LTG	100	55	20	**GT**	24 h 1.1	↑**CBZ epx**, ↓**VPA**
LTR	100	<10	>95	None	7 h 0.6	None
TPM	100	15	**85**	None	21 h 0.8	↑**PHT**, ↓**VPA**, BCP
GBP	60	0	>95	None	7 h 55	None
VGB	100	2	>95	None		↓**PHT**
TGB	90	**96**	2	CYP 3A4	7 h ?	↓VPA
ZNM	100	50	35	CYP 3A4	55 h 1.2	
OXZ	100	40	30	70% cytosolic system	9 h 0.7	
Lacosamide	100	15%	95%	CYP2C19	13h (and same cell, underneath)	0.6 L/kg, None

CYP, cytochrome P450; **VD,** volume of distribution; **epx, epoxide; theoph, theophylline.**

CBZ autoinduction takes about 2 weeks and **deinduction** about 4 days. After this "holiday," patients need to restart at a lower dose. **Antacids** decrease absorption of PHT and GBP but increase that of VPA. **Tube feedings** lowers absorption of PHT. **Hemodialysis** readily removes AEDs with low protein binding and barely those highly bound (as PHT). Bolus dose formula = VD × BW (kg) × (desired [concentration] − current [concentration]).

Classic AEDs	**Renal** metabolism, primarily	GBP, VGB, LTR, TPM
	Induce metabolism of other drugs	**PHT, PB, CBZ,** FBM, TPM
Newer AEDs	**Inhibit** metabolism of other drugs	**VPA,** FBM, TPM
	Significant protein binding	PHT, CBZ, VPA, TGB
	Reactive metabolites	CBZ epx, FBM, PHT, VPA

Although FBM decreases the levels of CBZ, it increases its epoxide (epx) metabolite: **CBZ toxicity** may be seen with **declining** levels of CBZ when combined with FBM. **High CBZ epx** level occurs when using CBZ in combination with FBM, LTG, and VPA in combination with PHT. Ideally, enzyme-inducing drugs in patients requiring combination AED therapy, especially VPA and LTG, should be avoided.

Mechanisms of Action of AEDs

- **PHT** and **CBZ** (and the prodrug OXZ) bind to the fast-inactivated state of the voltage-gated Na^+ channel reducing frequency of firing. OXZ and high-dose PHT reduce glutamate release presumably by presynaptic inhibition of Ca^{++} channels.
- **LTG** binds to the slow-inactivated state of the voltage-gated Na^+ channel. Blockade of Ca^{++} channels leads to reductions in glutamate release.
- **VPA** prevents fast frequency firing of the Na^+ channel and increases GABA by enhancing its production ($\uparrow$ GAD) and reducing its breakdown ($\downarrow$ GABA-T). T-type Ca^{++} channels are modestly blocked at high doses.
- **PB** (and **PRM** after its metabolism in the liver to PB) binds to the β subunit of the $GABA_A$ receptor prolonging Cl^- channel opening and neuronal hyperpolarization. **BZDs** bind to $GABA_A$ receptor through the α subunit increasing the frequency, and not duration, of Cl^-channel opening. The α subunits are present in the thalamus, explaining the efficacy of BZDs, unlike other selective GABAergic AEDs, against absence seizures.
- **ESM** inhibits the T-type Ca^{++} currents in thalamocortical relay neurons necessary for absence. **ZNM** also blocks T-type Ca^{++} as well as slow Na^+ channels while inhibiting the release of excitatory neurotransmitters.
- **TPM** has multiple actions, including blockade of voltage-gated Na^+ and Ca^{++} channels, potentiation of GABA effect, and inhibition of release of glutamate through the AMPA/kainate, instead of NMDA, receptor.
- **TGB** is a potent blocker of GABA reuptake by glia and neurons enhancing GABA-mediated inhibition. **VGB** irreversibly binds to GABA-T preventing the breakdown of GABA. **GBP** increases the synthesis and nonvesicular release of GABA and prevents its metabolism without interacting with GABA receptors or transporters. **FBM** also potentiates GABA while inhibiting the voltage-dependent Na^+ channels and the N-methyl-D-aspartate receptors (by preventing the binding of glycine to activate them).

Mechanism of action still uncertain for LTR.

- **Lacosamide** (recently approved for adjunctive treatment of partial-onset seizures) selectively enhances slow inactivation of voltage-gated sodium channels
- **Ezogabine (EZG, Retigabine [RTG])** (on Phase III studies for refractory partial epilepsy) acts on a group of voltage-gated potassium channels (Kv7.2-Kv7.5; corresponding genes *KCNQ2-KCNQ5*) stabilizing them in the open conformation, which increases conduction for potassium and hyperpolarizes the membrane.

SHARING HEPATIC METABOLISM (POTENTIAL DRUG-DRUG INTERACTIONS)

System	AED	Drugs That Inhibit the CYP System
CYP 3A4	CBZ, ESM, FBM, TGB, ZNM	Cimetidine, fluvoxamine, sertraline, nefazodone, diltiazem, fluconazole, omeprazole, propoxyphene
CYP 2C9	PHT PB	Fluoxetine, fluvoxamine, sertraline, warfarin
GT	VPA, LTG	

CYP, cytochrome P450; GT, glucuronosyl transferase.

EXTRA-CNS TOXICITY OF AED

System Affected	Side Effect	Mechanism	AED
Systemic	Weight gain	Dose-related	VPA, GBP
	Weight loss	Dose-related	TPM, ZNM, FBM
Hepatic	Hepatitis	Idiosyncratic	FBM and others
	↓ Fibrinogen	Dose-related	VPA
Renal	Kidney stones	Dose-related	TPM, ZNM
	Hyponatremia	Dose-related	CBZ, OXZ
Hematopoietic	**Aplastic anemia**	Idiosyncratic	**CBZ, FBM, PHT, VPA, ZNM**
	Hyponatremia	Dose-related	CBZ, OXZ
	Thrombocytopenia	Dose-related	VPA
Pancreas	Pancreatitis	Idiosyncratic	VPA
	↓ Insulin release	Dose-related	PHT
	↑ Insulin effect	Dose-related	TPM
Connective tissue	Gingival hyperplasia	Dose-related	PHT
	Lupus	Idiosyncratic	PHT
	Dupuytren's	Dose-related	PB
Skin	**Stevens-Johnson syndrome**	Idiosyncratic	**CBZ, FBM, PHT, ZNM** **LTG + VPA,** especially
	Minor rash	Dose-related	CBZ, PHT, PB, PRM
	Hair loss	Dose-related	VPA
	Hirsutism	Dose-related	PHT
Skeletal	Osteoporosis	Dose-related	**PHT,** CBZ, PB, PRM
Reproductive issues	Teratogenicity	Dose-related	**VPA,** CBZ, PB, PHT
	Polycystic ovaries	Dose-related	**VPA**
	BCP failures	Dose-related	All enzyme-inducing
	Reduced libido	Dose-related	PB
Gastrointestinal	Nausea, vomiting	Dose-related	CBZ, PHT, VPA
	Diarrhea	Dose-related	VPA

CBZ and OXZ may cause hyponatremia and edema because of antidiuretic hormone (ADH)-like action. They are known causes of the syndrome of inappropriate secretion of ADH (SIADH). **FBM may lead to aplastic anemia and hepatotoxicity** (20 times higher risk than that of CBZ) with use restricted to Lennoux-Gastaut syndrome. **VGB** may never be used given the complications of visual field constriction (25%) and psychosis.

PHT may cause mild dysmorphism (gingival hyperplasia, hirsutism, acne, facial coarsening) within months, whereas **folate deficiency, osteopenia, peripheral neuropathy, and cerebellar atrophy** are uncommon and take years to develop.

VPA is associated with dose-related tremor, weight gain, hair loss, menstrual irregularities (with potential for polycystic ovarian syndrome), pancreatitis, thrombocytopenia, and hepatotoxicity (1:20,000).

TPM and ZNM inhibit carbonic anhydrase, which may contribute to their side effects of nephrolithiasis (especially when calcium supplements and high-dose vitamin C are taken) as well as somnolence, confusion, and poor concentration.

Choice of AEDs According to Seizure Type

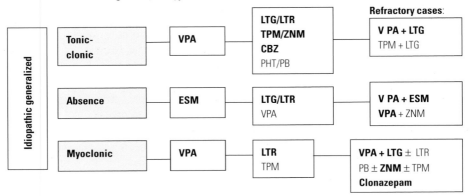

PHT, PB, and CBZ may worsen some primary generalized epilepsies
(Absence and myoclonic seizures); OXZ, TGB, and GBP are ineffective.

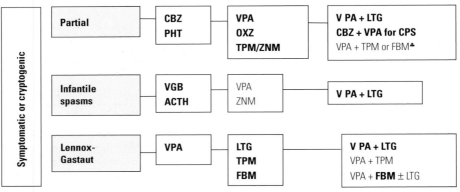

Most useful combinations are CBZ or PHT with GBP, TGB, TPM, or FBM (widely different mechanisms of action). Poor combinations are VPA-PHT (both compete for protein-binding sites) and CBZ-PHT (similar action, PHT induces CBZ metabolism). ♣ **Beware of the interactions between VPA and TPM and FBM**: VPA should be decreased or increased by one third at the time of FBM or TPM initiation, respectively.

Surgery for Epilepsy

Surgery may be the best treatment in many patients soon after two AEDs have failed to control their seizures. Structural epileptogenic lesions, especially **mesial temporal sclerosis,** are the most frequent and successful surgery indications. Surgically "privileged" seizure disorders have unilateral interictal epileptiform discharges on the EEG. Patients with refractory temporal lobe epilepsy are seven times more likely to be seizure-free after temporal lobectomy. The surgical risk of **cognitive worsening** (naming difficulty and verbal memory) is increased if the language-dominant hemisphere is resected, there is no mesial temporal lobe sclerosis on the side of surgery, and the functional measures made by the Wada test, PET scan, or MRS indicate higher performance on the side of surgery. Corpus callosotomy, vagus nerve stimulation, and multiple subpial transections are considered palliative surgery and may only ameliorate the seizure burden.

Status Epilepticus

SE is classically defined as the occurrence of two or more seizures without recovery of consciousness. Basic emergency measures should be ensured (airway patency, BP, cardiac rhythm). IV line is immediately set up. Thiamine (100 mg IV) and glucose (50 mL of D50 IV if glucose level unknown) are administered. Blood for AED levels, metabolic, and toxic screen is drawn.

Sequence of AEDs (assuming seizure persistence)

6–10 m

- **Lorazepam** 2 mg/min, repeating as necessary in 2-mg increments every 2 minutes, up to a dose of 10 mg or 0.1 mg/kg. If rapid IV access is not available, then give midazolam 10 mg IM or diazepam 20 mg PR (Diastat)
- **Fosphenytoin** 20 PE mg/kg IV at a maximum of 150 mg/min, with EKG and BP monitoring. Fosphenytoin is highly water-soluble and free of the PHT-related problems, namely, precipitation with dextrose-containing solutions and phlebitis.

10–60 m (intubation required)

- **Midazolam** 0.2 mg/kg load, repeating 0.2 mg/kg boluses every 5–10 minutes until seizures stop, up to a maximum total loading dose of 1 mg/kg, at a rate of 0.05–2 mg/kg/h. Titrate in increments of 0.05 mg/kg/h until seizures are controlled. If still seizing, add or switch to pentobarbital.
- **Pentobarbital** 5 mg/kg load, repeating 5 mg/kg boluses every 30 minutes, at a rate of 0.5–5 mg/kg/h. Titrate to burst-suppression on EEG in increments of 0.5 mg/kg/h.
- **Propofol** 5 μg/kg/min load (0.3 mg/kg/h) IV infusion for 5 minutes, then titrate in 5–10-μg/kg/min (0.3–0.6 mg/kg/h) increments every 5 minutes to achieve desired level of seizure control. The initial rate is 5–10 μg/kg/min with a range of 5–80 μg/kg/min. Burst-suppression on EEG is harder to maintain with propofol. Avoid using for more than 24–48 hours to minimize risk of propofol infusion syndrome (hyperkalemia, hepatomegaly, hyperlipemia, metabolic acidosis, myocardial failure, and rhabdomyolysis). CK, triglycerides, and acid-base status need monitoring.

Titration to EEG burst-suppression assumes that the "bursts" do not represent ictal discharges, although extensive spiking is acceptable in this setting. A general rule is to have ~50% of the EEG as suppression (e.g., 1–2 seconds of "burst" activity separated by 3–8 seconds of suppression).

Supplemental long-term seizure control can be accomplished with IV formulations first, with the following options: (1) IV levetiracetam: 1,000 mg load over 15 minutes. If still seizing, give an additional 1,000 mg over 15 minutes (maintenance: 1,000 mg bid); or (2) IV phenobarbital: 20 mg/kg IV load at 50 mg/min; or (3) IV valproate 20–40 mg/kg load over 10 minutes. If still seizing, give an additional 20 mg/kg over 5 minutes (maintenance: 15–20 mg/kg/d divided tid).

Epilepsy in Women

Epileptic women have a higher risk of developing **polycystic ovarian syndrome,** characterized by amenorrhea and infertility due to anovulatory cycles, and hirsutism, obesity, and acne secondary to hyperandrogenism. The risk increases to **60% with VPA** and 30% with CBZ.

Cautionary pearls during contraception:
- **All enzyme-inducing AEDs** (PHT, CBZ, OXZ, PB, PRM, FBM, and TPM) decrease the efficacy of oral, subdermal, and intramuscular contraceptive hormones by about 6%. Thus, oral contraceptives require higher concentration of estrogen (usually, 50 μg ethinyl estradiol instead of 30 μg) and progesterone (usually, 1 mg of norgestrel instead of 0.3 mg).
- **VPA, GBP, TGB, LTG, LTR,** and **ZNM** do not significantly alter estradiol levels or sex hormone binding globulin and are safer during contraception.

Cautionary pearls during pregnancy:
- **VPA, CBZ, PHT,** and **PB** have confirmed teratogenic potential and should be avoided in patients with family history of neural tube defects (NTDs).
- **All enzyme-inducing AEDs** can cause transient and reversible deficiency in vitamin K-dependent clotting factors in the newborn. This increases the risk of intracranial hemorrhage after a traumatic birth. Mothers should take 10 mg of vitamin K_1 daily for the last few weeks of pregnancy.
- **Monotherapy** is preferred over polypharmacy. If seizures have been absent for 2 years, careful reduction or withdrawal is suggested.
- **LTG, LTR,** and **TGB** do not have teratogenic potential and are preferred. However, if VPA is in use and has been effective, a change is deemed risky; instead, its total daily dose should be decreased to <1,000 mg/d.
- **Folic acid** at a dose of 0.4 mg/d should be used in all women of childbearing age to reduce the risk of NTD. A dose of 4 mg/d is recommended for those with family history of NTD.

Important drug-drug interactions: SSRIs amplify the inhibitory effect of some of the enzyme-inducing AEDs on the P450 system.

In experimental models, estrogen is proconvulsant; androgen and progesterone are anticonvulsant. The progesterone metabolite allopregnanolone is responsible for the antiseizure effects of progesterone. Changes in the balance between these hormones and AED concentrations during any component of the menstrual cycle may lead to an increase in seizure frequency (perimenstrual, periovulatory, or luteal *catamenial* seizures). **Acetazolamide,** a carbonic anhydrase inhibitor, at a dose of 250–500 mg/d, taken for 7–10 days before the menses and until cessation of bleeding, is an effective adjunctive therapy in catamenial seizures. **Progesterone** vaginal suppositories or lozenges (100–200 mg tid) during the phases of highest seizure frequency (days 15–25 of cycle) are promising in women with anovulatory or inadequate luteal phase cycles.

Neonatal and Pediatric EEG

CONCEPTIONAL AGE (wk)		BEHAVIORAL STATE	
		Awake	Asleep
<29	A	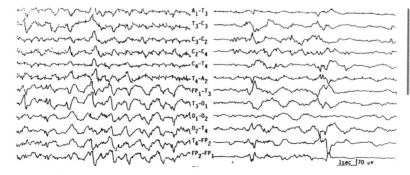	
30	B		
32	C		
36	D		
40	E		
44	F		
46	G		

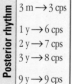

Sleep-wake differentiation begins at 30 weeks and is established by 36 weeks CA.

Sleep spindles (σ) appear at 46 weeks of CA. A delay suggests **hypothyroidism**

CA, conceptional age. Figure and EEG tracings courtesy of Dr. Omar Markand, Indiana University. (See following text for definition and discussion of TD, AM, TA, and CSWS.)

By 36 weeks, the **awake EEG is continuous,** low voltage, and shows mixed frequency background (*activite moyenne,* or AM) and quiet sleep discontinuity shifts from *tracé discontinu* (TD) to *tracé alternant* (TA), whereby the tracing alternates between high and low voltages, the latter being briefer (<4 seconds) and higher in amplitude than the interburst period of TD.

By 44 weeks, the immature discontinuous quiet sleep record begins to show *continuous slow wave sleep* (CSWS) or *high voltage sleep* (HVS). A complete transition from TA to CSWS occurs by 45 weeks. No more TA is seen thereafter.

At term, the following EEG patterns are seen during the sleep phases:

Active Sleep (AS)	Quiet Sleep (QS)
Low voltage irregular (LVI)	Trace alternant
Mixed	High-voltage sleep (HVS)

QS: High-voltage sleep   **QS**: Trace alternant

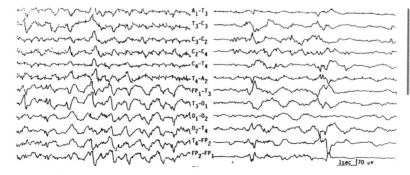

Posterior rhythm

3 m → 3 cps
1 y → 6 cps
2 y → 7 cps
3 y → 8 cps
9 y → 9 cps

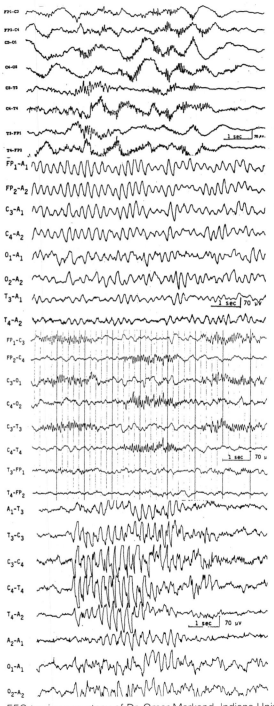

Delta brushes are a hallmark of premature EEG (26 wks-term): It is a combination of delta waves with a superimposed "buzz" of beta activity. This pattern can be seen both during sleep and wakefulness. Central (<32 wks) and occipital (older) are the predominant sites.

Hypnagogic hypersynchrony is the term used to describe high amplitude sinusoidal slow waves characteristic of the transient state between wakefulness and sleep in infants between 3 to 6 months. This pattern of drowsiness begins to drop after one year of life and becomes rare after 2 years of age.

Sleep spindles are asynchronous and "spiky" during infancy and become fully synchronous after the second year. They are located predominantly over the rolandic area and are one of the hallmarks of stage II Non-REM sleep. They are particularly long during the ages of 3-6 months.

Vertex sharp waves (VSW) and K complexes usually appear between 3-6 months of life. VSW are synchronous and symmetrical from the beginning. Because of their spiky appearance and asymmetry, especially during early stages of sleep, they are a common source of erroneous interpretation.

EEG tracings courtesy of Dr. Omar Markand, Indiana University.

Brainstem Auditory Evoked Potentials (BAEPs)

BAEP is of maximal utility in the evaluation of comatose patients, suspected demyelinating disorders, posterior fossa tumors, intraoperative monitoring of CN VIII, or in general audiologic evaluation. Seven waves are usually recorded in the first 10 ms following high-intensity clicks. Two-channel recordings are obtained: vertex (Cz) to ipsilateral ear and Cz to contralateral ear derivation. The BAEP is highly reproducible in a given subject, is **not affected by inattention to stimulus, alterations in the level of consciousness, or drugs.**

Parameters of interest when interpreting BAEP:
- Latencies of I, III, and V (the more consistent waves)
- Interpeak latencies (IPL) of I–III, III–V, and I–V
- Amplitude ratio of wave V to wave I (<0.66 is abnormal)
- Side to side variation in IPL is abnormal if <0.4 msec

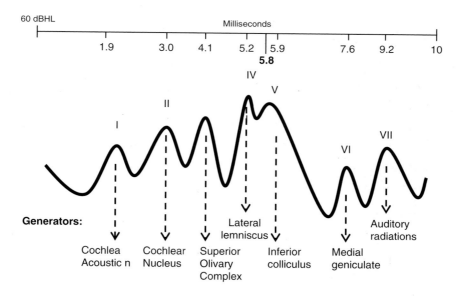

The absolute latency of the BAEP waves is dependent on the intensity of the click stimulus. Wave V is the most robust, still recognized at only 10 dB above hearing level. **At 70 dB above hearing level, all waves are identifiable.** Absence of all waves reflects a peripheral lesion (or a technical problem). In the presence of wave I, **absence of wave IV/V I indicates a lesion in CN VIII** and prolongation of the I-III or I-IV/V interval suggests a lesion of either CN VIII or brainstem. Acoustic schwannomas often show absence of all waves beyond wave I, or prolongation of I-IV/V latency.

Visual Evoked Potentials (VEPs)

Strong sedation abolishes the response. Very high amplitudes are seen in myoclonic epilepsy and startle syndromes. Side-to-side difference is abnormal if >10 msec.

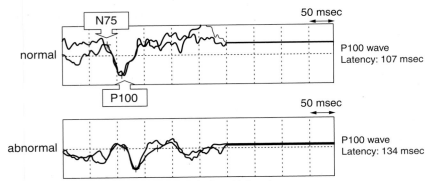

VEP tracings courtesy of Dr. Omar Markand, Indiana University.

Somatosensory Evoked Potentials (SSEPs)

SSEP WITH MEDIAN NERVE STIMULATION

Peak	Generator	Latency (ms)	IPL from N_9 (ms)	Side to Side Variation (L/IPL) (ms)
N_9	Erb's point	<11.5		<0.64
N_{13}	Spinal cord	<16.0	<5.0	<0.84/<0.84
N_{20}	Cortical	<21.5	<11.5	<1.5/<0.94

IPL, interpeak latency.

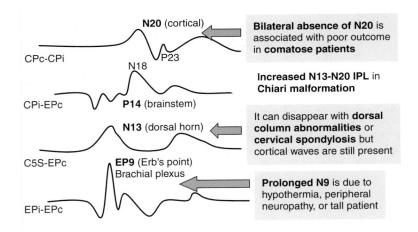

SSEP WITH TIBIAL NERVE STIMULATION

Peak	Generator	Latency (ms)	IPL	Side-to-Side Variation (ms)
N_7	Popliteal	<9.5	N_7–N_{22} <17.0	
N_{22}	Lumbar	<25.5	N_7–P_{37} <35.0	<1.5
P_{37}	Cortical	<44.0	N_{22}–P_{37} <22.0	<2.5

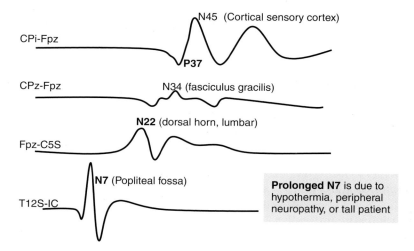

Prolonged N7 is due to hypothermia, peripheral neuropathy, or tall patient

SSEPs depend on the functional integrity of the fast-conducting, large-diameter group IA muscle afferent fibers and group II cutaneous afferent fibers, which travel in the **posterior column of the spinal cord.** Diseases of the dorsal columns in which joint position sense and proprioception are impaired invariably are associated with abnormal SSEPs.

One of the most important current uses of SSEP is in the **prediction of outcome in anoxic-ischemic coma.** Most studies show that the absence of cortical SSEP in the first week after cardiac arrest is the most reliable predictor of poor outcome. The proposed guidelines for patients with anoxic-ischemic coma include ascertainment of the following steps:

1. Presence of myoclonic status epilepticus
2. Absent pupillary and corneal reflexes on day 3
3. Motor response to pain no better than extension on day 3
4. Absent N20 cortical responses to SSEP, bilaterally, on days 1–3
5. Elevated serum neuron-specific enolase >33 g/L at days 1–3

In the presence of these parameters, with 100% specificity, the brainstem and cortical failure are permanent and further treatment can be deemed futile.

Myoclonic Encephalopathies

The most common causes of cortical myoclonus are posthypoxic myoclonus (Lance-Adams syndrome), spinocerebellar degeneration, Unverricht-Lundborg disease, mitochondrial encephalopathy, and celiac disease. Paradoxically, the pathologic findings are often concentrated in the **cerebellum** (mostly dentate nucleus, vermis, and superior lobes) and cerebellar pathways.

Typical Progressive Myoclonic Encephalopathies

PMEs are autosomal recessive, except hyperekplexia, DRPLA, and JME, which are autosomal dominant, and MERRF, mitochondrial in inheritance (see "Mitochondrial Encephalomyopathy Syndromes"):

- **Baltic myoclonus (Unverricht-Lundborg disease)** is a progressive resting, action, and stimulus-sensitive myoclonus (which worsens with phenytoin, as other primary generalized epilepsies) occurring between the ages 6 and 16 years, associated with **dementia** and a **vermian cerebellar syndrome** (loss of Purkinje cells). The mutation, **EPM1 (21q)**, causes loss of function in **cystatin B,** an inhibitor of intralysosomal cysteine proteases (cathepsins) involved in apoptosis. Early on, it may be difficult to distinguish from JME.

- **Mediterranean myoclonus (Ramsay-Hunt syndrome),** a variant of the former, is related to **celiac disease** with or without gluten-sensitive enteropathy. **Antigliadin antibodies** are found in the serum and CSF.

- **Sialidosis ("cherry-red spot myoclonus")** causes myoclonia precipitated by active and passive movements but not by light or sound, which persists during sleep. It is due to **neuraminidase** deficiency (**NEU1,** lysosomal sialidase, **6q**) **Urine oligosaccharides** are increased.

- **Neuronal ceroid lipofuscinosis (NCL)** leads to progressive motor and cognitive regression and **blindness** associated with lipopigment deposits. The most common types of NCL, excluding CLN1 (1p, *granular bodies*) can cause PME are CLN2 (late infantile, 11p, *curvilinear bodies*), CLN3 (juvenile or Batten disease, 16p, *fingerprint profiles*), CLN4 (adult), CLN5 (late infantile Finnish variant, 13q), and CLN6 (late infantile or early juvenile variant). **Adult NCL,** also known as **Kufs disease,** may present as PME (type A) or as dementia with cerebellar and/or extrapyramidal signs (type B). Visual deficits are rare if disease onset is over 30 years of age.

- **Lafora disease** consists of occipital seizures with **intense visual hallucinations,** cortical blindness; rapid progressive pyramidal and cognitive decline lead to death within 10 years after onset. The **Lafora bodies,** basophilic polyglucosan **PAS-positive neuronal perikarya inclusions,** are seen in the cerebral cortex, liver, muscle, and skin (mainly in eccrine, nonaxillary tissue). **EPM2A (6q)** encodes for **laforin,** a tyrosine phosphatase expressed mostly in the cerebellum and **EPM2B (6p)** encodes for **malin,** an E3 ubiquitin ligase. Laforin and malin interact to protect tissues from accumulating polyglucosans by regulating proteins involved in glycogen metabolism.

Atypical Progressive Myoclonic Encephalopathy

- **Juvenile gangliosidosis GM$_2$ (type III),** due to deficiency in *hexosaminidase A* activity in adults, may present as a progressive myoclonic encephalopathy, unlike the childhood phenotype (see "Lysosomal Disorders: Sphingolipidoses"). Other adult-onset GM$_2$ presentations include slowly progressive motor neuron disease, spinal muscular atrophy, and spinocerebellar degeneration. The latter, of juvenile onset, suggests Friedreich ataxia: ataxia, tremor, spasticity, dysarthria, optic atrophy, and dementia. The macular **cherry-red spot** (from ganglioside accumulation) is only seen in children who have no residual hexosaminidase A activity.

- **Juvenile Gaucher disease (type III),** due to deficient lymphocyte β-*glucocerebrosidase* activity, is recognized by the combination of ataxia, **horizontal supranuclear gaze palsy,** pyramidal dysfunction, and hepatosplenomegaly with lytic and necrotic bone lesions.

- **Biotin-responsive multiple carboxylase deficiencies:** skin rash, alopecia, hearing loss, hemianopsia, hemiparesis, and acidosis.

- **DRPLA** presents in childhood as PME and in adults as ataxia, chorea, and dementia. All groups end up with dementia, ataxia, and dysarthria.

- **Subacute sclerosing panencephalitis (SSPE)**

- Other: juvenile Huntington's disease, NBIA-1, Wilson disease, and bismuth toxicity

Myoclonic epilepsies (besides reflex myoclonic epilepsy and cerebral palsy)

- **Benign myoclonic epilepsy of infancy** is characterized by brief generalized myoclonic seizures with onset between 4 months and 3 years. Head drops or brief eye blinks without loss of consciousness occur in otherwise normal children. Development is normal after VPA therapy. EEG shows *ictal* diffuse irregular 3-Hz spike-wave or poly-spike-wave discharges.

- **JME** is a familial disorder beginning in the second decade suspected when **brief shoulders-and-arms myoclonic jerks with generalization occur after awakening** in ostensibly otherwise normal individuals. *Interictal* EEG demonstrates anterior-predominant generalized spike-wave or polyspike-wave discharges at a rate of about 3–5 Hz. Daily treatment with VPA may eventually not be necessary in one-third of patients.

- **Benign childhood epilepsy with centrotemporal spikes,** previously known as **benign rolandic epilepsy,** is a syndrome that occurs predominantly in males between 6 and 16 years of age. The **seizures usually occur during the first 2 hours of sleep** and are brief, simple focal motor seizures characterized by hemifacial **grimacing and twitching, speech arrest, and drooling,** which may generalize. EEG shows high amplitude unilateral or bilateral centrotemporal spikes during sleep. Treatment is usually unnecessary after the first or even the second seizure. CBZ and VPA are the drugs of choice. Antiepileptic medications are maintained up to 14–16 years of age, at which time the seizures spontaneously resolve.

Myoclonus and Renal Failure

The combination of myoclonus and renal failure raises an interesting differential diagnosis. When disturbance of consciousness is present, the following conditions need consideration:

- **Uremic encephalopathy** directly causing myoclonus, which is reversible with dialysis or transplantation
- **Dialysis encephalopathy** is caused by aluminium toxicity and is characterized by speech disturbance, seizures, and myoclonus. It is at least partially reversible if treated with complete absence of oral aluminium intake and elimination by desferrioxamine.
- **Drug toxicity in renal failure** may also present as a myoclonic encephalopathy. Myoclonus-inducing drugs in renal disease include acyclovir, ciprofloxacin, dobutamine, cephalosporins, and gabapentin.

Action myoclonus-renal failure (AMRF) syndrome should be suspected when myoclonus is *not* associated with an encephalopathic picture. Unlike uremic encephalopathy, in AMRF there is a clear sensorium and lack of improvement of neurologic features to dialysis or transplantation. Patients present in the second and third decades of life with renal, neurologic, or combined features, possibly with an autosomal recessive pedigree. **Tremor evolves into a progressively disabling action myoclonus,** coupled with cerebellar signs, infrequent generalized seizures, but preserved cognitive function. Renal disease presents as **proteinuria** and progresses to renal failure, requiring renal transplantation. Renal biopsy shows focal segmental glomerulosclerosis, which is more common in the setting of human immunodeficiency virus infection. EEG may demonstrate spike and spike-wave complexes. Brain autopsy shows extraneuronal lipofuscin accumulation. The neurologic manifestations precede renal involvement in about one-third of the cases. It is possible that cases with a predominantly renal presentation and later neurologic disease are misdiagnosed as uremic encephalopathy. It could actually represent a form of **cortical myoclonus,** as has been described in benign familial adult myoclonic epilepsy, or a variant of the newly recognized cortical tremor syndrome. The relatively pure syndromes of cortical tremor and cortical myoclonus are usually associated with discrete cerebellar cortical disease, often with disproportionate loss of granule cells. The latter may lead to diminished excitation of Purkinje cells, release of the cerebellar nuclei from tonic inhibition by Purkinje cells and consequent increased excitation of the cerebral motor cortex and cortical myoclonus or tremor.

May and White syndrome of **myoclonic ataxia and deafness** may also be associated with nephropathy, diabetes mellitus, infrequent seizures, and dementia. It is likely to be a mitochondrial cytopathy given the abundant ragged-red fibers that may be identified on muscle biopsy.

Galloway–Mowat syndrome is an autosomal recessive disorder of infantile onset associated with **proteinuria,** focal segmental glomerulosclerosis, **microcephaly,** and **cerebellar disease.**

Epileptic Encephalopathies with Myoclonus

- **Early infantile myoclonic encephalopathy (Ohtahara syndrome)** consists of refractory **tonic spasms, suppression-burst pattern** on interictal EEG, and psychomotor arrest and regression that begin before the age of 3 months. It often evolves into West syndrome between the ages of 3 and 6 months and into Lennox-Gastaut syndrome between the ages of 1 and 3 years. Ohtahara syndrome is often due to structural brain lesions but may be due to heterozygous mutations in *STXBP1* (syntaxin binding protein 1 gene).
- **West syndrome** corresponds to the triad of infantile spasms, arrest of psychomotor development, and **hypsarrhythmia** on EEG between 4 and 6 months of age. West syndrome is often symptomatic from various causes such as neonatal asphyxia, meningoencephalitis, tuberous sclerosis complex, and chromosomal abnormalities. Corticotropin is the treatment of choice. Other options include VPA and vigabatrin.
- **Lennox-Gastaut syndrome** typically develops after West syndrome as a collection of several seizure types (tonic, atonic, and atypical absences), diffuse cognitive impairment, and interictal EEG changes (frontally dominant interictal, 1.5–2.5-Hz slow spike-and-wave and ictal β bursts). VPA and CBZ are used in combination for atypical absence and tonic seizures. Corpus callosotomy has been advocated when drop attacks are prominent.
- **Landau-Kleffner syndrome** consists of acquired aphasia with word deafness (auditory agnosia) in 3–9-year-old children. Continuous 1–3 Hz multifocal spike and waves are seen during most of non-REM sleep **("status epilepticus of sleep").** Corticosteroids are more effective than AEDs.
- **Rasmussen syndrome** most commonly presents as epilepsia partialis continua in children between the ages of 3 and 15 years due to **antibodies to glutamate receptor subtype 3.** Intractability, even to steroids, makes hemispherectomy a required intervention.

Treatment of PME relies on traditional (VPA, clonazepam, and phenobarbital), newer AEDs (LTG, LTR, TPM, and ZNM), and other drugs, such as:
- **Piracetam** (7–24 g/d), a GABA-related compound previously used as a memory enhancer whose mechanism of action is unknown, is one of the best drugs for **action and stimulus-sensitive myoclonus** of cortical origin.
- **L-5-hydroxytryptophan (L-5HTP)** is a precursor of serotonin that aims at **restoring the serotonergic hypometabolism** in patients with PME (low concentrations of serotonin metabolites 5-HIAA and HVA). The benefits may disappear after long-term therapy. It should be taken with carbidopa to avoid peripheral metabolism. L-5THP is contraindicated in mitochondriopathies.
- **Lisuride** (0.1–0.15 mg/d IV), a postsynaptic dopaminergic and serotonergic agonist, decreases reflex and action myoclonus. Prior oral administration of domperidone prevents nausea and vomiting.
- **Thyrotropin-releasing hormone** has been used in intractable cases with improvements in gait, dysmetria, and myoclonus.
- **Baclofen** and *N*-acetylcysteine have been anecdotally shown to improve myoclonus, ataxia, and dysarthria.

Sleep Disorders

Sleep-wake cycles are established at 30–32 weeks gestational age and continue even during a persistent vegetative state. **Seizures** are more common during the first 2 hours of falling asleep. **Generalized epilepsy** is more common during the first hour after awakening.

Stage 1 (<5% of the night) consists of slow, roving eye movements, associated with a **drop of the alpha dominant rhythm** with or without **vertex sharp transients.** Frontal intermittent rhythmic delta activity (FIRDA) at sleep onset is a normal finding in the elderly. **Stage 2** (50% of the night) is made of **sleep spindles and K-complexes** with delta waves in <20% of the tracing. **Stages 3 and 4 (slow-wave sleep, SWS, non-REM)** (20% of total sleep) are restorative and associated with **high-amplitude delta waves** (1 cps) in >50% of the tracing. Disorders of arousals from sleep stages 3 and 4, present in 30% of children and 2% of adults, are of short duration and are minimally recalled:

	Precipitants	Other features
Sleepwalking	Other sleep disorders (e.g., OSA), shift work, sleep deprivation, alcohol, stress	Relatively calm behavior or activities that are more complex: dressing, cleaning, cooking. EEG shows **hypnagogic hypersynchrony**
Sleep terrors		Frightening events with head banging, body injury. If awakened: reports of terror, helplessness, and paralysis
Confusional arousals		Slow speech and mentation ("sleep drunkenness"), inappropriate behaviors. Antidepressants and sedatives can trigger.

REM sleep (20% of sleep) is mainly a cholinergic state in which arrhythmias and obstructive sleep apnea (OSA) may develop but seizures are unlikely. EEG shows **sawtooth waves and low-voltage mixed frequencies without vertex sharp transients.** There is phasic activity on EMG without muscle tone. REM sleep becomes progressively longer lasting, from 10 to 45 minutes, with each of the four or five sleep cycles. **Sleep-onset REM** (occurring within 15 minutes of sleep onset) is seen in 71% of narcoleptic patients but also with antihistamine withdrawal, severe depression, alcohol, barbiturates, and sleep deprivation. The REM changes with age are:

Neonate	Adult
REM sleep soon after onset	REM sleep after 90–120 minutes
50% REM	20% REM
30–70 minute sleep cycles	90 minutes
↑ Phasic activity during REM	↓ Phasic activity during REM
16 hours of sleep	8 hours at 20 years, 6 hours at 50

In the elderly, there is reduced sleep time and efficiency, and increased arousals. Stage 1 increases by 15%; stage 3 is reduced or even absent by 60 years, but REM remains unchanged.

Narcolepsy

Narcolepsy is excessive sleepiness due to **REM intrusion into wakefulness** that appears in the in the second or third decade of life in the form of cataplexy, sleep paralysis with sleep-onset REM, and/or hypnagogic hallucinations:

- **Cataplexy** are sudden and short-lived episodes (seconds to minutes) of muscle weakness with preserved awareness following strong emotions, commonly laughter. It may reach "status cataplecticus" if occurring often through the day. The atonia varies from facial sagging, slurred speech, to knee buckling. Respiratory and oculomotor muscles are not affected.
- **Sleep paralysis with sleep-onset REM** consists of inability to move while falling asleep or on awakening, often frightening.
- **Hypnagogic hallucinations** are dreamlike perceptions that occur while falling asleep or on awakening.

Narcolepsy is associated with the human leukocyte antigen (HLA) typing **HLA-DR2 DQw1** (6p), of which the **DQB1*0602** allele is positive in up to 95% of cataplectic narcoleptics, but also in 22% and 40% of normal white and black populations (low specificity). HLA-DQB1*0602-positive narcoleptic patients have loss of **hypocretin (Hcrt-1 or orexin)**, a peptide normally produced by neurons in the **perifornical and lateral hypothalamus.** Low CSF Hcrt-1 levels, **<110 pg/mL,** is highly specific (99%) and sensitive (87%) for the diagnosis. Multiple sleep latency test (MSLT) suggests narcolepsy when **sleep latency is < 8 minutes *and* at least two of four short-onset (<15 minute) REM periods** (SOREMPS). Similar MSLT findings may be present in OSA, PLMS, or REM sleep deprivation.

Symptomatic narcolepsies that need exclusion are MS with lesions involving the hypothalamic nuclei, craniopharyngioma removal complicated with hypothalamic infarction, hypothalamic tumors, sarcoid, tuberculosis, Whipple disease, and paraneoplastic limbic encephalitis (anti-Ma2, associated with germ cell tumors).

Kleine-Levin syndrome is a rare disorder of adolescents that consist of episodic attacks of daytime sleepiness associated hypersomnolence, compulsive eating, and hypersexuality. PSG shows reduced sleep efficiency and diffuse EEG slowing during episodes. **Lithium** may be the most effective drug.

Planned daytime naps and optimizing nocturnal sleep are the behavioral goals of treatment. **Modafinil** (alpha agonist without sympathomimetic activity), 200–400 mg every morning , is the usual first choice followed by **methylphenidate,** 10–20 mg every morning, which also treats cataplexy. Other "anticataplectics" are medications with anticholinergic properties such as **imipramine, clomipramine,** or SSRIs. **Sodium oxybate,** a gamma hydroxybutyrate analogue, is a novel hypnotic, probably a GABA$_B$ agonist, approved specifically for cataplexy. Selegiline (2.5–10 mg) and dexamphetamine (5–60 mg) are third-line agents. Abrupt discontinuation of tricyclic antidepressants and SSRIs (but not of sodium oxybate or the other agents) may cause **rebound cataplexy,** including status cataplecticus.

Other Disorders Causing Excessive Daytime Sleepiness

Obstructive sleep apnea (OSA)

OSA is the most common medical cause of daytime sleepiness. Bed partners commonly report loud **snoring, apneas,** and **restless sleep.** In addition to obesity, other risk factors for OSA include a narrow high-arched palate with **narrow pharynx, macroglossia, retrognathia,** and enlarged tonsils. Alcohol consumption prior to bedtime may increase the risk of OSA. An apnea-hypopnea index >5 is the PSG cutoff for OSA by most sleep experts. **OSA increases the risk of hypertension, right heart failure, and stroke** and exacerbates chronic headaches. Weight loss and alcohol avoidance should be tried before instituting **continuous positive airway pressure.**

REM Sleep Behavior Disorder (RBD)

RBD expresses as dream-enactment behaviors, potentially injurious, caused by loss of REM sleep atonia. RBD predates the onset of **synucleinopathies** (PD, MSA, and DLBD) by years or decades, more frequently in men. Damage to the **sublaterodorsal nucleus** of the pontine reticular formation can cause RBD. RBD worsens with SSRIs, tricyclic antidepressants, venlafaxine, mirtazapine, or chocolate. **Clonazepam** (0.5 mg every bedtime) is the treatment of choice. Melatonin may also restore normal EMG atonia. Dopaminergic drugs reduce RBD symptoms via suppression of REM sleep. A history of dream-enactment behavior represents "clinically probable" RBD; "clinically definite" RBD requires PSG confirmation of REM sleep without atonia during complex motor behaviors.

Evaluation of Sleep Disorders

- **Polysomnography (PSG):** Continuous monitoring of eye movements, one channel of EEG, EKG, and EMG (submental), respiratory parameters (airflow, effort, and oximetry), and, optionally, esophageal pH or penile tumescence, as indicated for gastroesophageal reflux disease or erectile function. Most common indications are excessive daytime sleepiness or insomnia and other cardiopulmonary etiologies (chronic obstructive or restrictive pulmonary disorders complicated by pulmonary hypertension, right heart failure, polycythemia, or morning headaches).
- **MSLT:** The same parameters as in PSG, which is performed in the preceding night, are monitored in four to five 20-minute nap opportunities offered at 2-hour intervals in order to (1) quantify sleepiness and (2) determine early-onset REM sleep. A mean latency of 5 minutes or less indicates severe excessive sleepiness.
- **Maintenance of wakefulness test (MWT)** is a measure of the ability to stay awake for a defined period, usually 40 minutes. Four 40-minute MWT trials are used to evaluate narcolepsy and response to treatment.
- **Ambulatory oximetry** is a screening tool to determine whether sleep desaturation is sufficient to explain biologic outcomes such as polycythemia, unexplained pulmonary hypertension, or congestive heart failure. Formal PSG and MSLT may be indicated afterwards.

Pharmacotherapy for Insomnia

Benzodiazepines

The newer drugs of this class of hypnotic agents (flurazepam, temazepam, estazolam, triazolam, and quazepam) promote sleep with greater margin of safety compared with older agents, although dependence and abuse are potential problems. Triazolam is a short-acting agent indicated primarily for sleep-onset insomnia but may cause marked rebound insomnia and anterograde amnesia. Temazepam and estazolam are intermediate-acting BZDs for sleep maintenance or combined sleep-onset and sleep-maintenance insomnia. Flurazepam and quazepam are long-acting agents rarely used because of risk of daytime sedation, gait unsteadiness, and cognitive impairment.

Nonbenzodiazepine Benzodiazepine-Receptor Agonists (NBBRA)

These hypnotic agents include zolpidem (Ambien), zaleplon (Sonata), and eszopiclone (Lunesta) bind to BZD-GABA receptor complex as benzodiazepines. Unlike them, NBBRAs have greater affinity for BZ_1 and BZ_3 receptors, pose lower risk of abuse and tolerance, and lack such properties of benzodiazepines as relaxation, anxiolysis, and anticonvulsant effects. The short-acting zolpidem and zaleplon are more effective in sleep-onset insomnia. The intermediate-acting eszopiclone is preferred for sleep-maintenance insomnia, whether or not sleep-onset insomnia is present. In contrast to short-acting benzodiazepines, little or no rebound insomnia occurs after discontinuation of zolpidem or zaleplon. Although amnestic reactions, including sleep-related eating, may occur occasionally with zolpidem, they are considerably less frequent than with triazolam.

Agent	Duration	Half-life (hr)	Dose (mg)
Zaleplon	Ultrashort	1	5–10
Zolpidem	Short	3	5–10
Eszopiclone	Intermediate	5–7	1–3

The U.S. FDA approved most BZDs and NBBRA for short-term use (7–10 days) with intermittent reuse. No limit has been recommended for eszopiclone. The short-acting agents indicated for sleep-onset insomnia are the BZD triazolam and the NBBRA zolpidem.

Antidepressants

Trazodone, a heterocyclic antidepressant, and the tricyclic amitriptyline, have been used in insomnia based on their sedative effects. Trazodone may cause orthostatic hypotension, arrhythmias, and priapism. Tricyclic antidepressants may lead to hypotension with syncope and ventricular arrhythmias.

Melatonin-Receptor Agonists

The hormone melatonin regulates circadian rhythms through stimulation of melatonin-receptors (MT1, thought to regulate sleep, and MT2, circadian rhythms), located in the suprachiasmatic nucleus. Ramelteon (Rozerem, half-life, 1–3 hours) has high selectivity and potency at the MT1 and MT2 receptors and decreases sleep latency on polysomnography but not wake time after sleep onset. Ramelteon may increase serum prolactin levels, especially in women.

Coma

This "state of unarousable unresponsiveness" (Plum and Posner, 1972) is caused by damage to the ascending reticular activating system (ARAS), the cerebral hemispheres, or the connection between them. Coma is to be distinguished from: (1) **persistent vegetative state** ("wakefulness without awareness") when it lasts more than 4 weeks, and sleep-wake cycles, autonomic functions, and response to painful stimuli are preserved; (2) **minimally conscious state,** when there is profound unresponsiveness but transient evidence of awareness, no matter how limited; (3) **locked-in syndrome,** when patients are awake and conscious but mute and motionless; and (4) **akinetic mutism,** a state of profound apathy due to mesial frontal lobes lesions.

GLASGOW COMA SCALE

Best Motor Response		Best Verbal Response		Eye Opening	
Obeying commands	6	Oriented	5	Spontaneous	4
Localizing to pain	5	Confused conversation	4	To speech	3
Withdrawing to pain	4	Inappropriate words	3	To pain	2
Abnormal flexion (decorticate)	3	Incomprehensible sounds	2	None	1
Abnormal extensor (decerebrate)	2	None	1		
None	1				

Brainstem reflexes required for assessment of comatose patients are the pupillary (CN II and III), corneal (V and VII), gag (IX and X), and vestibular (VIII, III and VI). The latter includes the **oculocephalic reflex** (doll's eye maneuver) and, with a stronger stimulus, the **cold water caloric testing** (irrigating the auditory canal with up to 120 mL of ice-cold water), in which there is a slow tonic deviation of the eyes toward the irrigated ear in the unconscious patient with intact brainstem function. The **ciliospinal reflex** tests midbrain structures: when the skin of the neck is pinched, the ipsilateral pupil should transiently dilate.

Prognostic indicators of poor outcome (American Academy of Neurology practice parameter)
1. Presence of myoclonic status epilepticus
2. Absent pupillary and corneal reflexes on day 3
3. Motor response to pain no better than extension on day 3
4. Absent N20 cortical responses to SSEP, bilaterally, on days 1–3
5. Elevated serum neuron-specific enolase >33 g/L at days 1–3

EXAMINATION FEATURES HELPFUL FOR PROGNOSIS

From coma onset	Clinical findings	LR of poor outcome
At 24 h	Absent corneal reflex	12.9 (2.0-68.7)
	Absent pupillary reflex	10.2 (1.8-48.6)
At 72 h	Absent motor response	9.2 (2.1-49.4)
	Absent pupillary reflex	3.4 (0.5-23.6)

From metanalytical study using cardiac arrest survivors' data (Levy et al, JAMA 2004) LR: likelihood ratio (95% CI). Composite Glasgow Coma Scale scores were not as predictive as individual brainstem reflexes.

In patients who lack pupillary and corneal reflexes at 24 hours and have no motor response at 72 hours, the chance of meaningful recovery is negligible.

Persistent Vegetative State

Persistent vegetative state (PVS) is the term applied to those who emerge from coma and seem **awake but without awareness** 1 month after acute traumatic, degenerative metabolic disorders or developmental malformations. **Impaired consciousness** is shown by the lack of sustained, reproducible, purposeful, or voluntary behavioral responses to visual, auditory, tactile, or noxious stimuli and absent language comprehension or expression. **Consciousness requires *awareness* (of environment and self) and *arousal* (wakefulness or vigilance).**

PVS patients have **normal sleep-wake cycles** and hypothalamic and brainstem autonomic functions, have bowel and bladder incontinence, and have variably preserved cranial nerve reflexes (pupillary, oculocephalic, corneal, vestibulo-ocular, and gag) and spinal reflexes. **Sustained visual pursuit is lacking** in most patients in a vegetative state. They do not fixate on, or track, visual targets, or blink to threat.

The circadian wakefulness in PVS is preserved by processing of sensory information by an **intact ascending reticular activating system** (ARAS). However, the precuneus, involved in self-referential processing and perceptual awareness, is impaired in PVS. Connectivity of ARAS (wakefulness) and precuneus (self-awareness) normally predict whether a somatosensory stimulus will be consciously perceived. Recent studies in PVS suggest there is hypermetabolism in the ARAS and **impaired functional connectivity between the ARAS and the precuneus.**

Cardiac arrest is among the most common causes of PVS among survivors. Reduction in gray matter volume has been identified among cardiac arrest survivors in the precuneus as well as the cingulate cortex, the dorsomedial thalamus, and the posterior hippocampus.

EEG in PVS show diffuse generalized **polymorphic delta or theta activity,** not attenuated by sensory stimulation. In most patients, the transition from wakefulness to sleep is associated with desynchronization of the background activity.

The mortality rate for adults in a PVS after an acute brain injury is 82% at 3 years and 95% at 5 years. Patients reach brain death state when neither the cerebrum nor the brainstem is functioning. Spontaneous cardiovascular activity remains, apnea persists in the presence of hypercarbic respiratory drive, and the only reflexes are those mediated by the spinal cord. Clinical observations compatible with brain death (not to be misinterpreted as evidence of brainstem function) include facial twitching, flexion at the waist, slow head turning, undulating toe movements, and shoulder abduction with arm flexion, even after brain death pronunciation or ventilator disconnection **(Lazarus sign).**

Brain Death

Brain death is a neurologic state of **irreversibly loss of all brain and brainstem reflexes** (pupillary, corneal, oculocephalic, oculovestibular, and gag) documented at repeated testing intervals up to 24 hours by two physicians on at least two separate occasions 12–24 hours apart. There must be **resolution of any mimicking disorders and possible confounding factors** such as severe electrolyte, acid-base, endocrine disturbances, severe hypothermia (core temperature ≤32°C), hypotension, drug intoxication, poisoning, or use of neuromuscular blocking agents.

Steps for determination of brain death:

- **Clinical examination** is focused on motor responses, pupillary responses, corneal reflexes, gag reflex, cough reflex following tracheal suctioning, and caloric stimulation. Because the brainstem reflexes are often lost in a rostrocaudal direction, medullary function may be retained the longest (there is normal BP, a cough reflex after tracheal suctioning, and tachycardia after the administration of 1 mg of atropine).

- **Apnea test:** Patients are preoxygenated (FIO_2 1.0 for 10 minutes) while ensuring that core temperature is ≥36.5°C, systolic BP ≥90 mm Hg, and fluid balance has been positive for 6 hours. The ventilator rate is disconnected once PaO_2 200 mm Hg and the $PaCO_2$ ≥ 40 mm Hg. Oxygen continues to be delivered at a rate of 6 L/m. Chest and abdominal wall are observed for respiration during 8–10 minutes while monitoring vital functions. *Apnea is confirmed when absence of respiratory drive persists despite a $PaCO_2$ of 60 mm Hg or 20 mm Hg above normal baseline values* and the pH <7.30.

Confirmatory laboratory tests

- **EEG** (≥8 electrodes, impedance of 100–10,000Ω, sensitivity ≥2 μV for 30 minutes, high-frequency filter ≥30 Hz and low-frequency filter ≤1 Hz) shows no reactivity to somatosensory or audiovisual stimuli.

- **SSEP** shows bilaterally absent cortical N20 responses within 1–3 days after cardiopulmonary resuscitation.

- **Serum neuron-specific enolase** levels are >33 μg/L at 1–3 days postcardiopulmonary resuscitation.

- **Cerebral angiography** demonstrates no intracerebral filling at the skull entry level of carotid or vertebral after high-pressure contrast injection in the aortic arch.

- **Transcranial Doppler ultrasonography** with bilateral insonation of the suboccipital window documents reverberating flow and small systolic peaks when the intracranial pressure is markedly increased.

- **Cerebral scintigraphy** with static images obtained soon after IV injection of technetium 99m hexametazime, at 30–60 minutes, and at 2 hours, shows no intracranial filling (hollow-skull sign).

Migraine and Other Headaches

Migraine is a form of neurovascular headache that affects 12% of the population and is three times more common in women, presumably because of menstrual-related estrogenic changes. Concordance rate of 25%–30% among monozygotic twins suggests that environmental factors contribute an important 70% to the risk.

Migraine with aura (25%) applies to an idiopathic, recurring headache disorder announced after a reversible aura (<60 minutes), localizable to a focal cortical or brainstem region. Headache, nausea, and/or photophobia last 4–72 hours. The aura in migraine is **visual** (95%, scintillating scotoma or fortification spectra) or **somatosensory** (5%, digitolingual or cheiro-oral paresthesias).

Migraine without aura (75%), similar to the preceding minus the aura, these attacks also last 4–72 hours with the following features: unilateral, pulsating, moderate, or severe intensity, aggravated by routine physical activities, and associated with nausea, photophobia and phonophobia.

Stimulation of the meningeal trigeminovascular afferents through the V1 division activates second-order dorsal horn neurons in the **trigeminal nucleus caudalis** and C1–C2. Impulses reach several thalamic nuclei and the caudal periaqueductal grey region. The activated trigeminovascular system releases substance P, **calcitonin gene-related peptide,** and neurokinin A ("sterile neurogenic inflammation") causing meningeal vasodilation, in part mediated by parasympathetic vasomotor efferents from the **superior salivatory nucleus.** Activation of the adjacent nucleus of the tractus solitarius induces nausea, vomiting, and dysautonomia. **Hypomagnesemia** (via excessive glutamate release), nitric oxide pathway dysfunction, and calcium channelopathy may cause CSD and migraine. **CSD** is a wave of cortical neuronal depolarization driving visual aura, leading to low rCBF and long-lasting neural suppression, which coincides with headache onset. The CSD-mediated reduction in rCBF may cause small regions of focal ischemia **(migraine with aura is a risk factor for ischemic stroke)** and increase in vascular permeability through elevation of MMP-9 (matrix metalloproteinases-9) during migraine attacks.

Familial hemiplegic migraine (FHM, caused by missense mutations in the **voltage-gated P/Q-type calcium channel** $\alpha 1_A$-**subunit gene _CACNA1A_,** highly expressed in Purkinje and granule cells, **19p** [with ataxia] **and 1q** [without ataxia]) manifests as typical migraine without aura, migraine with transient hemiparesis, ictal coma, or progressive cerebellar ataxia within the same families. CACNA1A gain-of-function mutation on calcium channel currents reduces threshold for CSD. Other genetic forms include FHM-2 (**_ATP1A2_,** $\alpha 2$-subunit of the Na^+/K^+-ATPase pump) and FHM-3 (**_SCN1A_,** voltage-gated Na^+ channel). The dominant CACNA1A mutation mechanisms are missense (FHM), deletions (EA-2), or polyglutamine toxicity (CAG expansion in SCA-6).

Abortive Migraine Treatment

Oral triptans, effective within 2 hours in 70% of mild-to-moderate attacks, **stimulate 5-HT1B and 5-HT$_{1D}$ serotonin receptors,** densely present in the hippocampus, dorsal raphe, and SN, and to a lesser extent in the cortex.

- Stimulation of **5-HT$_{1B}$** causes **vasoconstriction of meningeal vessels**
- Stimulation of **5-HT$_{1D}$** receptors **inhibits the neurogenic inflammation from trigeminal nerves** to dural peripheral projections and decrease the central nociceptive signals to the brainstem
- Inhibition of **5-HT$_{1D}$** has **antiemetic** action (ondansetron, metoclopramide)
- Stimulation of **5-HT$_7$** receptors cause **chronic vasodilation**
- Inhibition of **5-HT$_2$** receptors may provide **migraine prophylaxis**

EFFICACY OF MEDICATIONS USED FOR MIGRAINE

Best Efficacy	Good Efficacy	Statistical/Clinical Disparity
Triptans and ergots 5HT$_{1B/1D}$ Sumatriptan[Imitrex] SC/IN Rizatriptan [Maxalt]MLT 10 mg Zolmitriptan [Zomig] 2.5 mg Almotriptan [Axert] 12.5 mg Naratriptan [Amerge] 2.5mg Frovatriptan [Frova] 2.5 mg DHE SC/IM/IV/IN	Chlorpromazine[Thorazine] IM/IV Prochlorperazine[Compazine]IM/IR Metoclopramide IV Butorphanol IM Sodium valproate IV APAP/codeine, Fiorinal, Meperidine IM/IV, and Isometheptene [Midrin] lead to rebound headache and are discouraged.	Butalbital/ASA/caffeine [Fiorinal] Butalbital/APAP/caffeine [Fioricet] Ergotamine/caffeine [Cafergot] Metoclopramide IM/PR
Nonspecific: APAP/ASA/caffeine[Excedrin] Aspirin, Ibuprofen Prochlorperazine IV	Ketorolac IM Diclofenac Naproxen sodium Flurbiprofen	**Ineffective** **Acetaminophen** (APAP)

Onset of action: sumatriptan SC > sumatriptan NS > rizatriptan > zolmitriptan > naratriptan > frovatriptan. The latter has also the longest T½, (25 h) making it the agent with the lowest likelihood of recurrence. The *number needed to treat* (NNT) and *number needed to harm* (NNH) is 3.0 and 14.3 for oral sumatriptan (most effective) and 4.8 and 1,181 for naratriptan (safest), respectively. Sumatriptan formulations are 6 mg SC autoinjector, 5 or 20 mg NS, 25 or 50 mg tablets. *Maximum daily oral dosages* are, following the order from the table, 200 mg, 30 mg, 10 mg, 25 mg, and 5 mg, respectively.

The **Silberstein ER protocol** for management of acute migraine is as follows:
- **Metoclopramide** 10 mg IV or **prochlorperazine** 5–10 mg IV
- **DHE 0.5–1.0 mg IV,** 10–20 minutes following the previous pretreatment
- **DHE 0.5 mg IV,** additional to previous, if headache persists after 1 hour
- **Dexamethasone** 4 mg IV or **diazepam** 5–10 mg IV if headache persists
- **Ketorolac** [Toradol] 30–60 mg IM, **chlorpromazine** 0.1 mg/kg or narcotics

The suggested adjunctive antinausea treatment includes **metoclopramide** (Reglan), **domperidone** (Motilium), **promethazine** (Phenergan), and **ondansetron** (Zofran). The first two are favored for their additional prokinetic effect. Triptans are contraindicated in patients taking MAOIs or sibutramine (Meridia) or with history of coronary artery disease or severe hypertension. Rizatriptan requires a dose reduction when used along with propranolol. A 24-hour period should be allowed when switching from one triptan to another.

Rescue therapies are used after the maximum dose of a triptan, ergot, or NSAIDs has been achieved, 1 full hour has elapsed after the last dose of a triptan (triptan failure), and/or a third headache recurs within 4–5 days.

- **Butorphanol** nasal spray (1 mg/dose, repeating within 60–90 minutes if pain persists) has the greatest advantage among the **opioid** medications: onset of pain relief within 15 minutes, preferred delivery when nausea and vomiting are prominent, and mixed agonist-antagonist activity (low intrinsic μ-opioid receptor activity results in less potential for drug dependence).
- **Meperidine** (schedule II drug) has the disadvantages of a higher potential for abuse and a short half-life, which may result in headache recurrence.

Narcotics are the analgesic of choice for pregnant woman with severe intractable migraine. Patients with CDH or comorbid psychiatric disorders are at higher risk for abuse and dependence and are not good candidates for this class of drugs.

ORAL NARCOTICS PROVIDING RELIEF EQUIVALENT TO 10 mg OF MORPHINE

Drug	Doses (mg) Oral and Parenteral		Oral:Parenteral
Morphine	60	10	6:1
Hydromorphone	7.5	1.5	5:1
Meperidine	300	75	4:1
Methadone	20	10	2:1
Levorphanol	4	2	2:1
Codeine	200	130	1.5:1

Hydromorphone, meperidine, and codeine are most common drugs causing medication-overuse headache and their use is discouraged.

- **Dexamethasone** (4 mg IV) following **IV metoclopramide** may be effective in aborting refractory migraine. A tapering short course of prednisone (starting at 80–100 mg/d) or dexamethasone (starting at 8–20 mg/d) is also helpful. Corticosteroids are used only once a month in order to avoid adrenal suppression and steroid dependence.
- **Prochlorperazine** (5–10 mg IV) followed by **dihydroergotamine (DHE,** 0.5–1.0 mg IV) has been shown to be an effective rescue strategy for intractable migraine or status migrainosus. **Neuroleptics** in general (including haloperidol, thiothixene, chlorpromazine, and droperidol) are effective IV rescue medications but are associated with significant hypotension while they are administered and may potentially cause acute and tardive dyskinesia during long-term therapy.

Analgesic rebound headache: Daily or near-daily headache (CDH) resulting from the overuse of any abortive medications, especially ergotamine and caffeine-containing medications, may "reset" central pain control mechanisms in vulnerable individuals. Limiting the use of any single medication to <2 days per week prevents rebound headaches. The use of repetitive IV **DHE**), the drug with the least likelihood to cause rebound withdrawal headaches, or steroids helps detoxify from the offending agent(s).

Migraine Prophylaxis

Daily medication is used to reduce the frequency and intensity of the headache when (1) the patient has two or more attacks per month, (2) there is failure or intolerability of abortive agents, (3) aura that interferes with function, (4) menstrual migraine, or (5) presence of comorbid conditions. Good response to prophylaxis is defined, by consensus, as a 50% reduction in frequency or severity of attacks. The most common reason for prophylactic failure is the use of an agent at an insufficient dose during a relatively short length of time.

PROPHYLACTIC AGENTS ACCORDING TO LEVEL OF EVIDENCE AND SIDE EFFECTS

Best efficacy	Good efficacy	Good efficacy	Good efficacy
Good evidence	Limited evidence	Consensus	Good evidence
Mild to moderate side effects			**SE concerns**
Propranolol **Nadolol** Valproate **Amitriptyline** **Topiramate**	Metoprolol, atenolol, verapamil, nimodipine, gabapentin, fluoxetine, aspirin, ketoprofen, naproxen, vitamin B2	Cyproheptadine Diltiazem Nortriptyline Bupropion Paroxetine	Methysergide (no longer available in the United States)

SE, status epilepticus.
   Evidence indicates no efficacy over placebo: carbamazepine, lamotrigine, clonazepam, indomethacin, clomipramine, nifedipine, nicardipine, pindolol, and acebutolol.

Tricyclic antidepressants (TCAs) are preferred in the prevention of migraine in patients with coexistent tension-type headache, chronic daily headaches (CDH), and other chronic pain states. **Nortriptyline** has fewer adverse effects but is not as effective as amitriptyline. The side effects include sedation, dry mouth, weight gain, tremor, cardiac arrhythmias, aggravation of angle-closure glaucoma, and urinary retention.

Valproate may be chosen in those with associated mood disorders or epilepsy and those at risk for, or affected with, CDH. Adverse events include nausea, fatigue, weight gain, hair loss, tremor, liver dysfunction, and neural tube defects if taken during early pregnancy.

Beta-adrenergic blocking drugs are favored when migraine is accompanied by hypertension, angina, or anxiety disorders but at the potential cost of aggravating asthma, bradycardia, fatigue, depression, or masking the symptoms of hypoglycemia in diabetics. Patients on this drug should avoid concomitant use of triptans and ergot-derived medications. **Calcium channel blockers,** verapamil and occasionally diltiazem, are widely used despite the scant evidence of benefit. Their adverse effects include hypotension, atrioventricular conduction abnormalities, constipation, and peripheral edema.

Coxibs (selective inhibitors of cyclooxygenase-2) such as rofecoxib (Vioxx) and celecoxib (Celebrex), have not shown efficacy in migraine and other headaches, although they provide analgesia in pain of dental origin.

Cluster headache ("migrainous neuralgia," "erythroprosopalgia") refers to the 60–90-minute attacks recurring in *episodic* (7-day to 1-year periods separated by remissions ≥14 days) or *chronic* (periods >1 year and remission of <14 days) stereotypic and circadian clusters. Unlike migraine or trigeminal neuralgia, nocturnal attacks begin **at the onset of REM sleep.** The severe unilateral periorbital headache attacks reach a peak intensity within 5–10 minutes, radiate into the ipsilateral forehead and jaw, and are accompanied by lacrimation, conjunctival injection, rhinorrhea, facial flushing, and **Horner syndrome.** The patients are **restless** and prefer to **pace about** and remain awake and sober to prevent the REM sleep and alcohol triggers. Only one other trigeminal autonomic cephalgia also predominates in men: *s*hort-lasting *u*nilateral *n*euralgiform pain with *c*onjunctival injection and *t*earing **(SUNCT).** SUNCT and the indomethacin-responsive paroxysmal hemicranias (see following discussion) are distinguished from cluster headache by their higher frequency and shorter duration of individual attacks. The most rapid and effective relief for each attack is achieved with oxygen, SC sumatriptan, and IV DHE-45. Prednisone and dexamethasone are effective *transitional* prophylactic agents. Verapamil extended release (SR), at dosages of 80 mg tid or 240 mg, is the prophylactic drug of choice, followed by valproate and lithium.

Paroxysmal hemicrania consists of multiple (2–40 times), brief (2–45 minutes), unilateral, periorbital or temporal, daily painful attacks that persist unremittingly for years (chronic paroxysmal hemicrania) or occur after long remissions (rare episodic variant). One or more ipsilateral autonomic symptoms are present during attacks (conjunctival injection, lacrimation, nasal congestion, rhinorrhea, or ptosis). Neck movements may precipitate attacks. **Indomethacin** (25 mg tid, increased to 50 mg tid in 1 week) is the *diagnostic* treatment of choice.

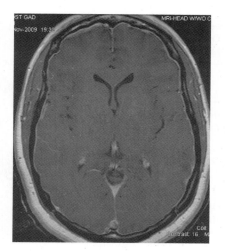

CSF hypotension (CSF volume depletion) is associated with very low or unobtainable CSF pressures due to spontaneous or traumatic CSF leak causing a positional headache aggravated by upright position and relieved with recumbency. Cranial or spinal surgery, post-traumatic CSF rhinorrhea, shunt overdrainage, and lumbar puncture are possible etiologies. Brain MRI shows diffuse pachymeningeal gadolinium enhancement, followed by "sinking" of the brain (including a secondary "Chiari I malformation"), subdural fluid collection, and decrease in size of the ventricles. CT dynamic myelography or radioisotope cisternography with indium[-111] helps localize the site of the leak. Epidural blood patch is often needed.

Call-Fleming syndrome is a rare, benign, recurrent thunderclap headache due to reversible multifocal segmental vasoconstriction of the cerebral arteries.

Idiopathic Intracranial Hypertension (Pseudotumor Cerebri)

IIH is a disorder of elevated CSF pressure (>200 mm H_2O or >250 mm H_2O if obese) usually in **obese women** of childbearing age presenting with the nonlocalizing deficits of headache, **transient visual obscurations** (not correlated with the severity of the **papilledema**), and diplopia due to bilateral CN VI palsy. Obstruction to CSF drainage (decreased flow through the arachnoid granulations or venous obstruction), **Addison disease,** steroid withdrawal, obesity, and **hypoparathyroidism** are clearly associated with IIH. **Vitamin A,** indomethacin, nitrofurantoin, and lithium have also been associated. Trauma, cerebral venous sinus thrombosis, or meningitis may cause IIH without papilledema.

Neuroimaging is normal but may show small (slitlike) ventricles or empty sella. Lowering raised ICP through **weight loss** is the most effective treatment with **acetazolamide** (250 mg bid gradually increasing up to 2 g/d) given optionally to help reduce CSF production. Repeated LPs have unproven efficacy. Surgical procedures include lumbar subarachnoid-peritoneal shunt and **optic nerve sheath fenestration,** which is the preferred method for reversing visual loss and protecting the optic nerve from further damage.

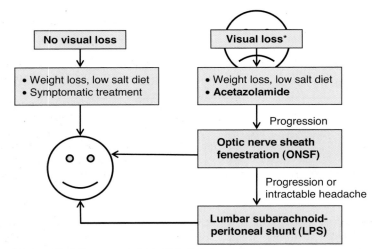

*Once papilledema occurs, **enlarged blind spots** are common
Management algorithm based on Wall M, *Neurol Clin* 1991;9:73–95)

Trigeminal Neuralgia

These paroxysmal shocklike electric jabs of unilateral pain, most commonly restricted to the V2 and/or V3 distribution of the trigeminal nerve, may occur in the setting of multiple sclerosis, basilar artery aneurysm, acoustic neuroma, meningioma, syringobulbia, and brainstem infarction. The neuralgic pain is triggered by stimulation of facial skin or oral mucosae. Carbamazepine is the first-line agent before phenytoin, baclofen, clonazepam, and newer AEDs.

Selected Secondary Headaches

Pheochromocytoma

Potentially associated with neurofibromatosis, von Hippel-Lindau disease, or multiple endocrine neoplasia type IIA or IIB, pheochromocytoma, is suspected in patients with hypertension who have headaches, palpitations, and sweating, with or without pallor, nausea, abdominal and chest pain, and tremor. Hypertension may be sustained or paroxysmal. The paroxysms last for a few minutes to a few hours and can be spontaneous or triggered by abdominal pressure (BP is higher in the sitting that in the supine position) or drugs such as tricyclic antidepressants, metoclopramide, and opiates. Most tumors are adrenal in origin and most extra-adrenal sites, known as *paragangliomas,* are abdominal (organ of Zuckerkandl, sympathetic ganglia, and the urinary bladder). Their excessive catecholamine secretion may cause:

- **Hemodynamic changes** from hypertension to **orthostatic hypotension** due to down-regulation of peripheral α receptors from chronic exposure to catecholamines and volume depletion caused by inhibition of the renin-angiotensin system
- **Hyperglycemia** due to inhibition of insulin secretion and stimulation of hepatic glucose output
- **Hypercalcemia** due to ectopic production of parathyroid hormone-related peptide by the tumor

The diagnosis is established by demonstrating increased levels of free catecholamines, metanephrines, or vanillylmandelic acid (VMA) in a 24-hour urine specimen. Plasma catecholamines have 90% sensitivity and 95% specificity for the diagnosis of pheochromocytoma. After a biochemical diagnosis, abdomen MRI and, if negative, [I^{131}] metaiodobenzylguanidine scan are used for tumor localization. **Phenoxybenzamine**, a nonspecific α-adrenergic antagonist, is used prior to the surgical excision of the tumor. **Paradoxical hypertension may be caused by the use of beta-blocker agents** presumably by abolishing the vasodilating effects of β2-receptor stimulation without interrupting the vasoconstricting α-1-receptor stimulation from excessive catecholamines.

> **Some hyperadrenergic and hyperadrenergic-like states** other than pheochromocytoma are anxiety attacks, hyperthyroidism, insulinoma, baroreflex failure, diencephalic seizures, subarachnoid hemorrhage, and cocaine abuse.

Paroxysmal Nocturnal Hemoglobinuria (PNH)

A condition that is neither paroxysmal nor nocturnal, PNH is suspected when the triad of headache, **venous thrombosis,** and **hemolytic anemia** is present. Thrombosis may occur in deep veins of legs and intracranial sinuses as well as hepatic (Budd Chiari syndrome) and dermal veins. Pancytopenia develops in about 20% of patients. PNH is diagnosed by ascertaining the **absence of CD59** membrane protein on red blood cells. The loss of this anchor protein for other complement-interacting proteins causes thrombogenesis and hemolysis.

3 Infectious Diseases

Although infectious diseases affecting the central nervous systems (CNSs) are plentiful, there is a subtle misperception that these may have become uncommon to pay much attention. Neuroinfectious disorders that would have been readily recognized by an expert clinician are increasingly sensed as rare. Regardless, many "classics" have always been fascinating.

Rabies is now effectively controlled with vaccination program in dogs and other pets, whose bites are the main sources of the virus. The literature sparked our interest with its similarities to vampirism. Spasms of the facial, laryngeal, and pharyngeal muscles give rise to hoarse sounds and the appearance of an "animal with teeth clinched and lips retracted." As saliva cannot be swallowed, there is frothing at the mouth and vomiting of bloody fluids. The spasms are generally triggered by some stimuli, such as air draughts (aerophobia), water **(hydrophobia),** light (photophobia), noises, odor, a minimal excitement, or "the sight of mirrors." A man was not considered rabid if he was able to stand the sight of his own image in a mirror.

Tabes dorsalis, now rarely seen because of comprehensive screening and treatment programs for syphilis, became readily recognizable with a simple neurologic examination maneuver. Moritz Romberg (circa 1840) reported the observation of increased postural sway upon eye closure in tabetics in what became known as the Romberg's sign. Subsequently, New York neurologist William Hammond (circa 1871) emphasized the sign's independence from muscle weakness and from cerebellar disease. Jean-Martin Charcot (circa 1888) considered the Romberg's sign as typical of tabes dorsalis but was the first to document it also in Friedreich's disease.

Postencephalitic parkinsonism (PEP) was a complication of **encephalitis lethargica** related to the influenza epidemic, described by Constantin von Economo (1917) and brought to the fore by the movie *Awakenings*. **Postpolio syndrome** was also a complication of **anterior poliomyelitis,** widespread in the 1940s–1950s. Both of these complications required extensive resources and long-term neurologic care but we had a giant with postpolio syndrome that steered Western democracies through the great depression and World War II.

Admissions to or consults by a busy hospital neurology service for any neuroinfectious disease accounts for <3% per year (*Neurology* 2008;71:1160–1166). About one-fourth of patients may have an HIV infection but almost one-third remain without an identifiable microbiologic etiology, require long hospitalizations, expensive diagnostic tests and treatments, and substantial posthospital rehabilitation and long-term care needs. The burden of recognizable and potentially curable conditions may be shortened by getting to the next few pages time and again while in rounds.

Cerebrospinal Fluid

CSF is formed in the ventricular choroid plexus at a rate of 500 mL/d. **Total volumes (and pressures in mm H_2O)** are 150 mL (180, 250 if obese) in adults, 60–100 mL (150) in children, and 30–60 mL (110) in neonates.

Hypoglycorrhachia (<45 mg/dL or a CSF:serum ratio of <0.6) can be seen in bacterial meningitis, HSV encephalitis, TB meningitis, fungal meningitis, carcinomatous meningitis, sarcoidosis, and hypoglycemia.

INFECTIOUS MENINGITIS

	Bacterial	**Viral**	**TB**	**Fungal**
OP	↑	Normal	↑	~Normal
WBC	↑:100→1,000 PMN*	↑: 300–400 lymphocytic[†]	↑: 10–500 lymphocytic	↑ lymphocytic (PMN: Blastomyces dermatidis)
Glu	↓: ratio <0.31	~Normal (↓ in LCMV)	↓: ratio <0.6 AFB smear	↓ CSF may be normal in up to 50% of HIV-infected individuals with
Prot	↑ (500–2,000)	~Normal	↑ (100–500)	↑ cryptococcal meningitis

OP = opening pressure; WBC = white blood cell count; Glu = glucose; Prot = protein.
*$\textbf{Lymphocytic pleocytosis}$ can be seen in bacterial meningitis when the WBC count is <1,000 cells/mm^3 and in bacterial meningitis due to *Listeria monocytogenes.*
[†]**PMN pleocytosis** typically indicates bacterial infections but may be seen within the first 24 hours in meningitis due to enteroviruses and arthropod-borne viruses (LaCrosse and St. Louis encephalitis), for which reverse transcriptase (RT) PCR and a fourfold increase in virus-specific IgG are diagnostic, respectively. **Persistent PMN pleocytosis** suggests HIV-associated CMV polyradiculomyelitis, as well as WNV meningoencephalitis; In HIV-1 meningitis, **mononuclear pleocytosis** occurs within 3–6 weeks of initial infection, when CD4$^+$ T-lymphocyte count is >400 cells/mm^3.

The latex particle agglutination test is useful for the detection of bacteria (*Haemophilus influenzae* type b, *Streptococcus pneumoniae, Neisseria meningitidis,* group B streptococcus, and *Escherichia coli* K1 strains) and fungus (cryptococcal antigen) in the CSF. Agglutination is more sensitive than India ink preparation for the diagnosis of cryptococcal meningitis.

Complement fixation antibody test is used for *Coccidioides immitis,* which may cause an eosinophilic meningitis in the southwestern United States. The **histoplasma polysaccharide antigen** can be measured in areas where *Histoplasma capsulatum* is endemic, especially the midwestern United States.

Syphilitic meningitis, or any of the neurosyphilitic syndromes, is confirmed with a reactive CSF VDRL test (false positives occur with blood-tinged CSF). A negative CSF VDRL test result does not rule syphilitic meningitis out, but a nonreactive CSF fluorescent treponemal antibody absorption (FTA-ABS) test or a nonreactive microhemagglutination-*T. pallidum* (MHA-TP) test definitively excludes the diagnosis. Interestingly, a reactive CSF FTA-ABS test or a reactive CSF MHA-TP test does not establish the diagnosis as they may result from the passive transfer of *T. pallidum*–specific IgG from the serum to the CSF.

Lyme disease (mononuclear or lymphocytic pleocytosis, elevated protein, and normal glucose in CSF) is demonstrated by the presence of specific antibodies against *Borrelia burgdorferi* in CSF. Both sera and CSF should be analyzed.

CSF of Encephalitis

	WBC	Glucose	Diagnosis	Other
HSV	5–500 cells, Lymphocytic	Normal to mildly low	HSV DNA (day 2–14) HSV antibody (8-30)	↑ RBC and/or xanthochromia
Arboviruses (Arthropod-borne)	PMN→lymph SLE→monocytic	Normal	Diagnosis is made by a fourfold virus-specific IgG increase in serum and/or by finding virus-specific IgM antibody	
Rocky Mountain spotted fever	Mild: <100 Lymphocytic	Normal	The indirect fluorescent antibody (IFA) and indirect hemagglutination tests are most sensitive and specific	
VZV	Mild: <250 Lymphocytic	Normal	VZV DNA PCR VZV antibodies	VZV can grow in CSF culture
Encephalitis to test in the setting of immunosuppression (besides VZV)				
CMV	Mononuclear	Low	CMV DNA PCR	CMV culture
EBV	Lymphocytic	Normal	EBV DNA PCR	IgM to VCA*
HHV-6	Lymphocytic	Normal	HHV-6 DNA PCR	HHV-6 culture
Enteroviral	PMN → Lymphocytic	Normal to mildly low	Enterovirus RT PCR	EV culture
Measles	Mononuclear or normal		Brain biopsy	Oligoclonal Ab

*VCA: Viral capside antigen; intrathecal synthesis of EBV-specific VCA antibody can be used for diagnosis of Epstein-Barr virus (EBV) meningoencephalitis. CSF may show atypical lymphocytes. EBV is rarely grown in CSF culture. Viral cultures are only worth the trouble for suspected VZV, CMV, HHV-6, and enteroviruses.

Fourfold IgG antibody increase between acute and convalescent sera is diagnostic for arboviruses, RMSF, EV, and HHV-6 (HHV-6 DNA is not sufficient since it may be due to latent infection). **Lymphocytic pleocytosis with low glucose** suggests the presence of fungus, TB, listeria, or sarcoidosis.

Eastern equine encephalitis, the deadliest of the arboviral encephalitis, may uniquely involve the *basal ganglia and thalami* early and cause xanthochromia and hyponatremia and raise the CSF leukocyte count above 1,000 (neutrophils). **The La Crosse virus** accounts for most cases of encephalitis in the pediatric age group. **Japanese B encephalitis virus** is the most common arthropod-borne human encephalitis worldwide, which does not show a July-to-October seasonal pattern of other arboviral encephalitis. The St. Louis encephalitis (SLE) and West Nile viruses (WNV) are discussed later.

MENINGOENCEPHALITIS AND RASH (RASH DISTRIBUTION, DIAGNOSIS, AND TREATMENT)*

RMSF *Rickettsia rickettsii*	Enteroviruses Coxsackie B5 and Echo 7,9,11,30	Meningococcemia *Neisseria meningitidis*
Palms and soles, centripetal Macular becoming petechial	Palms and soles, mostly vesicular	Trunk and legs, mostly petechial and ecchymotic
Skin biopsy of the rash	**RT PCR**	**Latex agglutination**
Doxycycline	Pleconaril	Penicillin

*Chickenpox and varicella from varicella zoster virus (VZV) may complicate their course with encephalitis and acute cerebellar ataxia, respectively. They develop 4–10 days after the onset of the typical rash. VZV encephalitis results from large (hemorrhagic infarctions) or small-vessel (ischemic and demyelinating) vasculopathy. The newest cause of rash and encephalitis is that caused by West Nile virus (see later).

Viral Encephalitis

HSV Is Responsible for 10% of Endemic Cases

Herpes simplex virus is responsible for 10% of endemic cases of viral encephalitis in the United States. (Japanese B encephalitis is the most common epidemic infection outside North America.) The typical focal abnormality on brain MRI is T2W-hyperintense signal in the orbitofrontal and temporal lobe. When bilateral destruction of the temporal lobes involves the anterior operculum and insular areas, a potential complication is the **opercular syndrome (Foix-Chavany-Marie syndrome).** It is characterized by loss of voluntary movements of the facio-pharyngo-glosso-masticatory muscles (anarthria, inability to move the tongue or swallow to commands) with preservation of reflex movements (intact cough and swallowing reflexes) and limb strength.

HSV type 2 is the major cause of benign recurrent lymphocytic meningitis **(Mollaret's meningitis).** Cowdry type A inclusion bodies are characteristic of HSV. (Negri bodies are of rabies.)

Varicella zoster virus (VZV), more common in immunocompromised patients, may or may not follow, by days to months, a zoster or varicella vesicular rash in a dermatomal distribution, though the rash can be absent in up to 40% of patients. VZV infects endothelial cells and oligodendrocytes, causing corresponding ischemic and hemorrhagic infarction and demyelination. **Anti-VZV IgG antibody in CSF** is the virologic test of choice for diagnosis. Negative VZV DNA PCR and negative anti-VZV IgG antibody in CSF most reliably excludes the diagnosis of VZV vasculopathy.

SELECTED CLINICAL CLUES PER ETIOLOGY

Myalgia and myocarditis	Coxsackie
Skin rash	Enteroviruses or HZV
Retinitis	CMV
Myelitis	WNV, SLE, VZV, HBV, HTLV, lymphocytic choriomeningitis virus (LCMV)
Parotitis and orchitis	Mumps
Paresthesias	Rabies, Colorado tick fever, LCMV
Tremor	Arboviruses (WNV, SLE, others)
Weakness	WNV, rabies
Arthralgia and lymphadenopathy	HIV
Hemorrhagic encephalopathy	Parvovirus

The three most common causes of viral meningitis and encephalitis in North America are **enteroviruses** (especially in infants and hypogammaglobulinemic patients), arboviruses (particularly WNV), and HSV. In adolescents and adults, herpes simplex virus 1 (HSV-1) more commonly causes encephalitis, whereas HSV-2 causes meningitis.

Preferential sites of involvement for selected viruses are the frontal and temporal lobes (HSV), the cerebellum (VZV and EBV), and the limbic system (rabies).

Imaging of Viral Encephalitis

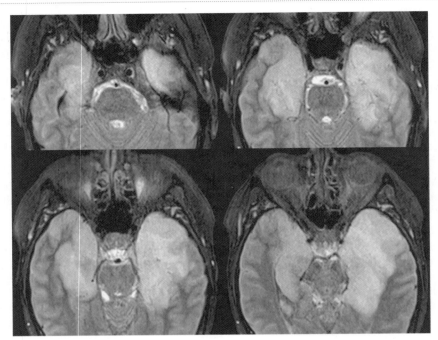

Herpes encephalitis: 63-year-old woman with a 2-week history of headaches and fever, followed by features suggestive of partial complex seizures (staring and tapping the dorsal aspect of her right hand with her left hand; repeating: "is OK, is OK"; calling a computer, "stove"). Brain MRI showed hyperintense T2/FLAIR signal abnormalities involving both anterior and medial aspects of the temporal lobes, left greater than right, and extending into the inferior left frontal lobe with some hemorrhage and enhancement. A similar pattern may be seen in some autoimmune (due to voltage-gated potassium channel or NMDAR antibodies) and paraneoplastic (limbic) encephalitis.

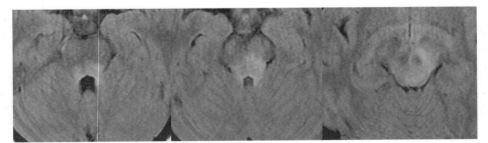

Rhombencephalitis: 28-year-old woman with 2-week history of flu-like symptoms and diplopia. CSF showed lymphocytic pleocytosis. She normalized after a 14-week course with Acyclovir. Etiology was not uncovered but viral entities associated with this presentation are arboviruses (St. Louis and West Nile), enteroviruses (Coxsackie), and adenoviruses. Rhombencephalitis is a form of encephalitis that affects primarily the brain stem and cerebellum (rhombencephalon), presenting with gaze palsy, diplopia, persistent hiccuping, central sleep apnea, or acute respiratory failure. *Listeria monocytogenes* infection has been a classical etiology. This imaging pattern has also been reported in the setting of paraneoplastic disorders due to anti-Hu, anti-Ri, and anti-Ma2 antibodies, lymphoma, vasculitic diseases (systemic lupus erythematosus, disease), Behçet disease, neurosarcoidosis, tuberculosis, multiple sclerosis, and acute disseminated encephalomyelitis.

Viral Meningoencephalitis with Neurologic Sequelae

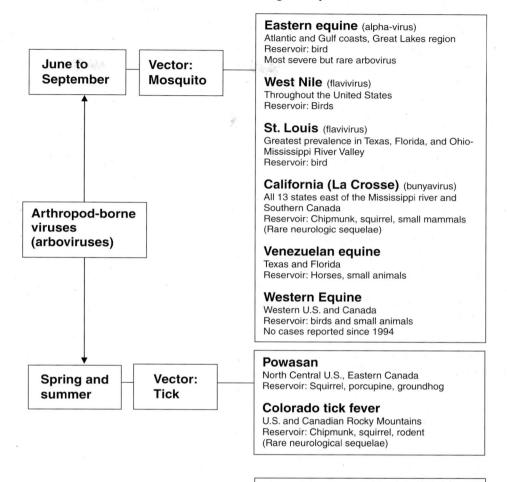

June to September — **Vector: Mosquito**

Eastern equine (alpha-virus)
Atlantic and Gulf coasts, Great Lakes region
Reservoir: bird
Most severe but rare arbovirus

West Nile (flavivirus)
Throughout the United States
Reservoir: Birds

St. Louis (flavivirus)
Greatest prevalence in Texas, Florida, and Ohio-Mississippi River Valley
Reservoir: bird

California (La Crosse) (bunyavirus)
All 13 states east of the Mississippi river and Southern Canada
Reservoir: Chipmunk, squirrel, small mammals
(Rare neurologic sequelae)

Venezuelan equine
Texas and Florida
Reservoir: Horses, small animals

Western Equine
Western U.S. and Canada
Reservoir: birds and small animals
No cases reported since 1994

Arthropod-borne viruses (arboviruses)

Spring and summer — **Vector: Tick**

Powasan
North Central U.S., Eastern Canada
Reservoir: Squirrel, porcupine, groundhog

Colorado tick fever
U.S. and Canadian Rocky Mountains
Reservoir: Chipmunk, squirrel, rodent
(Rare neurological sequelae)

Enteroviruses

Enteroviral meningitis occurring beyond the neonatal period in normal hosts is almost never associated with severe disease or subsequent neurological deficits. Enteroviruses may cause encephalitis in immunodeficient patients with agammaglobulinemia and in neonates.

Coxsackie A and B (A9, B3, B4, B5)
Echovirus (4, 6, 7, 9, 11, 18, and 30)
About 80% of late summer-early fall (aseptic) viral meningitis are non-polio enteroviruses. It is suspected, besides GI symptoms, in the setting of the enanthema of herpangina or the exanthema of hand-foot-mouth syndrome.

Paramyxoviruses

Measles
Mumps
Respiratory syncytial virus
Parainfluenza

St. Louis Encephalitis (SLE) and West Nile Virus Encephalitis (WNV)

The SLE (midwestern and southern United States) and WNV encephalitis (expanding from New York and northeast) are, respectively, the most common and most rapidly spreading **arboviral** infections during the late summer and early fall and have similar ecology and epidemiology. They belong to the Japanese encephalitis virus complex of antigenically related flaviviruses.

SLE and WNV encephalitis are **primarily avian infections** (reservoirs and hosts) that spread to humans via ornitophilic culicine mosquitoes (vectors). The WNV encephalitis was first identified in Uganda in 1937 and is endemic in the Middle East, Africa, and parts of Europe. It was initially mistaken as SLE in New York (August 1999) in two cases of **encephalitis associated with muscle weakness,** which were preceded by a fatal epizootic among American crows, *Corvus brachyrhynchos,* a species that remain a sentinel for the spread of this virus.

SLE typically causes mild to moderately severe illness, whereby 1 in 100 infected patients develop meningoencephalitis with myalgia requiring medical attention. Disease severity is worse in those older than 50 years, with tremor, seizures, and hyponatremia from inappropriate antidiuretic hormone **(SIADH)** complicating the course. **T2W hyperintensity in the substantia nigra** has been reported.

WNV infection causes a mild febrile illness in one out of five infected (3–6 days) with headache, **eye pain, nonpruritic macular rash,** and gastrointestinal problems. **Leukopenia with relative or absolute lymphopenia** is unusual in other viral encephalitides. Meningoencephalitis develops in 1 out of 150 infected and is often associated with **severe muscle weakness,** especially in the elderly or immunosuppressed. Parkinsonism, tremor, and myoclonus have also been reported. The predominant gray matter lymphocytic infiltration, causing T2W hyperintensity in deep brain and cerebellar nuclei, has the capability of affecting the entire neuroaxis and spinal roots.

The muscle weakness induced by WNV may present in two forms:
   Guillain-Barré type syndrome
   Poliomyelitis-like syndrome (affecting anterior horn cells)

Diagnosis of arboviral encephalitis can be relied upon the following tests:
- **Virus-specific CSF IgM** is confirmatory; **serum IgM** is suspicious. The latter requires a fourfold increase in **virus-specific IgG** in convalescent sera. IgM becomes detectable in 75% of patients with flavivirus encephalitis within the first 4 days of illness and may persist for one or more years after the infection.
- **Virus-neutralization tests** are used to distinguish the antigenically related WNV from SLE infections when serum specimens are available due to the serologic cross-reactions with other flaviviruses.
- Qualitative **rt-PCR** or quantitative PCR have poor sensitivity.

Aseptic Meningitis Syndrome

Infectious causes include enteroviruses, arboviruses, HSV-2, HHV-6, VZV, EBV, fungi, *Mycoplasma pneumoniae, Borrelia burgdorferi,* and *Treponema pallidum.* **Noninfectious** causes include sarcoidosis, carcinomatous meningitis, SLE, Wegener granulomatosis, Behçet disease, and drug-induced.

Tuberculous meningitis is suggested by low-grade fever, night sweats, and subacute meningismus in the setting of **lymphocytic pleocytosis and mild hypoglycorrhachia** on CSF. There may be cranial neuropathies, meningeal enhancement, or **progressive hydrocephalus**. Less than 50% of adults have a history of pulmonary TB. **Smears for acid-fast bacilli** are positive in only 10%–40% of cases of tuberculous meningitis in adults and <20% of cases in children. **CSF cultures** are positive in about 50% and may take up to 8 weeks. **PCR** for *Mycobacterium tuberculosis* is 80%–100% specific but only 25%–80% sensitive.

DRUGS FOR THE TREATMENT OF TUBERCULOSIS

Treatment	Dose	CNS Penetration/Action		Toxicity
Isoniazid	300 mg/d	Good with and without CNS inflammation/ bactericidal		Monitoring of LFT: liver toxicity
Pyrazinamide	30 mg/kg/d			
Rifampin	10 mg/kg/d	Poor. Require meningeal inflammation	Bactericidal	
Ethambutol	20 mg/kg/d		Bacteriostatic	Optic nerve
Streptomycin	1 g IM qd		Bacteriostatic	Vestibular

Pyrazinamide and ethambutol can be discontinued after 8 weeks and isoniazid and rifampin continued for 6 to 9 months. Streptomycin can be stopped if the susceptibility testing shows that the isolate is susceptible to the other agents. Pyridoxine (vitamin B₆), 50 mg/d, prevents the development of peripheral neuropathy. Dexamethasone for a short term is recommended only when hydrocephalus is present.

Neurosarcoidosis causes cranial neuropathy most frequently (especially facial nerve palsy) and recurrent aseptic meningitis. ACE levels are elevated in up to 70% of patients but false positives occur in the setting of CNS infections, malignant tumors, MS, GBS, and Behçet disease.

Leptomeningeal carcinomatosis may also lead to cranial neuropathy or spinal nerve root involvement: asymmetric reflexes and focal weaknesses are common. Repeated LPs increase the yield of CSF **cytology.** Immunophenotyping by **flow cytometry** has even lower sensitivity given the hypocellularity of the CSF.

Wegener granulomatosis is a necrotizing granulomatous small-to-medium vessel vasculitis of the respiratory and renal systems. Hemoptysis and epistaxis may be followed by cranial neuropathies (hearing loss, ophthalmoplegia, vision loss, and facial paresis) if the skull base is eroded by contiguous extension of granulomas. More than 90% of patients with active renal disease have a positive cytoplasmic antineutrophil cytoplasmic autoantibody (c-ANCA) in serum.

Drug-induced lymphocytic pleocytosis may be caused by NSAIDs, sulfa-containing antibiotics (especially TMP-SMX), intravenous immunoglobulin, and isoniazid. SLE, which may itself be a cause of aseptic meningitis, is the single most frequent underlying condition.

Postencephalitic Parkinsonism

Postencephalitic parkinsonism (PEP) represented a major neurologic sequel of the pandemic of **encephalitis lethargica** (von Economo's disease or "sleeping sickness," 1917–1927). Since then, other primary viral encephalitides have been recognized as potential causes of PEP. The classic phenotype was divided into three syndromes: *somnolent-ophthalmoplegic* (stupor and such oculomotor deficits as **oculogyric crises,** vertical supranuclear gaze palsy, eyelid opening apraxia, nystagmus, and ptosis), *hyperkinetic* (catatonic schizophrenia with motor restlessness and visual hallucinations), and *amyostatic-akinetic* (catalepsy or "waxy flexibility" and mutism). Parkinsonism developed following a **latency measured in months or even years** after the acute encephalitic illness. Other deficits in the classic and new PEP forms include dysarthria and palilalia, cervical and **facial dystonia** (particularly blepharospasm and jaw opening dystonia), motor tics, and obsessive-compulsive disorder.

Major criteria for diagnosis (Howard and Lees, 1987) are as follows: (1) signs of basal ganglia involvement, (2) oculogyric crisis, (3) ophthalmoplegia, (4) obsessive-compulsive behavior, (5) akinetic mutism, (6) central respiratory abnormalities, and (7) somnolence and/or sleep inversion.

Bilateral substantia nigra hyperintensity on T2W and FLAIR MRI sequences characteristically occur within days of the acute encephalitic illness.

> The newer cases of PEP differ from those from Von Economo's encephalitis mainly by the **shorter latency** of the parkinsonism, the **less common oculogyric crises**, and the **gradual improvement** rather than continued deterioration after the initial viral encephalitic insult. **Oculogyric crises** may also occur as an idiosyncratic reaction to metoclopramide and phenothiazines.

VIRAL ENCEPHALITIDES ASSOCIATED WITH PARKINSONISM (LATENCY, 2–20 DAYS)*

Affecting Mainly Substantia Nigra	Affecting Basal Ganglia and/or Thalami
Japanese B encephalitis	Japanese B encephalitis
St. Louis encephalitis	Eastern equine encephalitis
Coxsackie B3 and B4	Measles and mumps
Postmeasles vaccination	ECHO virus 25 (hemichorea)

*Although Japanese B encephalitis (the most common arthropod-borne human encephalitis worldwide) may equally involve the substantia nigra and the basal ganglia and thalami, no full parkinsonian syndrome has been reported when combined lesions, especially substantia nigra and thalamus, are present.

Perivascular lymphocytic infiltration with diffuse neuronal loss, neurofibrillary tangles, and astrocytic reaction is observed in the brainstem and, less commonly, the spinal cord and the cerebral cortex. The presence of these tau-positive neural and glial fibrillary tangles are indistinguishable from those found in such tauopathies as progressive supranuclear palsy and parkinsonism-dementia complex of Guam, suggesting a possible common pathogenesis.

HIV/AIDS-Related Infectious Disorders

CMV infection may occur when $CD4^+$ lymphocyte count drops below $100/mm^3$:

- **Meningoencephalitis and ventriculitis** are indistinguishable from the **AIDS-dementia complex** except that they develop rapidly over 2 weeks with or without cranial neuropathies. **Retinitis** occurs in up to 40% of patients.
- **Polymyeloradiculitis** is recognized by myelopathic deficits with sensory loss especially common in the S4 and S5 dermatomes.

Treatment is based on **Ganciclovir** (deoxyguanosine analogue like acyclovir but 50 times more active against CMV *in vitro; Neutropenia* and *thrombocytopenia* are possible complications) and **Foscarnet** (a pyrophosphate analogue).

HIV AND DIFFUSE MENINGEAL ENHANCEMENT OR HYDROCEPHALUS (BESIDES CMV)

Cryptococcal meningitis	Neurosyphilis (aseptic meningitis)
Most common fungal meningitis in AIDS (Histoplasmosis in the midwestern United States)*	Most common forms in HIV are ocular, meningeal, and meningovascular[†]
Lymphocytic pleocytosis; reactive CSF cryptococcal antigen (95% sensitive and specific) is diagnostic	*Monocytic* pleocytosis; reactive CSF VDRL establishes the diagnosis (65% sensitive and 100% specific)
India ink is positive in 60%–80% of patients	*T. pallidum* DNA PCR is experimental
Amphotericin B (+ Fluconazole, as maintenance against cryptococcus)	Penicillin G 2–4 million units IV every 4 hours for 10–14 days

*Multiple **unenhanced** pseudocysts in the basal ganglia and prominent Virchow-Robin spaces can be seen in cryptococcal meningitis. Histoplasma polysaccharide antigen diagnoses *Histoplasma capsulatum* (whereby **abscesses** are common).

[†]Early neurosyphilis may manifest in eit her of three forms: *ocular* syphilis, which may lead to iritis, uveitis, or optic neuritis; *meningovascular* syphilis, which may lead to strokes and myelitis; and the *meningeal* form, which may lead to hydrocephalus, seizures, and cranial neuropathies. Late neurosyphilis occurs more than 10 years later as dementia, Argyll-Robertson pupils, and tabes dorsalis.

HIV AND MULTIFOCAL MASS LESIONS (ALSO SEE FUNGAL INFECTIONS, NEUROPATHOLOGY)

Toxoplasmosis	Primary CNS lymphoma	PML
Most common cause of **multiple** enhancing lesions with surrounding edema	Frontal or periventricular **single enhancing** lesion with prominent edema	**Single unenhanced** lesion (**no mass effect**) becomes multifocal/confluent
Reactivation of latent infection occurs in 95% of cases	Reactivation of EBV infection is main cause	Reactivation of latent infection with JC virus
CD4 count <100 cells/mm^3		CD4 count <200 cells/mm^3
Anti-Toxoplasma IgG is present in up to 100% of cases*	**EBV DNA PCR** in CSF is present in up to 100% of cases	**JC virus DNA PCR** in CSF is present in 99% of cases
Pyrimethamine + sulfadiazine or clindamycin (sulfa allergy)	**Sensitive to radiation therapy; corticosteroids** shrink the lesion size	Highly aggressive antiretroviral therapy (**HAART**)

*__Toxoplasma gondii__ PCR in CSF/serum is specific but not sufficiently sensitive (62%); anti-Toxoplasma IgG has a higher diagnostic value. Toxoplasmosis reactivates more likely in those *not* taking TMP-SMZ (Bactrim), used for primary prophylaxis against PCP, toxoplasmosis, nocardiosis (*Nocardia asteroides* [gram-positive weakly acid-fast bacillus]), and listeriosis (*Listeria monocytogenes* [gram-positive intracellular rod]). Nocardia and, more rarely, Listeria, are uncommon causes of **multiple multilocular abscesses** and **cerebritis with perivascular microabscesses** in patients with HIV, respectively. The latter is also known for its tropism for the brainstem, leading to the underrecognized syndrome of *Listeria rhombencephalitis*.

Opportunistic infections in AIDS based on imaging and CSF findings

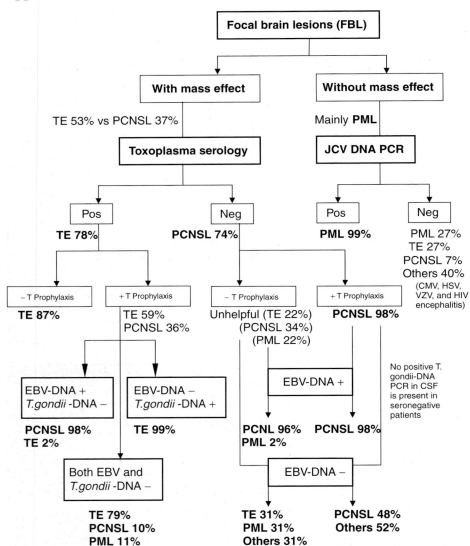

TE: toxoplasmic encephalitis; PCNSL: primary CNS lymphoma; PML: progressive multifocal leukoencephalopathy. In patients with mass effect and high risk for herniation, LP is contraindicated and empiric anti-Toxoplasma trial administered. Otherwise, diagnostic PCR in CSF discriminates TE from PCNSL. (Adapted from data published by Antinori et al. Neurology 1997;48:687–94.) Multiple lesions on imaging and presence of contrast enhancement did not fully discriminate between TE and PCNSL. Only TE was more likely to affect the basal ganglia. Toxoplasma seronegative patients with FBL should have a diagnostic LP only in the absence of a prophylactic regimen to assess for EBV-DNA. If this not detected, anti-Toxoplasma treatment trial and/or brain biopsy is recommended. (Adapted from data published by Antinori et al. Neurology 1997;48:687–694.)

Neuroimaging of Abscesses

MRI shows a central core of restricted diffusion (hyperintensity) on diffusion-weighted sequences and a thin rim of low signal on T2W sequences.

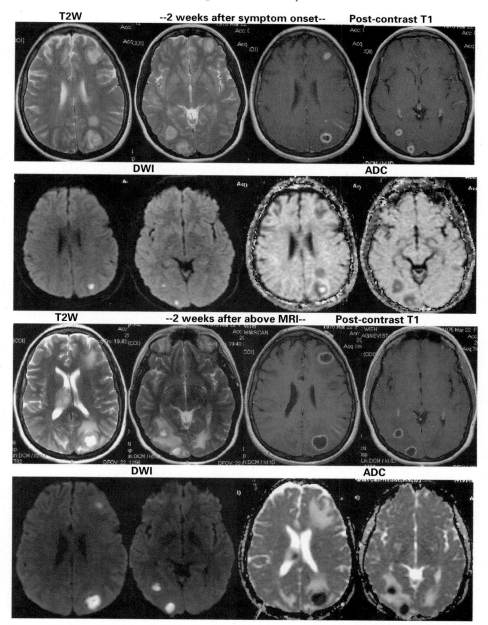

Images kindly provided by Dr. Rob Neel, University of Cincinnati, taken from a patient with abscesses due to Fusobacterium and Streptococcus milleri as a complication of traumatic periodontal procedure.

Neurosyphilis

Neurosyphilis may present as a low-grade chronic meningitis. Patients may experience chronic headaches, mild meningismus, and occasional cranial nerve palsies. **Acute syphilic meningitis** may lead to hydrocephalus, seizures, and cranial neuropathies. Ocular changes include iritis, uveitis, or optic neuritis.

Meningovascular syphilis leads to strokes and myelitis. Two types of vascular involvement have been described: Heubner endarteritis and Nissl-Alzheimer endarteritis. The most common Heubner endarteritis involves medium-sized vessels. Nissl-Alzheimer endarteritis affects the small intracranial vessels. The predilection of syphilitic inflammation for medium- and small-sized vessels may result in various classic brainstem eponymous syndromes, such as **Foville** (dorsal pontine tegmentum: face-sparing contralateral hemiplegia, ipsilateral peripheral CN VII palsy, and gaze palsy); **Millard-Gubler** (ventro caudal pons: contralateral hemiplegia and ipsilateral CN VI and VII palsy); **Benedikt** (midbrain stroke; ipsilateral CN III palsy with contralateral ataxia); **Weber** (midbrain stroke; ipsilateral CN III palsy with contralateral hemiplegia); and **Wallenberg** (lateral medullary syndrome; hypesthesia to pain and temperature below the neck in the contralateral body and ipsilateral face; ipsilateral Horner's).

INTERVAL BETWEEN PRIMARY INFECTION AND SYMPTOMATIC
NEUROSYPHILIS BY TYPE

0–0.5 Year	0.5–5 Years	1–20 Years	5–30 Years
Meningeal syphilis	Meningovascular syphilis	"General Paresis"	Tabes dorsalis (tertiary syphilis)

Late or tertiary neurosyphilis occurs with the cluster of dementia, Argyll-Robertson pupils (light-near dissociation), and tabes dorsalis. **Tabes dorsalis** due to **posterior cord involvement** presents as a sensory ataxia. There may be unusual patterns of decreased sensation in the so-called Hitzig zones (central face, around the nipples, medial forearms, lateral legs, and perianal area). Lightning pain may occur in the lower limbs and abdomen. **Aortitis** is characteristic and aortic regurgitation a common complication.

Syphilis and HIV may coexist in the same population. Genital ulcerations caused by syphilis may increase the risk of HIV infection. Coinfection does not alter the course of disease or make it more refractory to treatment.

CSF confirmation of infection is obtained through a reactive VDRL, *not* a serum fluorescent treponemal antibody absorption test (FTA-ABS) or microhemagglutination assay for ***Treponema pallidum*** (MHA-TP). However, as the VDRL test result is often normal in tertiary syphilis, infection can be ascertained by FTA-ABS or MHA-TP. Both tests remain reactive indefinitely, regardless of treatment. The reported false-negative rate for CSF VDRL test is 39%–60%. Seroconversion of VDRL in CSF may be delayed by up to 8 weeks in meningeal syphilis. Finally, a blood-tinged CSF sample results in a false-positive VDRL.

Lyme Disease (Neuroborreliosis)

Erythema migrans around a tick bite (first diagnosed in children from Lyme, Connecticut, in the late 1970s) usually appears within 7–10 days after the bite and must reach 5 cm for definitive diagnosis. It looks like a target lesion with central clearing or the erythema, reflecting outward spread of the **spirochete *Borrelia burgdorferi.*** Infected ticks of the genus Ixodes are the vectors of Lyme disease. *Ixodes scapularis* and *Ixodes dentatus,* abundant in the Eastern United States, become active during the warmer months from May to October. The risk of transmission to humans is directly proportional to the prevalence of infected ticks in a given region and the length of tick feeding. If the tick is removed within 24 hours, the risk of infection is negligible.

The classical neurological features of early infection are as follows:
- **Unilateral or bilateral facial palsy** or other cranial neuritis
- **Headache** as a sign of **lymphocytic meningitis**
- **Painful radiculoneuropathy** or, rarely, encephalomyelitis

The hallmark of early neuroborreliosis is meningitis or meningoradiculitis, a syndrome previously termed lymphocytic meningoradiculitis following tick bite (Bannwarth's syndrome). **A Guillain-Barré type picture** (ascending paralysis without albumino-cytologic dissociation) may also be part of the spectrum of Lyme disease ("tick paralysis"). Extraneurological symptoms include atrioventricular conduction defects, myocarditis, and joint swelling.

> Isolated unilateral or bilateral facial palsy in children from endemic regions must raise suspicion of neuroborreliosis. There is no evidence that facial palsy in adults without previous erythema migrans is caused by *B. burgdorferi.*

Chronic or late neuroborreliosis may express as persistent chronic meningitis, meningoradiculitis, and progressive radiculomyelitis or encephalomyelitis (which may lead to strokes and epilepsy). Pain is not a prominent feature. Asymmetrical axonal polyneuropathy and **acrodermatitis chronica atrophicans** may develop.

Laboratory evidence must include the following:
- Lymphocytic pleocytosis with normal glucose in the CSF; and
- DNA PCR of **B. burgdorferi** from tissue or body fluid; or
- Antibodies against the spirochete using enzyme-linked immunosorbent assay and, if positive, Western blotting for confirmation.

IgG antibodies appear 1 month after the onset of illness. IgM seropositivity is persistent, rendering serology useless in monitoring treatment. CSF antibodies without pleocytosis exclude active early or late neuroborreliosis and may reflect previous subclinical infection or a false-positive test.

Oral doxycycline may be as effective as intravenous penicillin G in early infection, but **intravenous ceftriaxone** (2 g/d) for 2–4 weeks is the first line of therapy.

Progressive Multifocal Leukoencephalopathy (PML)

PML is an **acquired leukoencephalopathy** of immunosuppressed adults, caused by a reactivation of a **polyomavirus,** the **JC virus** (after the index case), which remains latent in the lymphatic system and kidney of immunocompetent adults. JC virus infects oligodendrocytes and astrocytes in the CNS, inducing non-inflammatory demyelination and necrosis. Up to 86% of adults have antibodies against JC virus, detectable by PCR in the urine of 30% of the normal population. PML occurs in approximately 4% of adult patients with AIDS and is the heralding AIDS-defining illness in approximately 1% of all HIV-infected persons. Their CD4 count is usually <200 cell/mm^3. It presents with rapidly progressive focal neurologic deficits, especially visual loss. It has been recently described in patients with β-1a (Avonex) and natalizumab (Tysabri).

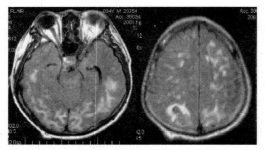

"Moth-eaten" appearance on axial FLAIR brain MRI

Confluent white matter lesions are bilateral but asymmetric. The posterior centrum semio-vale is the most common site. **T2W** brain MRI shows **hyperintense lesions** with involvement of the **U-fibers. Cavitation** may be observed. Enhancement occurs in only 10% of the cases, and suggests better prognosis. **Mass effect is absent.**

Acquired leukoencephalopathies associated with immunosuppression, besides PML, are, primary CNS lymphoma, herpes infection, and AIDS-dementia complex (diffuse and periventricular demyelination). Meningeal disease predominantes in CMV, cryptococcal meningitis, and neurosyphilis.

Clinical diagnosis is achieved by documenting a positive **JC virus DNA PCR in CSF** and typical radiologic features. Definitive diagnosis requires demonstration of the JC virus on brain biopsy, suggested by the presence of ballooned or **giant oligodendrocytes with intranuclear eosinophilic inclusions.** Other CSF findings may be mild pleocytosis (<20 cells/mm^3) and slightly elevated protein levels. Hypoglycorrhachia is observed in fewer than 15% of the cases.

Better prognosis (longer survival) occurs in those whose PML is the initial manifestation of AIDS, who have higher CD4 counts (>300 cells/mm^3), and who show contrast enhancement on imaging. Treatment is based on cytosine arabinoside **(Ara-C),** which inhibits JC virus replication but does not prolong survival. Highly aggressive antiretroviral therapy improves both neurologic conditions and survival in individuals with AIDS-associated PML. **Cidofovir** is an antiretroviral with considerable activity against all polyomavirus, including JC, which is being studied on a large scale given its anecdotal benefits.

Parasitic Diseases of the Nervous System

Neurocysticercosis (Tapeworm *Taenia solium*)

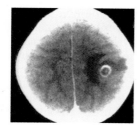

This fecal-oral and contaminated water-transmitted helminthic infection can, as **cysticerci**, reach the brain parenchyma (especially cortex and basal ganglia), subarachnoid space (basal cisterns), ventricular system (choroid plexus, fourth ventricle), and spinal cord. Symptoms occur when the **immune tolerance** to the parasite is replaced by an inflammatory response. **Seizures** occur in more than 70% of cases, but any focal neurologic signs may occur, as a direct mass effect or from **hydrocephalus**. The **hole-with-dot** (cyst with scolex in center) is the only pathognomonic finding on imaging.

Extra-CNS symptoms include sudden blindness due to subretinal cysticerci and muscular pseudohypertrophy caused by massive infestation of skeletal muscles.

Management depends on the location of the parasites and the disease activity:
- Calcified lesion: symptomatic treatment
- Parenchymal or subarachnoid cysts:
  - **Albendazole** (15 mg/kg/d for 1–2 weeks) if two or more brain lesions
  - **Praziquantel** (100 mg/kg in three doses in 1 day) if single lesion
- Ventricular lesion: endoscopic removal or albendazole
- **Cysticercotic encephalitis: avoid cysticidal drugs** (exacerbate edema); dexamethasone (16 mg/d) and mannitol (100 mL every 6 hours) are recommended for the treatment of intracranial hypertension.

Cerebral Malaria (Protozoa *Plasmodium falciparum*)

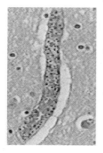

Acquired by inoculation of sporozoites during a **female *Anopheles* mosquito** blood meal, malaria (3 million fatalities per year) causes diffuse brain swelling and small ring hemorrhages from endothelial damage and **vascular plugging** by clumped, parasitized erythrocytes. Rapid progression to stupor and coma occur along with other systemic complications such as disseminated intravascular coagulation, pulmonary edema, and acute renal failure.

Given the prevalence of chloroquine-resistant strains of *P. falciparum,* **quinine** and **artemether** are the drugs of choice for treating cerebral malaria. Anticonvulsants, sedatives, osmotic diuretics, and blood transfusions may also be needed.

Thick blood smears with Giemsa stain demonstrates the gametocyte or ring forms. Repeated examinations may be needed given the cyclic parasitemia. Dipstick **antigen-capture assay** using a monoclonal antibody against *P. falciparum* (ParaSight-F test) may be of use in those with low levels of parasitemia.

Chagas Disease (Protozoa *Trypanosoma cruzi*)

Most common in South America, Chagas is transmitted by the feces of the "kissing bugs" arthropods *Triatoma infestans* and *Rhodnius prolixus* as they sting or by blood transfusion. Acutely, there are subcutaneous swelling developing at the port of entry (**Romaña's sign** if in the orbital region) as well as **chagasic encephalitis** (multiple areas of hemorrhagic necrosis and granulomas) and myocarditis. The chronic manifestations in survivors are **megaesophagus, megacolon, and dilated cardiomyopathy,** which may lead to **cardioembolic stroke** from arrhythmias or ventricular aneurysms.

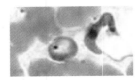

Thick blood of CSF smears with Giemsa stain demonstrates *T. cruzi* trypomastigotes in acute but not chronic disease. Blood *T. cruzi* PCR can be used for congenital or reactivation cases. **Benznidazole** (Rochagan) is the treatment of choice for patients with active disease. **Anticoagulation** for secondary stroke prophylaxis is recommended for patients with stroke and cardiomyopathy.

Schistosomiasis or Bilharzia (Trematodes *Schistosoma* sp)

These parasites, released from infected freshwater snails, penetrate the skin as larva (cercariae) and migrate to the mesenteric veins first and to the spinal cord or cerebral vasculature later. The lower spinal cord is especially affected.

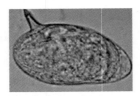

S. japonicum causes, in the acute stage, **diffuse *meningoencephalitis*** (Katayama fever) with visual loss, whereas chronic disease leads to seizures and focal deficits from **intracranial hypertension** or, less often, **intracranial hemorrhages** from the development of parenchymal brain granulomas and blood vessels injury, respectively.

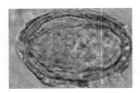

S. mansoni and *S. haematobium* most commonly lead to ***transverse myelitis*** **with radicular lumbar pain** from inflammatory necrosis of the spinal cord. The parasite may also occlude the anterior spinal artery.

Stool or urine search for schistosomal eggs is specific but poorly sensitive. Most patients with spinal cord involvement have specific antibodies detected by ELISA. **Praziquantel** is effective for patients with brain and spinal cord involvement. Oxamniquine is used for praziquantel-resistant cases.

Strongyloidiasis (Nematode *Strongyloides stercoralis*)

After *S. stercoralis* enters through the skin as filariform larvae and migrates to the lungs and intestine (where eggs are transformed into infective larvae in the process of **autoinfection,** unique to this helminthic infection), disseminated disease occur during immunosuppression (**hyperinfection syndrome** from poor control of chronic autoinfection) leading to **arachnoiditis,** granulomas or **brain abscesses** (ring-enhancing lesions), and **cortical infarcts.** CSF may show *S. stercoralis* larvae as well as neutrophilic pleocytosis with normal glucose. **Thiabendazole** is the drug of choice for treating disseminated disease.

Neurosarcoidosis

CNS involvement, especially of the **hypothalamic-pituitary** system, is among the least frequent manifestations of sarcoidosis (<10% of patients of which two-thirds may spontaneously remit). Most patients with sarcoidosis only have **abnormal chest radiograph** or, less often, ocular symptoms, skin changes (erythema nodosum), or lymph node enlargement. **African Americans** are up to 20 times more frequently affected than Caucasians. Chinese Asians are the least affected. Sweden has the highest documented rate of sarcoidosis (64/100,000). The peak incidence occurs around 30 years. The rare childhood (<15 years) sarcoid shows the triad of **cutaneous nodules, arthritis,** and **uveitis**.

Adult neurosarcoidosis is characterized by the following:
- **Facial palsy,** frequently bilateral, may result from compression by the enlarged parotid gland. The addition of uveitis to cranial neuropathy and parotiditis has been referred to as **Heerfordt's syndrome** (1909).
- **Diabetes insipidus** (polydipsia and polyuria) occurs in patients with hypothalamic-pituitary sarcoidosis. Somnolence, changes in temperature and appetite regulation, impotence, and amenorrhea are other symptoms. **Hypopituitarism** may result in gonadotropin, thyroid-stimulating hormone, and ACTH deficiencies as well as pituitary dwarfism, infantilism **(Frohlich's syndrome),** and fatal hypoglycemia.
- **Meningeal invasion** leads to alteration in mental status, photophobia, and nuchal rigidity. Space-occupying lesions are less common.
- **Other cranial neuropathies,** likely from meningeal invasion of nerve roots, manifest as vertigo, sensorineural deafness, facial numbness, dysphagia, dysphonia, and impaired taste and smell.
  - **Papilledema and optic atrophy** may complicate the invasion of the meningeal covering of the optic nerves
  - **Peripheral neuropathies** ranging from symmetric peripheral neuropathy to mononeuritis multiplex can be seen

Muscle biopsy shows sarcoid tubercles in over half of patients with sarcoidosis despite the absence of myopathic deficits. Pathology shows large, **non-caseating, epithelioid cell granulomatous tubercles** with sparse lymphocytes and variable number of giant cells.

MRI FLAIR sequences increase the yield of abnormal findings. Enhancement can be seen. **Presence of pituitary calcification is evidence against the diagnosis.** High serum **ACE, calcium,** immunoglobulins, and alkaline phosphatase are common. CSF shows mononuclear pleocytosis and increased protein (with hypoglycorrhachia seen in meningeal form) along with increased ACE, lysozyme, and beta2-microglobulin levels. Oligoclonal bands have also been reported. **Responsiveness to steroids** is typical.

Whipple Disease

Whipple disease (WD) was first reported as **"intestinal lipodystrophy"** in a patient with arthritis, diarrhea, abdominal pain, and weight loss (George Hoyt Whipple, 1907). This syndrome of malabsorption was later known to occur from infection with the gram-positive **actinomycete *Tropheryma whippelii*.**

WD occurs in about 1 in 100,000 people, of whom only 5%–10% develop CNS involvement. There is a clear **male** preponderance. *T. whippelii* is believed to be a commensal ubiquitous organism (present in saliva in 35% of normal subjects).

The extraintestinal WD may present exclusively with neurologic deficits:

- **Oculomasticatory myorhythmia** are the pathognomonic rhythmic movements of palatal, tongue, and mandibular muscles, synchronized with **convergent-divergent nystagmus** oscillating at about 1 Hz.
- **Skeletal myorhythmia or rhythmic myoclonus** (often in the absence of an oculomasticatory component), ophthalmoplegia, and dementia form a classic triad, although they occur in combination in only 10% of cases.
- **Supranuclear ophthalmoplegia** may occur without oculomasticatory myorhythmia but when the latter is present, supranuclear vertical gaze palsy is always present. The earliest deficit is slowness and hypometric upward saccades without restriction in the range of ocular movements.
- **Parkinsonism with abnormal vertical gaze,** which can be mistaken as progressive supranuclear palsy.
- **Hypothalamic involvement** (insomnia, hyperphagia, and polydipsia) is among the rare manifestations of WD along with ocular disorders (uveitis, retinitis, and optic neuritis) and a sarcoidosis-like syndrome with lymphadenopathy involving the mediastinal nodes

A duodenal or jejunal biopsy demonstrates periodic acid-Schiff positive, diastase-resistant **foamy macrophages** in the lamina propria on light microscopy and the characteristic **intracellular rod-shaped bacilli** on electron microscopy.

PCR of the bacterial 16 S ribosomal RNA of *T. whippelii* can be identified in most affected tissues (pleural, synovial, vitreous, and neural), nondiagnostic intestinal biopsy specimens, CSF, and peripheral blood. The current guidelines for diagnosis allow for *definite* CNS WD if *either* oculomasticatory myorhythmia *or* positive duodenal/jejunal biopsy *or* positive PCR is documented. In up to 50% of cases, brain MRI may show **high signal within the middle cerebellar peduncles** or, less commonly, temporal lobe, hypothalamus, mammillary bodies, cerebral peduncles, and, rarely, spinal cord.

Trimethoprim-sulfamethoxazole for 6–12 months is the treatment of choice for initial therapy and relapses of neurologic WD.

Subacute Sclerosing Panencephalitis

Subacute sclerosing panencephalitis (SSPE) is a delayed inflammatory and neurode-generative encephalitis of children and young adults related to the **measles** (rubeola) virus. The median latency period from the acute infection to the onset of SSPE is about 8 years. The incidence of SSPE among nonimmunized children is 200 times higher than among those previously immunized.

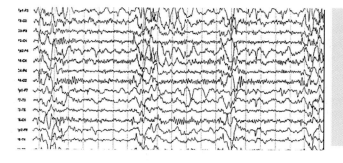

Typical EEG of SSPE: Periodic synchronous and symmetrical high-amplitude delta waves associated with the myoclonus every 5–10 seconds, suggesting a **burst-suppression** type of pattern.

Measles spreads to the brain causing either of three different outcomes:
(1) **Acute** measles encephalitis (AME), occurring during convalescence
(2) **Subacute** measles encephalitis (SME), mostly in immunosuppressed patients with **epilepsia partialis continua** and focal neurologic deficits
(3) **Subacute** sclerosing panencephalitis (SSPE)

Length of latency is the distinguishing factor: days to weeks in (1), months in (2), and years in (3). The differences in latency of the otherwise similar SME and SSPE may be immune mediated: immunosuppression is related to shorter disease latency and greater severity.

Four stages are proposed: (1) **behavioral and personality changes;** (2) cognitive decline, **myoclonus,** choreoathetosis, seizures, and **monocular blindness** from papilledema, chorioretinitis, homonymous hemianopsia, and/or cortical blindness; (3) **autonomic instability, rigidity,** and decreasing level of consciousness; (4) quadripa-resis, **akinetic mutism,** startle response, and coma.

The viral spread causes **demyelination** and neuronal loss, perivascular inflammatory infiltration, glial proliferation, and **neuronal and glial intranuclear (Cowdry A) and intracytoplasmic inclusions.** The occipital lobes, thalamus, and putamen are the structures with the greatest burden of pathology.

EEG (burst suppression) and CSF (antimeasles IgG antibodies and **oligoclonal bands)** are the critical tests. Brain MRI is often normal in early stages. The risk of developing SSPE is higher if acute measles occurs in the first 2 years of life. In 10% of patients, the disease lasts 10 years, whereas 10% die within 3 months (with most dying within 10 years). Early childhood immunization against rubeola remains the only preventive measure.

Prion Diseases

Prions or transmissible spongiform encephalopathies refer to *pro*teins with *in*fectious capability that result from posttranslational changes from a normal α-helical structure (**PrP^C**, *cellular*) to a β-pleated insoluble and protease-resistant pathogenic isoform (**PrP^sc**, *scrapie*), which aggregates within neurons. Prion diseases can be inherited (mutations in the *PrP* gene [**PRNP,** 20p]), acquired (contaminated neurosurgical instruments, tissue grafts or human cadaveric pituitary hormones), or sporadic. Sporadic Creutzfeldt-Jakob disease (sCJD) makes up to ~85% cases of all prion diseases. Prion diseases occur worldwide with an incidence of $1/10^6$ population/year. A polymorphism at **codon 129 of PRNP** leading to methionine or valine homozygosity increases the risk of CJD. **Gray matter vacuolation** is the pathologic hallmark.

CJD is a **rapidly progressive dementia** with **myoclonus** (and pathologic startle), **cerebellar ataxia, pyramidal or extrapyramidal dysfunction,** and **cortical blindness.** Progression to akinetic mutism and death may occur in 2–3 months (70% of patients die in <6 months). Raised CSF 14-3-3 protein, neuronal-specific enolase, and S-100 are helpful but nonspecific findings. The EEG may show **pseudoperiodic sharp wave discharges** in ~70% of cases. Atypical forms of CJD may have a prolonged clinical course (>2 years) or an ataxic rather than cognitive presentation. The Heidenhain variant of CJD refers to cases of cortical blindness with predominant occipital lobe involvement.

	Sporadic CJD (sCJD)	Variant CJD (vCJD)*
Age at onset	**Older** (mean 60)	**Younger** (mean 26)
Course	**Rapid**, various deficits	**Slower**, stereotypical
14-3-3	Positive >90%	Positive <50%
EEG	Periodic discharges, 80%	Periodic complexes, absent
Codon 129 of PRNP	Met/Met: rapid dementia Val/Val: slower ataxia	Met/Met: all cases
Pathology	**Spongiosis** with few or no PrP-amyloid plaques	"**Daisy plaques**" (dense core PrP-plaques)
T2W MRI	**Basal ganglia** hyperintensity	**Pulvinar** bright signal

*Psychiatric presentation with painful sensory symptoms is common in vCJD, which is an acquired prion disease caused by exposure to BSE. Lymphatic infiltration allows for diagnosis with tonsil biopsy.

Gerstmann-Sträussler-Scheinker disease is a slower (2–10 years) familial disorder presenting with ataxia and dysarthria followed by pyramidal and extrapyramidal deficits and late dementia, without EEG changes, in relatively young individuals (<50 years). Pathologically, NFT and PrP-amyloid plaques with minimal spongiform changes may be confused with Alzheimer's disease.

Fatal familial insomnia is a rapidly progressive disorder (death in 1–2 years) associated with insomnia, ataxia, dysautonomia, and pyramidal and extrapyramidal deficits with late dementia. Neuropathology shows **thalamic gliosis** with minimal or no spongiform change.

Differential Diagnosis in Prion Diseases

Given the wide variation in presentation and symptoms, prion diseases should be considered in any adult patient with dementia, movement disorder, or late-onset psychiatric symptoms, especially when the rate of progression is fast.

Among the specific diseases that should be considered in the differential are
- **Alzheimer's disease,**
- **Dementia with Lewy bodies,**
- Frontotemporal dementias,
- **Adult ceroid lipofuscinosis** (Kufs disease),
- Huntington disease and **HD phenocopies,**
- **AIDS-dementia complex,** and
- Primary progressive MS.

The rapid progression suggests the following categories of disease:
- **CNS vasculitis** (excluded by normal brain MRI and cerebral arteriogram)
- **Wernicke-Korsakoff syndrome**
- **Infectious encephalopathies:** cryptococcal meningitis, CMV, progressive multifocal leukoencephalopathy, herpes simplex encephalitis, and
  - WD caused by the gram-positive actinomycete Tropheryma whippelii has a neurologic presentation in 5% of cases. **Oculomasticatory myorhythmia** is pathognomonic of WD. Dementia, **supranuclear gaze palsy,** and rhythmic myoclonus are the classic but infrequent triad. Parkinsonism and hypothalamic dysfunction may occur. Systemic symptoms such as weight loss, lymphadenopathy, steatorrhea, arthralgias, and hyperpigmentation are important clues. Left untreated, WD is fatal within 1 year.
- **Toxic encephalopathies**
  - **Bismuth toxicity** may present as subacute **dementia** and/or psychosis along with myoclonus, ataxia, tremor, and seizures. It has been erroneously mistaken for Alzheimer's disease. Bismuth is widely used as an over-the-counter medication for dyspepsia.
  - **Mercury toxicity** causes a **progressive cerebellar syndrome** occasionally associated with choreoathetosis and parkinsonism.
  - **Lithium toxicity,** when severe, leads to tremor, choreoathetosis, ataxia, hyperreflexia, opisthotonos, seizures, and even coma. Periodic complexes are found on EEG.
- **Hashimoto encephalopathy** is a steroid-responsive encephalopathy associated with autoimmune chronic lymphocytic thyroiditis (aka, "nonvasculitic autoimmune meningoencephalitis") consisting of **relapsing** alterations in consciousness, involuntary movements (myoclonus or tremor), and epileptic or psychiatric symptoms. **Antithyroid antibodies** (thyroperoxidase [formerly, antimicrosomal] and antithyroglobulin) are present.
- **Paraneoplastic limbic encephalitis**

Pathology of Infectious Diseases

PATHOLOGY OF VIRAL INFECTIONS

Cowdry type A 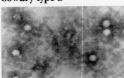	**Large, solitary, nuclear eosinophilic inclusion** surrounded by prominent halo dominates nuclear architecture.	**CMV**: predilection for ependymal cells. **Herpes simplex**: hemorrhagic necrosis of the temporal lobes. **Varicella zoster**. **Measles** (SSPE): demyelination.
Cowdry type B 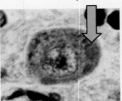	**Small, multiple,** no halos, no effacement of nuclear architecture.	**Poliomyelitis** (acute): anterior horn cells of spinal cord affected.
Negri bodies "Lyssa bodies" 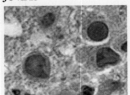	**Intracytoplasmic eosinophilic** inclusions in **Purkinje** cells and **pyramidal** cells of hippocampus.	**Rabies** results from transdermal viral inoculation by an animal bite. 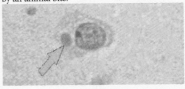
JC virus	**"Ballooned" oligodendrocytes** have enlarged dark pink "ground glass" inclusions containing viral antigen.	**Progressive multifocal leukoencephalopathy** causes typical demyelination, which is immunopositive for p53.

Differential diagnosis of **hemorrhagic basal frontal/temporal lobes**:
- Acute contusion
- **Herpes simplex** encephalitis
- **Rhinocerebral mucormicosis**
- **Naegleria** amoebic encephalitis

PATHOLOGY OF FUNGAL INFECTIONS

Aspergillus 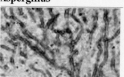	**HYPHAE**	**Angioinvasive** and commonly CNS focal infection in immunosuppressed patients with organ or bone marrow transplantation. **Branching of 45 degrees**, septate hyphae of uniform diameter.
Mucormycosis 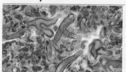		**Angioinvasive** and potentially lethal infection in **immunosuppressed** and patients with diabetes. **Branching of 90 degrees, nonseptate hyphae** of nonuniform diameter.
Cryptococcus 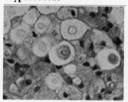	**YEAST**	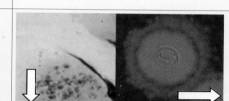 **Indian ink** finding **Small cysts** within underlying cortex and within deep nuclei are seen in chronic cryptococcal meningitis.
Coccidioidomycosis 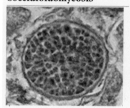		**Coccidioides immitis** is found in arid regions of the southwestern United States, Mexico, and South America. **Arthrospores** are inhaled from soil dust and cause lung infection, followed by secondary CNS spread in immunocompromised patients. **Necrosis and multinucleated giant cells** are seen along the **large spherules** with thick, refractive capsule (compared with the thin-walled toxoplasma cyst).
Histoplasmosis 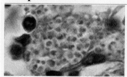		**Obligate intracellular** fungus, residing in **macrophages**, which have a clear zone around a central blue nucleus giving the cell membrane the appearance of a capsule.
Blastomycosis 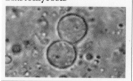		**Immunocompromised patients** are primary target but it is not an AIDS-defining condition. Most prevalent in Mississippi, Ohio, and St. Lawrence river basins, the Great Lakes area, and the southeastern United States. **Intracranial or spinal abscesses** or meningitis is the clinical presentation. Treatment with amphotericin B.
Candida 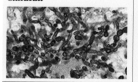	**BOTH**	**Immunocompromised** patients are primary target. Budding cells **(yeasts) and pseudohyphae** are both present.

PATHOLOGY OF PROTOZOAN INFECTIONS

Acanthamoeba	**Granulomatous amoebic encephalitis** forms **cysts**. *Naegleria fowleri* is an uncommon cause of severe **meningoencephalitis** (fulminant, rapidly fatal), which does not form cysts but creates **hemorrhagic lesions in the olfactory bulbs and basal frontal lobes**. Infection occurs via nasal mucosae from swimming in stagnant fresh water ponds.
Toxoplasmosis	**Immunocompromised** patients are primary target (AIDS-defining disease). Cysts will rupture and release free-living forms (**tachyzoites**). Lesion is often necrotic. Cysts are easier to spot than tachyzoites.
P. falciparum	**Cerebral malaria** ("salt and pepper"). 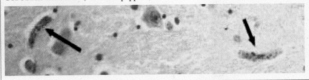

PATHOLOGY OF METAZOAN INFECTIONS

Taenia solium	**Ova of striated edge** are about 35 μm in diameter.	**Cysticercosis** from pork tapeworm (T. solium) develops by ingesting cystercerci from the **muscle of infected animals**. **Single or multiple cysts** are seen in parenchyma, ventricles, or basal subarachnoid space cisterns. Praziquantel is treatment of choice.

PATHOLOGY OF PRION DISEASES

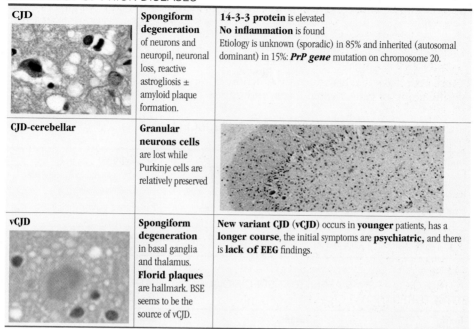

CJD	**Spongiform degeneration** of neurons and neuropil, neuronal loss, reactive astrogliosis ± amyloid plaque formation.	**14-3-3 protein** is elevated **No inflammation** is found Etiology is unknown (sporadic) in 85% and inherited (autosomal dominant) in 15%: **PrP gene** mutation on chromosome 20.
CJD-cerebellar	**Granular neurons cells** are lost while Purkinje cells are relatively preserved	
vCJD	**Spongiform degeneration** in basal ganglia and thalamus. **Florid plaques** are hallmark. BSE seems to be the source of vCJD.	**New variant CJD (vCJD)** occurs in **younger** patients, has a **longer course,** the initial symptoms are **psychiatric,** and there is **lack of EEG** findings.

4 Neurotoxicology

Most neurotoxic agents cause dysfunction or destruction of subcellular structures, specific group of cells, axonal tracts, and diffuse neuronal or myelin dysfunction.

NEUROTOXIC AGENTS AFFECTING SPECIFIC SUBCELLULAR STRUCTURES OF THE PNS

Toxin	Target	Key Deficits
Diphtheria	Schwann cell nucleus	Acute demyelinating polyneuropathy
Hexachlorophene	Myelin sheath	Peripheral neuropathy
Marine toxins (CTX, TTX, saxitoxin)	Voltage-gated sodium channels	Paresthesias, paralysis, respiratory failure
Organophosphates, carbamates	Acetylcholinesterase enzyme	Cholinergic paralysis See *Toxic gases*

NEUROTOXIC AGENTS AFFECTING SPECIFIC SUBCELLULAR STRUCTURES OF THE CNS

Toxin	Target	Key Deficits
Ketamine, PCP	NMDA receptors	Psychosis
Cyanide, CO, 3-NPA	Mitochondria	Coma, seizures
Tetanus toxin Strychnine	Glycine release Glycine receptors*	Spastic paralysis See *Toxic weakness*
Amphetamines, cocaine	(+) Dopamine and NE reuptake inhibitors	See *Psychostimulants*
Domoic Acid (amnestic shellfish toxin)	(+) Kainate receptors, esp. in hippocampus	Amnesia, seizures, hemiparesis, and coma

NMDA, *N*-methyl-D-aspartate.

* **Glycine** receptors are parts of Cl⁻ channels in spinal inhibitory interneurons; **strychnine** blocks glycine receptors (postsynaptic); **tetanus** toxin inhibits release of glycine (presynaptic): both of these toxins cause spastic paralysis from failure to inhibit spinal and brainstem interneurons.

NEUROTOXIC AGENTS USED AS MODELS OF HUMAN DISEASES

Toxin	Target	Human diseases
β-*N*-oxalyl-amino-L-alanine (BOAA)	(+) AMPA receptors, corticospinal tract, cortical neurons	HSP, PLS
Quinolinic acid	Caudate nucleus, cortical neurons	Huntington disease
n-Hexane, acrylamide	Spinocerebellar tract, axons	Spinocerebellar degeneration, distal axonopathies
Doxorubicin	Dorsal root ganglion	Sensory neuronopathy
Methyl-phenyl-tetrahydro-pyridine (MPTP), 6-OH-dopamine	Substantia nigra (also sympathetic ganglion for 6-OH-DA)	Parkinson disease
Elapid toxin immunology	Neuromuscular junction	Myasthenia gravis

Manganese Toxicity

Sources of manganese exposure include mining, **welding,** .ferromanganese smelting, industrial and agricultural work, chronic liver failure **(acquired hepatolenticular degeneration),** total parenteral nutrition, and ingestion of Chinese herbal pills. A relatively new form of manganese toxicity, "ephedronic encephalopathy," results from the addictive use of **methcathinone** (also known as ephedrone), which can be synthesized by combining pseudoephedrine (Sudafed), a common over-the-counter cold remedy, and potassium permanganate. Manganese typically enters the body by ingestion or inhalation. As manganese uses the same transporter for absorption in the gastrointestinal tract, iron deficiency increases its absorption. **Manganese is eliminated almost exclusively via biliary excretion.** Hence, hepatic excretion mechanisms are crucial in preventing excess blood manganese from crossing into the blood–brain barrier and selectively concentrating in the striatum.

Manganese intoxication may cause a levodopa-resistant parkinsonism with marked axial deficits in the form of early dysarthria, dysphagia, and postural impairment. This form of parkinsonism is also distinguished from Parkinson's disease (PD) by its symmetry, a tremor with postural but no resting component, poor to no response to levodopa, and a **"cock walk" gait** (walking on toes with arms flexed and erect posture) with freezing and tendency to lean backward. The most important finding is the presence of **pallidal T1W hyperintensity with normal T2W** signal on brain MRI. Normal fluorodopa PET scans suggest an intact nigrostriatal system. On pathology, unlike PD, there are no Lewy bodies or direct involvement of the substantia nigra pars compacta; instead, the internal segment of the globus pallidus is predominantly involved. Epidemiologic studies have failed to establish a cause–effect relationship between manganese exposure and PD or that such exposure accelerates the development of PD.

> **Abnormal T1– *and* T2-weighted signal in the globus pallidum** moves the differential diagnosis away from manganese toxicity (T1W-only hyperintensity) to Wilson's disease, neurodegeneration with brain iron accumulation 1, melanoma, neurofibromatosis type 1, calcification, hyperglycemia, blood products, and fat.

Management of manganese toxicity is dependent on the source of exposure. Welders are advised to have adequate ventilation and personal respiratory protection during welding. **N-acetylcysteine** may be used in cases of potassium permanganate poisoning. Manganese supplementation should be kept below 0.018 μmol/kg/d in total parenteral nutrition to prevent toxicity. Liver transplantation may be necessary in cases of liver cirrhosis-induced acquired hepatolenticular degeneration. **Iron deficiency increases the gastric absorption of manganese** and needs to be corrected. Chelation with ethylene-diamine-tetra-acetic acid (EDTA) may result in modest improvements. Permanent sequelae are likely.

Botulism

Botulism is a paralyzing disease caused by a powerful toxin, lethal at the small dose of 0.05 μg, produced by an anaerobic, spore-forming, soil-dwelling gram-positive bacteria *Clostridium botulinum*. The bacteria can generate **heat-resistant spores** and eight immunologically distinct **heat-labile** (A, B, C1, C2, D, E, F, and G) **exotoxins.** When ingested, **heat-resistant spores** are responsible for infant botulism. Recovery time from type A poisoning is longer than from type E. The toxin blocks the release of **acetylcholine** (ACh) by binding to the presynaptic terminal and entering into the cell by endocytosis. The two main protein enzymatic cleavages needed for prevention of exocytosis of ACh depends on the specific toxin: A, C, and E cleave the protein synaptosome-associated protein **(SNAP-25);** B, D, F, and G cleave the synaptobrevin vesicle-associated membrane protein **(VAMP-2).**

Classic Botulism

Botulinum toxin types A, B, and E are the most common cause of food-borne or classic botulism. The most common source is contaminated fish and seafood (type E). It leads to symmetric **cranial nerve dysfunction,** especially ptosis, diplopia, dysarthria, and dysphagia, within 12 to 48 hours from the ingestion of contaminated food, and is followed by **"descending paralysis,"** including respiratory weakness. There are no sensory abnormalities, no preceding fever, and no mental status changes, but prominent gastrointestinal (cramping, early nausea and diarrhea) and autonomic **(dry mouth,** urinary retention, constipation, hypotension, and bradycardia) symptoms. **Fixed dilated pupils and normal reflexes** in a pattern of descending weakness are most suggestive. Besides seafood, other important historical clues are "skin popping," heroin use, and unsterile wound. Repetitive stimulation studies show decrement of the CMAP amplitude in at least two muscles with postexercise or tetanic facilitation (>20%) for at least 2 minutes, with no postactivation exhaustion. The only other condition with similar electrophysiology is **hypermagnesemia.** When high-frequency repetitive stimulation (50 Hz) causes facilitation >100%, the differential diagnosis should include Lambert-Eaton myasthenic syndrome (LEMS). Other neuromuscular disorders must be in the differential diagnosis such as myasthenia gravis, Miller-Fisher variant of Guillain-Barré syndrome (areflexia, descending weakness, GQ1b autoantibodies), tick paralysis, and diphtheric neuropathy (tonsillar exudate). Antitoxin, catharsis, forced vital capacity monitoring, and symptomatic support are recommended.

Infant Botulism

Spores (rather than preformed toxin) are ingested and germinate in the intestinal tract of an infant, which lacks protective bile acids and bacterial flora. The toxins generated cause early constipation, weak cry, difficulty feeding, and bulbar and limb weakness. Over 1–3 days, there is **loss of head control,** hypotonia, tachycardia, hypotension, and **dry mouth.** Most infants recover within weeks or months with supportive care. Botulism immune globulin (BIG) appears to shorten the duration of respirator dependence, but its use is not yet widely accepted.

Nonbotulism Causes of Toxic Weakness

Diphtheria is rare due to widespread immunization.

Tetanus Poisoning

The anaerobic spore-forming rod *Clostridium tetani* forms **tetanospasmin,** one of the most potent toxins, which is retrogradely transported from the neuromuscular junction, adjacent to seemingly insignificant wounds, to the upper motor neurons and by transcytosis to the inhibitory Renshaw cells. The thermolabile tetanospasmin then cleaves the vesicle-associated membrane protein (VAMP), blocking the **presynaptic release of glycine and γ-aminobutyric acid (GABA)** from spinal and brainstem inhibitory interneurons. Early manifestations include rigidity of the masseter muscles **(trismus or lockjaw),** neck or face **(risus sardonicus),** and painful abdominal wall rigidity and **opisthotonus** with relative sparing of distal muscles and preservation of consciousness. Painful reflex spasms and autonomic dysfunction (sweating, hyper-salivation, tachycardia, labile hypertension) are common. The severity of symptom reaches a peak in 2 weeks and begins to recede at 4 weeks. Tetanus toxoid as a prophylaxis is part of the five doses of tetanus-diphtheria toxoid (DPT) given during childhood immunization up to the age of 6 years. DPT boosters are recommended every 10 years.

Strychnine Poisoning

Available from rodenticides and pesticides, strychnine poisoning can mimic tetanus except by its faster onset (within 1 hour from ingestion), less abdominal rigidity, and lack of trismus. Strychnine competitively **blocks the *postsynaptic* glycine receptors** by modulating Cl⁻ permeability in the spinal cord and motor neurons.

Curare

Curare is a plant-derived toxin of the *Strychnos* species, like strychnine, used traditionally as arrow poisons in the South American rainforest. Curare introduced directly into the bloodstream competes with acetylcholine for the receptor and thus **blocks neuromuscular transmission** and causes progressive paralysis of striated muscle and eventual respiratory failure.

Lathyrism

It refers to the development of a purely motor hypertonic paresis, affecting the legs more than the arms, resulting from the consumption of a variety of toxic chickpea named *Lathyrus*. The chickpea poison responsible for the paraparesis is the excitatory glutamate analogue β-*N*-oxalyl-amino-L-alanine (L-BOAA), a powerful agonist of the AMPA glutamate receptors. The clinical picture is similar to HTLV-related tropical spastic paraparesis.

Lytico-Bodig

Lytico-Bodig applies to the combination of motor neuron disease and parkinsonism present in the Chamorro people in Guam, one of the Mariana Island in the Pacific Ocean, presumed to be caused by the excitotoxin β-methyl-amino-L-alanine (BMAA). The mode of poisoning occurs via the ingestion, for food and medicine, of the cycad seed plant, which contains BMAA and cycasin, as well as the fruit bat, which feeds on cycad seed.

Envenomations

Spider envenomation occurs after the bite of the female **black widow spider,** *Latrodectus mactans*, which injects the potent **latrotoxins.** Latrotoxins activate **presynaptic calcium channels** allowing massive influx of calcium, rapid release of acetylcholine at the NMJ, and excessive muscle depolarization. Latrodectism manifests as **muscle spasm with restlessness, hypertension, diaphoresis, and salivation,** evolving into **seizures** and, rarely, death. Calcium gluconate with or without methocarbamol or dantrolene are used as first-line treatments for muscle spasms. *Latrodectus* antivenin is reserved for severe envenomation.

Tick paralysis results from the inoculation of toxin contained in the saliva of a fertile female tick at the time of a blood meal. The neurotoxin is produced by the Rocky Mountain wood tick (*Dermacentor andersoni*), American dog tick (*Dermacentor variabilis*), and Australian marsupial tick (*Ixodes holocyclus*). Like botulinum toxin, these neurotoxins **block presynaptic acetylcholine** release. Patients exhibit an **acute ascending paralysis** with few sensory symptoms, **reminiscent of the Guillain-Barré syndrome.** Disengagement or active removal of *Dermacentor* ticks ends neurological toxicity within 24 hours.

Scorpion stings occur after accidentally touching or stepping on these arthropods. The **Mexican Durango scorpion** (*Centruroides suffuses*) causes 200,000 envenomations and almost 1,000 deaths annually. Only one scorpion species in the United States is medically relevant, the **Arizona bark scorpion** (*Centruroides sculpturatus*). Regional paresthesias at the sting side give way to a **hyperparasympathetic syndrome** (salivation, lacrimation, urinary incontinence, defecation, gastroenteritis, and emesis **[SLUDGE syndrome]**). Scorpion stings cause **abnormal eye movements** (ptosis, nystagmus) **and neuromuscular hyperactivity** ("restless child with roving eyes"), particularly fasciculations. Ataxia, myoclonus, dystonia, rigidity, clonus, and opisthotonus have been reported.

Toxic mushroom poisoning occurs when toadstools (*Amanita phalloides*, **gyromitrin, muscarine,** and psilocybin) are confused with truffles (edible mushrooms). *Amanita* consumption causes toxicity directly from its heat-stable α-**amatoxin** or indirectly as brain edema from **liver failure.** Muscarine mushroom toxin causes the **SLUDGE syndrome** without any CNS symptoms, as it does not cross the blood–brain barrier. **Gyromitrin mushroom poisoning** may cause nystagmus, ataxia, tremor, and rarely seizures in the setting of liver failure.

Buckthorn (also called Tullidora, wild cherry, Capulin tullidor, or coyotillo) is an invasive poisonous plant from Mexico, southern United States, Central America, and the Caribbean whose ingestion causes a Guillain-Barré–like disorder with gastrointestinal symptoms.

Snake envenomation by Mohave rattlesnake (*Crotalus scutulatus*; southwest United States and central Mexico) may cause myokymia, cranial nerve palsies, weakness, rhabdomyolysis, myoglobinuria, renal failure, and respiratory paralysis.

Lead Poisoning

Plumbism results from exposure to **inorganic** lead. The common ways of absorption are transdermal, inhalation, or ingestion. Ingested lead is only 10% but is the most common mechanism of toxicity in children with compulsive lead-based paint chewing **(pica).** Inhaled lead gets into the bloodstream at a 40% rate and represents the usual mechanism for occupational exposure in adults, especially those involved in painting, printing, pottery, glazing, lead smelting, and battery manufacturing. **Inhalation of gasoline fumes** in workers of gasoline storage tanks causes **organic** lead intoxication with tetraethyl and tetramethyl lead. **Calcium and iron deficiency increase absorption and the risk of lead poisoning.** Long-term storage occurs in the skeletal system and recirculation of bone-bound lead may be increased during enhanced bone resorption (e.g., pregnancy, lactation, menopause, osteoporosis, etc.).

Children have predominantly CNS symptoms. Brief but intense exposures (lead levels, 50–70 μg/dL) are reminiscent of acute intermittent porphyria, with an **encephalopathy and acute abdomen.** Anorexia is followed by vomiting and irritability, **tremor,** fatigue, hallucinations, and headache with depressed sensorium. **Wrist drop** from radial and other focal palsies may occur. The degree of neuropathy does not correlate with lead level or length of exposure.

SYMPTOMS AND SIGNS OF CHRONIC LOW-LEVEL LEAD EXPOSURE

Children: irritability, hyperkinetic behavior, distractibility, impulsiveness, and anemia	**Adults**: chronic renal failure, hypertension, arthralgias, teratogenesis, and impotence

Adults show predominantly PNS symptoms. Encephalopathy is rare but **colic, anemia,** and **peripheral neuropathy** are common. A **gingival lead line** may develop. In these cases, insomnia, irritability, delusions, and hallucinations, associated with a maniacal state define the clinical picture. No hematological abnormalities are found, and chelating agents are of no value.

Basophilic stippling of red cells with **microcytic hypochromic anemia,** leukopenia, hemolysis, and renal insufficiency are serologic markers. **Lead lines** at the bone metaphyses suggest the diagnosis. High excretion of **urinary coproporphyrin** (UCP) and of **δ-aminolevulinic acid** (ALA) confirms it.

Chelation therapy is recommended when blood lead levels are >45 μg/dL: 2,3-dimercaptosuccinic acid (DMSA) or parenteral calcium disodium ethylene-diamine-tetraacetic acid (CaNa$_2$EDTA). When levels are >70 μg/dL, British anti-Lewisite (BAL) should be administered before CaNa$_2$EDTA to prevent the latter from increasing the distribution of lead into the brain. **Mannitol** can be used in cases of cerebral edema. Intravenous diazepam is preferred for control of seizures. Renal function should be monitored because a **nephrotoxic reaction** may develop.

Mercury Intoxication

The three major current sources of exposure are fish consumption, dental amalgams, and vaccines, each causing a distinctive syndrome of intoxication.

Route	Inhalation	Oral	Parenteral
Main source	Dental amalgams	Fish	Vaccines*
In these forms	Mercury vapor	Methyl mercury	Ethyl mercury
Manifesting as	Peripheral neuropathy, erethism, and tremor	Ataxia, visual constriction, and acral paresthesia	Ataxia, visual and hearing loss, and paresthesia
Other features	Stomatitis, gingivitis, proteinuria		Tubular necrosis, acrodynia[†]
Treatment	DMSA: Meso-2,3-dimercaptosuccinic acid[‡]	Chelators not effective	Chelators not effective

* **Ethyl mercury** is the active ingredient of the preservative *thimerosal*, used in vaccines.

[†] **Acrodynia** was a childhood hypersensitive reaction to inorganic mercury consisting of painful redness of hands and toes; photophobia, irritability, anorexia, and hypertension.

[‡] **DMSA** (2,3-dimercaptosuccinic acid) **is preferred over penicillamine** (antagonist of mercuric chloride) as the treatment of choice because it induces greater mercury excretion. Further, DMSA can almost completely inhibit the uptake of methyl mercury by RBCs and hepatocytes. Since organic mercury is mainly located in erythrocytes, **whole blood rather than urine is required to test for methyl mercury** exposure. Urinary mercury correlates with elemental or inorganic mercury, not methyl mercury.

Methyl mercury enters the aquatic food chain and reaches the highest concentration in long-living predatory fish, such as swordfish and shark in the oceans and pike and bass in freshwater. Chronic exposure to methyl mercury causes a **progressive cerebellar syndrome** and widespread tremor of the extremities, tongue, and lips, occasionally associated with choreoathetosis and parkinsonism. Neuropathological examination shows regional loss of neurons in the cerebellar granule cells (with sparing of Purkinje cells) and visual cortex. MRI shows cerebellar vermis atrophy and increased T2W signal in the visual cortex.

Minamata disease was the term coined for the **epidemic chronic mercurialism** experienced by villagers living in **Minamata Bay**, Kyushu Island, Japan, between 1953 and 1956, who were exposed to fish contaminated with industrial waste containing methyl mercury. Nearly 150 tons were discharged into Minamata bay during four decades. The main deficits were **concentric constriction of the visual fields, hearing loss, cerebellar ataxia, postural and action tremors, and stocking-glove hypesthesia.**

Mercury vapor inhalation is suggested by the triad of intention **tremor, gingivitis, and erethism,** which alludes to the behaviors of excessive shyness and aggression (said to have affected the Mad Hatter in *Alice in Wonderland*, probably a victim of occupational mercury intoxication).

Ethyl mercury is more potent, has a shorter half-life than methyl mercury (7–10 days versus 50 days), and is metabolized more rapidly to inorganic mercury, which causes kidney damage before any neurologic deficits can develop. As there is no accumulation of mercury, thimerosal in vaccines is deemed safe.

Other Heavy Metals

Arsenic poisoning may occur with exposures to herbicides, insecticides, or rodenticides containing copper arsenate. Arsenic in seafood is a nontoxic organic compound but may raise levels if consumed within days prior to testing. A gastrointestinal illness is followed by an **encephalopathy, hemolysis,** endothelial damage, and vasodilation, which may cause rapidly progressive **shock and rhabdomyolysis.** Patients may complain of a **metallic taste** and have a **garlic breath.** Following these acute symptoms, an ascending weakness **resembling Guillain-Barré** may evolve over days to weeks. **Chronic arsenicalism** may present with symptoms reminiscent of **Wernicke-Korsakoff encephalopathy.** Dermatologic changes with chronic exposure include **Mees lines** and **hyperkeratosis** of the palms and soles. Increased levels of arsenic are found in urine (months) and hair (years). Blood changes include pancytopenia, **basophilic stippling,** increased hepatic transaminases, and renal insufficiency. Urine excretion of >0.1 mg/L (or 100 μg/24 h) is abnormal. Although it may not prevent progression of acute arsenic neuropathy, **parenteral chelator** such as British anti-Lewisite (BAL) or dimercaptopropane-sulfonic acid (DMPS) is indicated for symptomatic patients.

Bismuth-induced encephalopathy presents with subacute changes in mental status and memory, psychosis, and depression, associated with myoclonus and ataxia, and occasionally spike-wave complexes on EEG and seizures. Patients can be **misdiagnosed as having Alzheimer's disease or Creutzfeldt-Jakob disease.** Bismuth subsalicylate (Pepto-Bismol), used in the treatment of gastric ulcers, diarrhea, and *Helicobacter pylori* infection, is a common culprit. A blood–bismuth concentration during chronic therapy of 50–100 μg/mL is of concern. Head CT shows hyperdensities in the basal ganglia and cerebral cortex.

Aluminum-induced dialysis dementia also causes a similar myoclonic encephalopathy (myoclonus associated with dysarthria, dysphasia, apraxia, personality changes, and, occasionally, seizures) when aluminum hydroxide is used as a phosphate binder in patients undergoing prolonged dialysis. **Deferoxamine** is the preferred chelator.

Zinc toxicity can induce a picture of **subacute combined degeneration** similar to that of nitrous oxide toxicity, due to B_{12} deficiency. This **copper-deficiency myeloneuropathy** can occur in patients in postgastrectomy and other malabsorption states as well as those undergoing chronic hemodialysis, treated with **parenteral zinc supplementation.** There is increased T2W signal in the dorsal column by spine MRI and low ceruloplasmin in serum. Oral copper supplementation prevents neurologic deterioration and reverses some deficits.

Thallium, used in the electronics industry and cardiac imaging, poisoning presents as rapidly progressive and **painful sensory polyneuropathy,** optic atrophy, and occasional ophthalmoplegia, followed in 2–3 weeks by diffuse alopecia. The use of potassium chloride by mouth may hasten thallium excretion.

Toxic Gases

Carbon monoxide toxicity due to smoke inhalation in an enclosed vehicle, gas from the kitchen stove, and a house's leaky gas heater causes an acute self-resolving encephalopathy, which may be followed, after about 1 month, by axial-predominant, tremorless **parkinsonism,** retropulsion, cognitive impairment, psychotic behaviors, and incontinence. **Bilateral pallidal necrosis** is the imaging hallmark. The parkinsonism may actually be related to the diffuse white matter hyperintensity and may stabilize or slowly improve. Response to levodopa is suboptimal due to damage to postsynaptic nigrostriatal dopamine receptors. Chorea and dystonia as sequelae are alternative phenotypes. Hyperbaric oxygen shortly after the exposure may prevent delayed parkinsonism.

Nitrous oxide toxicity results from inhalation of this gas employed as anesthetic during surgical or dental procedures (anesthesia paresthetica) or from chronic use of cartridges of whipped cream dispensers for which nitrous oxide is used as propellant. Nitrous oxide (NO) irreversibly oxidizes methylcobalamin (MCbl) and leaves methionine synthase without its cofactor. This B_{12} deficiency from a deficit of its active form, MCbl, leads to a progressive **myeloneuropathy** or sensory ataxia suggestive of subacute combined degeneration of the spinal cord as well as to **hyperhomocysteinemia**-induced vascular injuries. Acute effects may include **finger and perioral paresthesias,** tinnitus, and sensitivity to sound and heat sensation. Acute NO exposure (<2 months) may suffice for myeloneuropathy to develop among those with preexistent subclinical B_{12} deficiency. Initial clinical features may be acral paresthesias and a **"reverse" Lhermitte's sign,** vibration and position sensory loss, and leg hypo- or arreflexia. Nerve conduction studies show an axonal sensorimotor neuropathy. Serum B_{12} may be normal or reduced; homocysteine and methylmalonate are often elevated. Most patients improve following elimination of the NO exposure, but B_{12} and methionine supplementation are used in those with residual deficits.

Methyl bromide toxicity (an insecticidal fumigant gas at room temperature; liquid in cool temperature) acutely may cause visual disturbances **(horizontal diplopia),** **tremor, myoclonus, dysarthria, ataxia,** and seizures; chronically, neuropsychiatric, pyramidal, and cerebellar dysfunction. Brain MRI may show high T2W signal in the inferior olives, dentate nuclei, dorsal pons and midbrain, and periaqueductal region, suggesting **Wernicke encephalopathy.**

Organophosphate poisoning from insecticide exposure produces a cholinergic storm by its anticholinesterase properties, with vomiting, sweating, abdominal cramps, salivation, wheezing, miosis, fasciculations, and weakness. Atropine and pralidoxime reverse these symptoms. Intermediate symptoms (24–96 hours) may be respiratory insufficiency, which can be fatal. Symmetrical sensorimotor polyneuropathy is a delayed symptom (2–5 weeks after exposure). The intermediate and delayed symptoms do not respond to atropine or other drugs.

Toxic Solvents and Other Chemicals

n-Hexane and methyl-*N*-butyl ketone are hexacarbons commonly used in industrial solvents and household glues, which may be intentionally inhaled for intoxication. Their metabolism in the liver produces **2,5-hexanedione,** directly responsible for the neurotoxicity. Repeated exposure causes a peripheral neuropathy **(glue-sniffer neuropathy),** which may be associated with bluish acral discoloration, reduced limb temperature, and **Mees' lines.** A potential presentation is the **Guillain-Barré syndrome.** Continued progression may occur for weeks ("coasting"), despite cessation of exposure.

Acrylamide is a crystalline vinyl monomer used in ore processing, wastewater management, and gel chromatography. **The axon terminal is the primary site of acrylamide toxicity.** Acute neurotoxicity is characterized by gait ataxia and encephalopathy, followed by delayed neuropathy. Chronic toxicity leads to progressive, distal symmetric, **large-fiber axonal sensorimotor neuropathy.** Gait impairment is disproportionate to the weakness and sensory loss.

Carbon disulfide is used as a solvent in perfumes and varnishes, as an insecticide, and as grain fumigant. Inhalation-based occupational exposure produces the **copper- and zinc-chelating dithiocarbamate metabolite,** responsible for the encephalopathy of acute exposure and the extrapyramidal, cerebellar, behavioral, and neuropathic changes of chronic exposure.

Ethylene glycol is used as automotive antifreeze and hydraulic brake fluids. Its metabolites, glycolic and oxalic acid, may cause **seizures, optic neuropathy,** and coma, with anion-gap metabolic acidosis, **hypocalcemia, oxaluria** (oxalate crystals), and renal failure. **Fomepizole,** approved by the FDA for the treatment of ethylene glycol toxicity, is also effective in methanol poisoning.

Methanol (methyl alcohol, wood alcohol), the active ingredient in windshield wiper fluid and household cleaners, may be accidentally ingested, resulting in severe **anion-gap metabolic acidosis** due to oxidation of **methanol to formic acid.** Epileptic encephalopathy with unreactive mydriasis and **large symmetrical central scotomas** due to retinal ganglion cells destruction follows within hours. The characteristic MRI finding is **putaminal infarcts or hemorrhage.** Administration of **ethanol,** a competitive substrate of alcohol dehydrogenase, may have some benefit in reducing the formation of formic acid.

Isopropyl alcohol (water and propene combination), through its metabolite acetone, causes headache, lethargy, and coma but without metabolic acidosis.

Toluene (methylbenzene) may cause a permanent encephalopathy with cerebellar, brainstem, basal ganglia, and cranial nerve dysfunction after chronic exposure. At high concentrations, toluene may cause bone marrow suppression. Brain MRI may show T2W **thalamic and red nuclei hypointensity.**

Marine Biotoxins

Thermostable ingested **polyether toxins** (ciguatera, puffer fish, shellfish) **activate sodium channels** of peripheral nerves and muscle membranes, creating **paradoxical sensory disturbances,** especially to temperature (hot feels cold or vice versa). **Sodium channel modulation** (e.g., PHT, CBZ, OXZ, LTG, TPM, ZNM, lidocaine, and mexiletine) reduces toxin-induced pain.

Thermolabile contact **toxins** (jellyfish, anemones, venomous fish, and stingrays) **and envenomation** (sea snakes, cone snails) **act via** *peptides* to bite, sting, kill prey, or protect against aggressors. **Heat denatures peptides** and reduces their effects on sodium and calcium channels.

The **most common marine biotoxin syndromes** result from the consumption of thermostable toxins, unaffected by cooking, freezing, or salting.

Ciguatoxins (CTX) accumulate in the viscera of fish with the dinoflagellate *Gambierdiscus toxicus.* **Ciguatera, from** CTX-containing tropical reef fish or their predators, such as barracuda, is the most common seafood poisoning. It begins within 24 hours after ingestion with **headache and vertigo** followed by **perioral and limb centrifugal paresthesias, paradoxical reversal of temperature sensation, metallic taste,** pruritus, arthralgias, myalgias, and dental pain. Hypotension, bradycardia, **diarrhea, insomnia, and hypersalivation** are the common dysautonomic symptoms. **Scaritoxin,** a CTX from parrotfish, may produce a **delayed tremor-ataxia syndrome** 5 to 10 days after symptom onset. **Mannitol 20%** is helpful if administered within 10 hours after onset of symptoms.

Brevetoxin (BTX) is a ciguatera-like toxin from **shellfish** polluted with the dinoflagellate *Karenia/Gymnodium* from the subtropical waters of the Gulf of Mexico, Caribbean Sea, and northern New Zealand. BTX acts only at the **slow sodium channels** on sensory but not motor axons.

Tetrodotoxin (TTX) poisoning begins within a few minutes of eating **puffer fish,** with initial **euphoria and circumoral paresthesias,** which is the allure of eating puffer fish **(fugu)** in Japan, where over 150 intoxications and 20 deaths occur annually. Paresthesias generalize and an **arreflexic bulbar and limb paralysis** develops within 20 minutes. **Saxitoxin** is a TTX-like toxin ingested from **shellfish** living in temperate waters with red tides (paralytic shellfish poisoning).

Domoic acid (DA) poisoning ("amnesic shellfish poisoning") from ingestion of **anchovies, mussels, and Dungeness crab** contaminated with the diatom microorganism *Pseudonitzchia*, is the only ingestible marine toxicity associated with an acute epileptic encephalopathy (amnesia, seizures, and hemiparesis). DA excites glutamate and kainate CNS receptors, particularly in the hippocampus. Birds symptomatic from DA-contaminated crab are the basis for Hitchcock's *The Birds.*

Substance Abuse Disorders

Substance dependence refers to a maladaptive pattern of substance use and unsuccessful efforts to discontinue, despite knowledge about its consequences, which leads to clinically significant impairment or distress.

- **Physical dependence** is based on the evidence of tolerance or withdrawal associated with the inability to discontinue substance use
- **Psychological dependence** is defined by the chronic craving and drug-seeking behavior, which can occur without tolerance (dose escalation)

Substance abuse is defined as **recurrent substance use** within a 12-month period, with failure to fulfill major responsibilities, use during hazardous activities, recurrent substance-related legal problems, and routine social or interpersonal problems caused or exacerbated by the effects of the substance.

The dopaminergic neurons of the midbrain ventral tegmental area projecting to the nucleus accumbens and other limbic structures are the basis of the mesocorticolimbic "reward circuit" activated during the administration of cocaine, morphine, or ethanol.

In the acute setting, a distinction must be recognized between:

Substance Intoxication	Substance Withdrawal
Reversible substance-specific syndrome due to recent ingestion or exposure to a substance	Reversible substance-specific syndrome due to the cessation or reduction in substance use that has been heavy and prolonged

Although the symptoms of intoxication and withdrawal may be relatively similar, their complications and treatment can differ greatly.

The **CAGE questionnaire**, whose name is an acronym for its four questions, is validated instrument to screen for alcohol dependence. Two "yes" responses warrant further evaluation.

1. Can you **c**ut down on your drinking?
2. Are you **a**nnoyed when asked to stop drinking?
3. Do you feel **g**uilty about your drinking?
4. Do you need an **e**ye-opener drink when you get up in the morning?

Seizures and Drug Abuse

True alcohol withdrawal seizures rarely occur more than once every 12 months, although ethanol-related seizures increase with age and cumulative exposure to alcohol, consistent with the same kindling phenomenon of psychostimulant-induced seizures. **Cocaine, on the other hand, leads to seizures on the first exposure in 40% of cases.** Normeperidine is the toxic metabolite of meperidine responsible for lowering the seizure threshold. Its half-life is extended in renal failure. **Marijuana and heroin are the drugs with the lowest risk for developing new seizures.** Anticonvulsant maintenance therapy is not necessary for drug and ethanol-related seizures because of the dangers of poor compliance in persistent abusers and the futility of these drugs in abstainers.

Alcohol and Sedatives Abuse and Withdrawal

Acute intoxication, similar for sedatives and alcohol, causes **anterograde memory impairment, behavioral disinhibition,** slurred speech, ataxia, nystagmus, and impaired consciousness. Unconsciousness usually develops with an alcohol level of 500 mg/dL and death when the level is 600–800 mg/dL.

Withdrawal syndrome begins 2–7 days after drinking cessation, peaks at 72 hours, and lasts 3–7 days. Seizures from barbiturates occur 72 hours after last use and from long-acting benzodiazepines may take a week or more. Symptoms reflect reduced GABA$_A$ and increased glutamate (NMDA) neurotransmission.
- **Stage 1:** hyperadrenergic syndrome (anxiety, agitation, sweating)
- **Stage 2:** above, plus **tremor and visual or auditory hallucinations**
- **Stage 3: seizures** (often within 48 hours of last drink)
- **Stage 3: acute confusional state (delirium tremens), fever**

Alcohol withdrawal responds to the following therapies:
- Long-acting benzodiazepines such as **chlordiazepoxide** (Librium) 50–100 mg rqid, or **diazepam** (Valium) 5–10 mg q2-4h, as needed
- Anticonvulsants such as **carbamazepine, valproate,** or **magnesium** given its antagonism of the NMDA receptors
- Adjunctive agents such as **beta-blockers** (atenolol, propranolol), which relieve craving and improve vital signs, and **alpha-agonists** (clonidine), which decrease severity of withdrawal symptoms

Barbiturate withdrawal can be treated or prevented with a short-acting barbiturate such as **pentobarbital,** at a dose of 200–400 mg q6h, tapered after 2–3 days by ≤100 mg/d to avoid reemergence of symptoms.

Benzodiazepine overdose, which can lead to coma, can be treated with the rapid-onset but short-acting antagonist **flumazenil.** Compared to most sedatives and hypnotics, benzodiazepines do not produce anesthesia at high doses, are much less likely to cause respiratory depression, have less addictive ability, and have a larger margin between therapeutic doses and physical dependence.

> **Disulfiram (Antabuse)** is used in the treatment of chronic alcoholism. It **disrupts the metabolic breakdown of acetaldehyde** by irreversibly binding aldehyde dehydrogenase. The resulting **acetaldehyde poisoning** produces very unpleasant symptoms, such as headache, nausea, and anxiety, for up to 2 weeks after ingestion discouraging alcohol intake. Other effects may be cardiac arrhythmias, psychosis, tremor, seizures, and hepatitis.

Alcoholic cerebellar degeneration from chronic alcoholism results in a low-frequency (3 Hz) leg tremor best seen as a slow "bobbing" of the body when the patient stands with feet together and knees half bent, or as a kicking movement when the patient is recumbent with legs elevated.

Alcoholism

This is a chronic disease characterized by uncontrolled cravings for, and physical dependence on, ethanol as well as tolerance to its intoxicating effects. The different actions of alcohol are a reflection of the actions of different transmitters.

The mechanisms underlying euphoria or pleasure, which leads to reinforcing action by alcoholic individuals, is mediated by increases in dopamine in the nucleus accumbens as well as **up-regulation of opioid receptors μ and δ** (the antagonists **naloxone** and **naltrexone** reduce relapse during abstinence) and **5-HT$_2$ receptors,** in type 2 or early-onset alcoholics. Type 1 or anxious alcoholics have excess 5-HT activity and benefit from the use of **buspirone,** an agonist at presynaptic 5-HT$_{1A}$ receptors, which reduces 5-HT release.

At low alcohol concentrations, GABA$_A$ inhibition mediates anxiolysis, sedation, and ataxia through the γ_2 receptor subunit. Higher levels produce excessive Cl$^-$ influx independent of GABA. Chronic alcoholism causes GABA$_A$ decrease and tolerance to ethanol, benzodiazepines, and barbiturates.

At high alcohol concentrations (>100 mg/dL), NMDA channel blockade mediates amnesia through a reactive increase in the number of receptors. Eventual "normalization" of glutamate and calcium function occurs and tolerance develops. Inhibition of NMDA receptors in hippocampus causes alcoholic blackouts.

Alcohol withdrawal is associated with hyperexcitability from a relative excess of NMDA function, excessive calcium influx, and **hypomagnesemia.** A natural glutamate antagonist, magnesium may be more effective than benzodiazepines in alcohol withdrawal seizures. Chronic alcoholism causes decreased GABA$_A$ receptor activity and may contribute to the symptoms of withdrawal and tolerance to benzodiazepines. **Acamprosate,** a new NMDA modulator, reduces the conditioned aspects of drinking learned through NMDA receptor.

Gamma-hydroxybutyric acid (GHB), a GABA$_B$ receptor agonist formed by the dehydrogenation of one of its precursor 1,4-butanediol, a commercially available solvent contained in compact disc and printer cleaners, can enhance the effects of alcohol in "rave" parties and as a date-rape drug. When alcohol is ingested with large doses of 1,4-butanediol, a **severe myoclonic encephalopathy with hallucinations and seizures** (unlike what occurs with isolated alcohol toxicity) is followed by transient improvement as alcohol is metabolized, followed by a relapse once 1,4-butanediol is dehydrogenated to GHB. Treatment is supportive with benzodiazepines for seizures and atropine for bradycardia. Due to its short half-life, GHB toxicity usually resolves within 6 hours. It should be noted that, despite being a drug of abuse, GHB has found clinical use in the treatment of narcolepsy and, paradoxically, alcoholism. More recently, GHB has been used to treat alcohol-responsive drug-refractory posthypoxic myoclonus.

Alcoholism Complications

Wernicke-Korsakoff syndrome (WKS) is a nutritional disorder of thiamine (vitamin B_1) deficiency seen in chronic alcoholics, hyperemesis gravidarum, anorexia nervosa, prolonged starvation, renal insufficiency, and gastrectomy. Pathology shows symmetric demyelination, petechial hemorrhages, and gliosis around the third ventricle, cerebral aqueduct, and fourth ventricle. The main affected areas are the **mammillary bodies,** the **dorsomedial thalamus,** hypothalamus, vestibular nuclei, and superior cerebellar vermis.

- **Wernicke encephalopathy** combines ataxia, ocular motor abnormalities (nystagmus, gaze palsies), and global confusion. Tachycardia, hypotension, or hypothermia indicates hypothalamic involvement.
- **Korsakoff amnestic syndrome** is characterized by anterograde, and to a lesser degree, retrograde amnesia along with impairment in attention shifting, presumably from frontal lobe damage.
- **Dry beriberi** is characterized by sensorimotor neuropathy of the legs.
- **Wet beriberi** (cardiovascular thiamine deficiency) presents as edema and congestive heart failure.

Thiamine is required as a cofactor by several enzymes involved in carbohydrate metabolism, such as pyruvate dehydrogenase. Hence, a high carbohydrate diet or glucose is harmful in the presence of thiamine deficiency since the metabolic demands are increased. Thiamine deficiency differs from Leigh syndrome in the invariable involvement of mamillary bodies and sparing of the substantia nigra. Thiamine stores are depleted within 1 month since body storage is minimal. **Parenteral thiamine replacement** (100 mg/d) improves ocular abnormalities within hours to a few days. Confusion and ataxia have slower improvement rates. About 25% of amnestic syndrome patients will not recover.

Alcoholic cerebellar degeneration refers to the loss of Purkinje cells in the anterior and superior cerebellar vermis, which leads to truncal and lower extremity ataxia. Thiamine deficiency, with or without direct toxicity from ethanol, is responsible for the selective atrophy.

Central pontine myelinolysis (CPM) applies to bilateral symmetrical focal demyelination of the ventral pons with involvement of corticobulbar and corticospinal tracts. Locked-in syndrome may occur in severe cases. **Aggressive correction of hyponatremia** is the major, but not necessary, precipitant factor. Extrapontine myelinolysis may be found in the lateral geniculate body and cerebral and cerebellar white matter.

Marchiafava-Bignami disease is a demyelinating disorder of the corpus callosum, centrum semiovale, and occasionally the middle cerebellar peduncles, resulting in abulia, **apraxia** (as part of an isolated hemispheric disconnection syndrome), prominent frontal release signs, and spasticity or rigidity. High T2W signal in the corpus callosum is seen in the acute stage on brain MRI.

Alcoholic myopathy is the most prevalent muscle disease in North America, characterized in the acute phase by proximal weakness, muscle pain, tenderness, and cramps, and associated with **rhabdomyolysis and myoglobinuria,** which can lead to renal failure, hyperkalemia, and death. The chronic form is usually painless and blood CPK levels are normal. Pelvic girdle muscles are atrophied. Coexistent cardiomyopathy may lead to congestive heart failure. The myopathy usually improves 2–3 months after drinking cessation.

> **Toxic painful myopathies with rhabdomyolysis** include those due to alcohol, amphetamines, alkaloidal cocaine ("crack"), HMG-CoA reductase inhibitors ("statins"), isoniazid (INH), cyclosporine propofol, lithium, and zidovudine.

Fetal alcohol syndrome refers to the mentally retarded or hyperactive children from alcoholic pregnancies, with **microcephaly,** growth failure, **midfacial hypoplasia,** upturned nostrils, and thin upper lip. They may have congenital heart defects (ventricular septal defect, atrial septal defect) and skeletal abnormalities (joint anomalies, altered palmar crease patterns, and small distal phalanges). **Migrational brain defects** are common neuropathologic findings.

Hepatic encephalopathy in chronic alcoholism consists of **asterixis,** tremor, chorea, myoclonus, dystonia, and hyperreflexia in the setting of an acute confusional state. **Hyperammonemia** and **triphasic waves** are seen in plasma and EEG, respectively. An **increased T1W signal in the globus pallidum** on brain MRI, presumably due to manganese accumulation, **correlates with the plasma ammonia** or bilirubin levels but not with the degree of encephalopathy.

Acquired hepatolenticular degeneration applies to those with chronic hepatic dysfunction who develop mild to moderate dementia with or without a movement disorder. Cerebral atrophy with cortical laminar necrosis, microcystic basal ganglia, and cerebellar degeneration are seen in this condition. **Alzheimer's type II cells** are the pathologic correlate of persistent hyperammonemia.

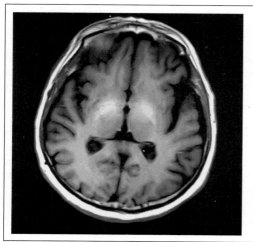

The **differential diagnosis for symmetric basal ganglia** *T1W* **hyperintensities on MRI** is small. The known causes are hepatic encephalopathy, acquired hepatolenticular degeneration, long-term TPN (possibly caused by manganese toxicity), neurofibromatosis, and calcifications.

Pallidal MRI T1-weighted hyperintensities in a 79-year-old man with alcoholic liver cirrhosis admitted with cognitive impairment and asterixis of both hands.

Psychostimulants: Cocaine and Amphetamine

Cocaine is used intranasally or parenterally as cocaine hydrochloride or smoked as alkaloidal cocaine ("crack"); dextroamphetamine is used for alertness or weight loss and illegally injected or smoked ("ice").

Cocaine and amphetamine are **monoamine reuptake inhibitors**, increasing the synaptic concentration of dopamine and norepinephrine. The amphetamine derivative 3,4-methylenedioxy-meth-amphetamine (**MDMA, Ecstasy**) is a potent serotonin releaser. Repeated cocaine use reduces postsynaptic D2 receptors.

Cocaine intoxication, due to its sympathomimetic effects, leads to **mydriasis,** tachycardia, hypertension, fever, and arrhythmias, associated with euphoria, **hypersexuality,** grandiosity, and insomnia. Neurologic manifestations may include **seizures, strokes, chorea, and dystonia.** Intermittent, slow limb movements, often associated with a sensation of restlessness or akathisia, can follow acute cocaine exposure for 2–6 days and is often referred to as "**crack dancing**" among addicts. Chronic use leads to **psychosis,** especially **tactile hallucinations** and **delusional parasitosis;** aggressive behavior, and weight loss. Use in pregnancy causes prematurity, placenta previa, and abruptio placenta. Some teratogenic effects include microcephaly, intracerebral hemorrhage, and urinary tract abnormalities.

Treatment hinges on abrupt withdrawal followed by supportive interventions. Tricyclics agents (such as desipramine), amantadine, and carbamazepine may decrease craving. Methylphenidate, an indirect dopamine agonist, does not decrease cocaine use but allows longer treatment retention.

Amphetamine intoxication also causes hyperactivity and euphoria, but chronic amphetamine users have greater propensity to **hallucinations and delusions. Ecstasy** users experience disorientation, a sense of personal enlightenment, and **masseter spasm with tongue and cheek biting** for 4–6 hours (baby pacifiers are relied upon by experienced users). **Chewing and tooth-grinding** are recognizable features of amphetamine abusers. MDMA may cause seizures, autonomic lability (with hypo- or hypertension, arrhythmias), malignant hyperthermia, and alteration in the level of consciousness, features suggestive of **serotonin syndrome.**

Treatment also consists of abrupt withdrawal and supportive interventions, particularly antipsychotics (if not MDMA-induced toxicity) and benzodiazepines. **Succinylcholine is to be avoided** in MDMA toxicity because it tends to cause masseter spasms, hyperkalemia, and hyperthermia.

Withdrawal of cocaine and amphetamines results in a **"crash period"** for the first 9 hours to 14 days and consist of insomnia, agitation, anorexia, and severe depressive symptoms. Anhedonia and fatigue can persist for 2 weeks. **Increased appetite, vivid dreams, delusions, paranoid ideation, and stereotyped behaviors** are more common in amphetamine withdrawal.

Marijuana, Hallucinogens, and PCP

THC, obtained from the hemp plant *Cannabis sativa*, is usually smoked with a "joint." It has antinociceptive effects (which has encouraged used for pain of neuropathic origin) and antiemetic effects.

Marijuana (tetrahydrocannabinol [THC]) acts in the brain by modulating GABAergic synaptic transmission through CB_1 **cannabinoid receptors** predominantly located in the hippocampus, amygdala, and cerebral cortex. Like other euphoria-inducing drugs, THC selectively activates dopaminergic neurons in the ventral tegmental area. THC intoxication begins with a transient tingling sensation of the head and body and is followed by euphoria, relaxation, jocularity, conjunctival injection, tachycardia, **hyperphagia,** and distorted perception or dream-like state (which translates into paranoid ideation, **delusions, hallucinations,** and depersonalization). Judgment and motor impairment are affected for up to 24 hours. **Flashbacks** may occur days or weeks after the last dose. Chronic use may result in smaller testicles and azoospermia, COPD, and bronchial carcinoma.

Psychological dependence may develop but existence of physical tolerance is controversial. Because overt withdrawal symptoms are rare in most users, THC was not considered a drug of addiction in the past. However, a reported **human cannabis withdrawal syndrome** consists of craving, decreased appetite, sleep difficulty, and weight loss, sometimes accompanied by anger, aggression, irritability, and restlessness.

Phencyclidine (PCP, "angel dust") eaten, snorted, or injected, inhibits NMDA receptors and induces delirium and frank psychosis (with "negative" symptoms of schizophrenia such as loss of ego boundaries and autism, unlike the "positive" ones resulting from cocaine and amphetamines), hyperacusis, decreased pain sensitivity, fever, and diaphoresis. Important findings are **miosis, nystagmus,** ataxia, hyperreflexia, myoclonus, muscle rigidity, hypertension, and tachycardia. Seizures and coma may develop at very high doses.

Depression may occur on withdrawal. Lacking a PCP antagonist, the treatment is mainly supportive with benzodiazepines and antipsychotics. Phentolamine may be used to treat serious hypertension. Drugs with anticholinergic side effects (phenothiazines) should be avoided to prevent potentiation of the anticholinergic properties of PCP. Urine acidification hastens drug excretion.

Hallucinogens such as LSD and mescaline produce vivid formed hallucinations with alteration of alertness, attention, memory, and orientation, unlike most other drugs of abuse. After a short period of dizziness and blurred vision, **visual distortions, palinopsia** (prolonged afterimages), and **synesthesias** (mixing of sensory inputs) appear, followed by visual hallucinations and a sensation of derealization and depersonalization with preservation of insight and memory. Physical findings include **mydriasis** with preserved pupillary light reflex, tremors, ataxia, tachycardia, diaphoresis, and palpitations. No physical addiction or withdrawal syndrome occurs. Management only requires calm reassurance.

Opioids Intoxication and Withdrawal

Heroin is the most commonly abused opioid. When combined with cocaine it is called "speedball," which can be dissolved in water and injected intravenously ("mainlining") or subcutaneously ("skin-popping"). Opioids include naturally occurring opium and morphine, semisynthetic heroin, and synthetic hydromorphone (Dilaudid), meperidine (Demerol), methadone, propoxyphene (Darvon), and codeine. Opioids are used therapeutically as analgesics, anesthetics, antidiarrheal agents, and cough suppressants.

Intoxication may acutely cause euphoria followed by **miosis**, postural hypotension, constipation, urinary retention, and eventually **respiratory depression** and coma. **Withdrawal** causes **mydriasis** and **influenza-like symptoms: myalgias, lacrimation, rhinorrhea, sneezing, piloerection** ("gooseflesh"), yawning, sweating, nausea, vomiting, and diarrhea. Intensity of withdrawal syndrome is greatest with opiates of short half-life such as heroin.

"Chasing the dragon" is a smoking technique for heroin (heating the drug on metal foil and "chasing" the resulting vapor with a tube or straw), which causes gait and limb ataxia and dysarthria, followed by spastic quadriparesis. T2W and FLAIR brain MRI reveal a **progressive spongiform leukoencephalopathy** in the form of symmetric white matter hyperintensities in the posterior limb of the internal capsule, splenium of the corpus callosum, cerebellum, and brainstem.

Meperidine may cause tremor and myoclonus. Methadone may cause tremor and chorea. Mixed agonist-antagonists butorphanol (Stadol), pentazocine (Talwin), and buprenorphine (Buprenex) may cause visual hallucinations. No seizures or hallucinations develop with heroin intoxication or withdrawal.

After Last Dose of:	Symptoms Begin	Symptoms Peak	Symptoms End
Heroin	8–12 hours	2–3 days	7–10 days
Methadone	12–24 hours	4–5 days	>14 days
Buprenorphine	8–12 hours	2–3 days	7 days

Heroin crosses the blood–brain barrier more rapidly than morphine and is metabolized to it (3 mg heroin = 10 mg morphine).
Buprenorphine symptoms are less severe and slightly shorter than heroin. Rifampin, phenytoin, carbamazepine, and barbiturates (but not valproate) accelerate methadone metabolism and can precipitate withdrawal symptoms in patients receiving methadone maintenance therapy.

Treatment of opioid withdrawal relies on **Naloxone** (Narcan), 2 mg IV, IM, or SQ given immediately (and repeatedly up to 20 mg) to patients with respiratory compromise. When used for rapid detoxification, it requires using a combination of buprenorphine, clonidine, and naltrexone for the management of the resulting withdrawal symptoms. **Methadone** (Dolophine), 20–35 mg/d, is a long-acting orally active opioid whose chronic administration produces tolerance to opiate-like drugs, **blocking the euphoric effects of heroin.** Methadone, however, can induce choreic movements in a dose-dependent fashion in individuals receiving it for heroin addiction, especially when rapidly titrated. **Clonidine** (0.1-0.3 mg qid for 10 days) suppresses autonomic symptoms as an adjunct to methadone. Clonidine can mask early symptoms of alcohol or sedative withdrawal, preventing the use of appropriate seizure prophylaxis.

Toxic Leukoencephalopathies

These refer to the white matter (myelin) damage that results from exposure to a wide variety of agents, as outlined below. Any patient who presents with an acute or chronic neurobehavioral deficit, especially changes in mental status with apathy, depression, or anxiety, should raise the index of suspicion for a toxic leukoencephalopathy. **Language, praxis, and cortical sensation are usually not affected** at least in the early stages since the cortical gray matter is unaffected.

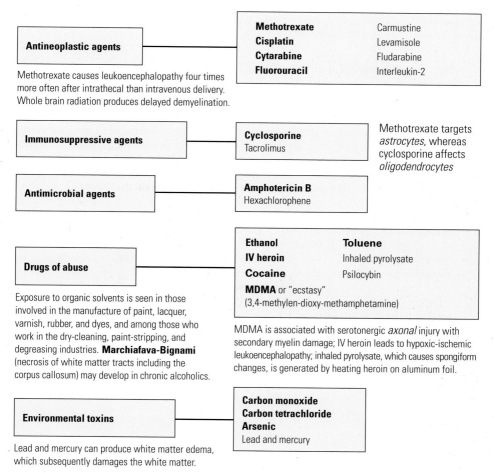

Antineoplastic agents

Methotrexate	Carmustine
Cisplatin	Levamisole
Cytarabine	Fludarabine
Fluorouracil	Interleukin-2

Methotrexate causes leukoencephalopathy four times more often after intrathecal than intravenous delivery. Whole brain radiation produces delayed demyelination.

Immunosuppressive agents

Cyclosporine
Tacrolimus

Methotrexate targets *astrocytes*, whereas cyclosporine affects *oligodendrocytes*

Antimicrobial agents

Amphotericin B
Hexachlorophene

Drugs of abuse

Ethanol	Toluene
IV heroin	Inhaled pyrolysate
Cocaine	Psilocybin
MDMA or "ecstasy" (3,4-methylen-dioxy-methamphetamine)	

Exposure to organic solvents is seen in those involved in the manufacture of paint, lacquer, varnish, rubber, and dyes, and among those who work in the dry-cleaning, paint-stripping, and degreasing industries. **Marchiafava-Bignami** (necrosis of white matter tracts including the corpus callosum) may develop in chronic alcoholics.

MDMA is associated with serotonergic *axonal* injury with secondary myelin damage; IV heroin leads to hypoxic-ischemic leukoencephalopathy; inhaled pyrolysate, which causes spongiform changes, is generated by heating heroin on aluminum foil.

Environmental toxins

Carbon monoxide
Carbon tetrachloride
Arsenic
Lead and mercury

Lead and mercury can produce white matter edema, which subsequently damages the white matter.

The Digit Span and Serial Sevens, Three-Word Delayed Recall, clock drawing, and alternating motor sequences, respectively, can assess deficits in attention, recent memory, visuospatial skills, and executive dysfunction. The MMSE is relatively insensitive since it relies heavily on language.

Toxicology screens detect alcohol and cocaine if the exposure is recent. Toluene toxicity requires analysis of 24-hour urine collection. Screening of urine for heavy metals detects cases of chronic arsenic, lead, and mercury poisoning. Testing for *carboxyhemoglobin* quantifies the exposure to carbon monoxide. T2W MRI is the sequence of choice to evaluate the white matter, although FLAIR MRI may be more sensitive in ethanol intoxication cases.

Neuroleptic Malignant Syndrome (NMS)

This iatrogenic and idiosyncratic iatrogenic effect of treatment with neuroleptic drugs (dopamine D_2 receptor blocking agents), consists of **encephalopathy, fever** (from hypothalamic D2 receptor blockade), **dysautonomia** (hypertension, diaphoresis, or incontinence), **and generalized lead-pipe rigidity and tremor** (increased calcium release from the sarcoplasmic reticulum). Less common causes include lithium and abrupt dose changes of dopaminergic agonists and levodopa. The main complications are **rhabdomyolysis,** myoglobinuria, and subsequent acute renal failure. **Creatine kinase (CK)** elevations may range from 200 to 10,000 IU/L. No other test is helpful for reaching this clinical diagnosis.

> **Nonantipsychotic neuroleptic drugs** include the antiemetic phenothiazines thiethylperazine and **prochlorperazine** as well as the substituted benzamides **metoclopramide** and clebopride.

Treatment is based on discontinuation of the offending agent and aggressive rehydration with urine alkalinization. **Bromocriptine** 2.5–5.0 mg tid (maximum, 30 mg/d) and **dantrolene** (sequesters calcium in the sarcoplasmic reticulum) 1–3 mg/kg IV qid (maximum, 10 mg/kg, cumulative) are helpful. **Risk of recurrence can be up to 80% if reexposure to neuroleptics occurs within 2 weeks.**

NMS-like disorders include:
- **Malignant hyperthermia** (from halogenated inhaled anesthetics used alone or in conjunction with succinylcholine or other depolarizing muscle relaxants) manifests tachycardia, cyanosis, and hemodynamic instability.
- **Serotonin syndrome** (from excessive activation of $5\text{-}HT_{1A}$ and $5\text{-}HT_2$ receptors) consists of severe **leg-predominant rigidity,** dysautonomia (*diarrhea,* excessive lacrimation), and encephalopathy with **myoclonus, hyperreflexia, and seizures. Mydriasis** and hyperactive bowel sounds are clues. Severe cases progress to rhabdomyolysis, myoglobinuria, and renal failure. Cyproheptadine may be helpful.

DRUGS CAUSING SEROTONIN SYNDROME

Inhibitors of serotonin reuptake	SSRI, TCA, dextromethorphan, dexamphetamine, cocaine, meperidine, opiates (except morphine)
Inhibitors of serotonin metabolism	MAO-B inhibitors (selegiline), MAO inhibitor antidepressants
Enhancers of serotonin synthesis	L-tryptophan
Enhancers of serotonin release	MDMA (Ecstasy), amphetamines, cocaine, fenfluramine
Serotonin agonists	Sumatriptan, ergotamine, buspirone
Nonspecific serotonin enhancers	Lithium, electroconvulsive therapy (ECT)

- **Anticholinergic toxicity** (from tricyclic antidepressants and cocaine) causes dry skin and mouth, mydriasis, urinary retention, and arrhythmias. Rigidity is absent. Physostigmine should be given during drug withdrawal.
- **Tyramine cheese reaction** from ingestion of tyramine-containing food or sympathomimetic agents when already taking nonselective or MAO-A inhibitors. **Phentolamine** is recommended for the hypertensive crises.

Movement Disorders   5

Cerebellar ataxias are investigated in a rational manner by the use of an algorithm that includes mode of inheritance and MRI pattern of atrophy:

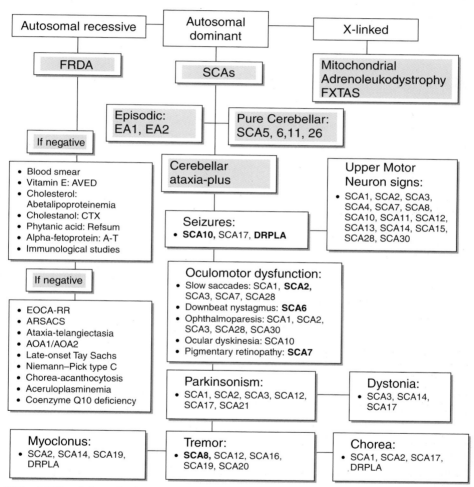

MSA, anti-GAD cerebellar ataxia, gluten ataxia (celiac disease due to antigliadin antibodies), Miller-Fisher syndrome, paraneoplastic cerebellar degeneration, and ILOCA are sporadic entities considered in the differential of ataxias. MSA is the most common nonhereditary degenerative ataxia. ILOCA (idiopathic late-onset cerebellar ataxia) is considered when the patient exhibits a sporadic progressive degeneration of the cerebellum for which the underlying cause remains unclear. Age of onset is usually between 40 and 55 years. FRDA, Friedreich ataxia; SCA, spinocerebellar ataxia; AVED, ataxia with vitamin E deficiency; CTX, cerebrotendinous xanthomatosis; A-T, ataxia telangiectasia; EOCA-RR, early-onset cerebellar ataxia with retained tendon reflexes; ARSACS, spastic ataxia of Charlevoix-Saguenay; AOA1-2, apraxia-oculomotor apraxia. Maternal, X-linked ataxias are discussed later.

INHERITED ATAXIAS WITH IDENTIFIABLE BIOCHEMICAL ERRORS

Disorder	Clinical Clues	Tests	Treatment
Episodic ataxias (except channelopathies EA-1, EA-2)			
Urea cycle defects: **OTC deficiency**	Encephalopathy, **ophthalmoplegia,** episodic headache	↑ NH3, orotic acid, ↓ citrulline	Protein restriction, benzoate
X-linked ataxia with lactic acidosis	Dysarthria and lethargy triggered by infection/stress	↑ Lactate between attacks; ↑ pyruvate during attacks	**Thiamine,** High-fat diet, Acetazolamide
Intermittent **Maple syrup** urine disease	Brain edema, occ. **ophthalmoplegia, ketoacidosis**	BCAA and BCKA in urine, ↓ BCKA dehydrogenase	Thiamine BCAA-free diet
Hartnup disease	Photosensitive **rash** and headache	Tryptophanuria, aminoaciduria	Nicotinamide
Chronic ataxias			
Multiple carboxylase deficiency	**Rash,** recurrent **ketoacidosis, motor regression**	↑ Propionate, ↑ glycine, ↓ biotin	Biotin
Biotinidase deficiency	**Rash, alopecia,** seizures, DD, hyperventilation	↑ Pyruvate, ↑ CSF >serum lactate, ketoacidosis	Biotin
Hyper-tryptophanemia	**Rash** (pellagra-like), MR, ataxia	↑ Tryptophan	Tryptophan-free diet
Vitamin E deficiency	FA phenotype, retinitis pigmentosa	α-Tocopherol level (mutation in Chr 8)	Vitamin E
Abetalipo-proteinemia	FA phenotype, retinitis pigmentosa	Vit E, β-lipoprotein acanthocytes, low cholesterol	Vitamin E
Vitamin B$_{12}$ deficiency (pernicious anemia)	**Sensory ataxia,** Romberg sign	Megaloblastic anemia, B$_{12}$ level, **homocystinuria**	Cobalamin
Refsum disease	Deafness, polyneuropathy, retinitis pigmentosa	↑ **Phytanic acid**	Restrict dietary phytanic acid
CTX: Cerebrotendinous xanthomatosis	**Cataracts,** spasticity, tendon xanthomas	↑ **Cholestanol**	**Chenodeoxycholic acid**
Coenzyme Q10 deficiency (familial cerebellar ataxia)	Cerebellar ataxia, **pyramidal signs,** and **seizures** and/or myoclonus	CoQ10 in muscle and cultured skin fibroblasts	**Coenzyme Q10**

OTC, ornithine transcarbamylase; BCAA, branched chain amino acids; BCKA, branched-chain alpha-ketoacid; DD, developmental delay; CSF, cerebrospinal fluid; MR, magnetic resonance; CTX, cerebrotendinous xanthomatosis.

Screening tests: lactate, pyruvate, NH$_3$, vitamin E, lipoproteins, amino acids, urine organic acids, and cholesterol.

HEREDITARY ATAXIAS—AUTOSOMAL DOMINANT INHERITANCE

	Chromosome	Mutation	Repeats	Clinical Features Besides Ataxia
SCA1✚	**6p**	CAG expansion Ataxin 1	N: 6–44 A: 39–82	**Spasticity** (with bulbar weakness), **parkinsonism,** dystonia, chorea, and terminal **amyotrophy** (peripheral neuropathy) with late **slow saccades** (causing ophthalmoparesis).
SCA2✚ Most common in Asians	**12q**	CAG expansion Ataxin 2	14–32 34–64	**Upper limb areflexia** (peripheral neuropathy). **Slow saccades** with eventual gaze paresis (pons atrophy). **Dementia** is seen in early onset. **Myoclonus,** action tremor or, rarely, chorea. **Parkinsonism** is uncommon.
SCA3✚ **(MJD)** Most common in Portugal	**14q**	CAG expansion Ataxin 3	12–40 56–86	**Dystonia, parkinsonism,** and **hyperreflexia** (with bulbar weakness) appear early with **slow saccades, areflexia,** diplopia, and **"bulging eyes"** (eyelid retraction) later. In older onset, sensory neuropathy, **fasciculations** and **facial myokymia**
SCA4	**16q**	Unknown		**Sensory neuropathy,** proprioceptive loss, generalized **areflexia.**
SCA5✚	**11p**	SPTBN Nonrepeat mutations		Pure cerebellar ataxia (referred to as the "Lincoln family ataxia")
SCA6✚ Relatively common in Japan, UK Germany	**19p**	CAG expansion **α-CACNL1A/** Cav2.1	4–18 21–30	Older onset, "benign" course, normal life span. Diplopia and **downbeat nystagmus** *without slow saccades.* Parkinsonism, pes cavus, and sphincter disturbance can occur. It is allelic with **episodic ataxia type 2.**
SCA7✚	**3p**	CAG expansion Ataxin 7	4–35 37–>200	**Upper motor neuron signs** are among first signs. **Seizures, dementia,** and **slow saccades** with or without supranuclear gaze palsy are common in early onset. **Macular degeneration** causes visual loss.
SCA8✚	**13q**	**CTA/CTG** expansion ATXN8OS	107–127	Relatively pure cerebellar syndrome. Severe **truncal titubation** is common. Mild **athetosis with myoclonic component** may be seen. Reduced penetrance suggests an AR disorder.

SCA, spinocerebellar ataxia; MJD, Machado-Joseph disease; AR, androgen receptor.

SCA9 has not yet been characterized. No single clinical feature is exclusively predictive of a given SCA, except for macular pigmentary degeneration in SCA7. In addition, there is significant intrafamilial phenotypic variability in any given SCA. Isolated cerebellar atrophy is most consistent with SCA5, SCA6, SCA10, SCA14, and EA-2. SCA2 and SCA4 have no upper motor neurone signs (only lower motor neurone). Parkinsonism can arise within SCA2, SCA3, SCA8, and SCA17, or in mild form in SCA6, usually considered "pure" ataxia.

✚, Commercially available.

(Continued)

Chromosome		Mutation	Repeats	Clinical Features
SCA10* Second most common in Mexico after SCA2	22q	**ATTCT** expansion ATXN10	10–29 >800	**Generalized motor seizures** occur in some but abnormal EEG in all. Ophthalmologic features include nystagmus and hypometric saccades or even ocular flutter or "dyskinesias".
SCA11*	15q	TTBK2 Tau tubulin kinase		Benign, late onset cerebellar ataxia with mild pyramidal signs
SCA12* Common in India	5q	CAG expansion	<29 66–78	***Head and hand tremor,*** associated with upper motor neuron signs and cortical as well as cerebellar atrophy
SCA13*	19q	**KCNC3** Kv3.3		**Mental retardation** with slow/early ataxia, dysarthria, and hyperreflexia
SCA14*	19q	**PRKCG** mutation		**Axial myoclonus** with tremor of head and limbs in early onset (<27 y); pure cerebellar ataxia in onset >35 y.
SCA15/SCA16 Allelic SCAs	3p	**ITPR1** IP3 receptor		***Head and hand tremor*** in one third of cases; **pure cerebellar ataxia** with slow and benign course in most
SCA17*	6q	TBP (TATA binding protein)	25–42 45–63	**Epilepsy with absence seizures, dementia, parkinsonism** and **chorea**
SCA18	7q	Unknown		Sensory loss, pyramidal tract signs, muscle weakness
SCA19	1p	Unknown		Cognitive impairment, **myoclonus,** and low frequency **postural tremor**
SCA20	11p	Unknown		**Palatal tremor,** dysphonia, and dentate nucleus calcification
SCA21	7p	Unknown		**Parkinsonism,** postural tremor, hyporeflexia, cognitive impairment
SCA22	1p	Unknown		**Predominantly cerebellar** with hyporeflexia
SCA23	20p	Unknown		No published information available
SCA24	19	Unknown		Likely recessive. Saccadic intrusions, **increased saccadic speed,** sensory neuropathy, and **myoclonus**
SCA25	2p	Unknown		Sensory neuropathy
SCA27*	13q	FGF14		**Hand tremors** in childhood followed by ataxia and cognitive problems

SCA, spinocerebellar ataxia; EEG, electroencephalogram. PRKCG, protein kinase C gamma gene.

SCA1, SCA3/Machado-Joseph disease, SCA7, SCA13, and dentatorubropallidoluysian atrophy (DRPLA) may have childhood onset. Anticipation is more prominent in SCA2, 7, 17, and DRPLA (average increase of four repeats for paternal transmission). Expanded CAG repeats coding for **polyglutamine** tracts cause SCA1, 2, 3, 6, 7, and 17. SCA8 and 12 are caused by **noncoding** expansions in CTG and CAG, respectively. SCA 10, seen almost exclusively in Mexicans, results from an unstable expansion of a pentanucleotide repeat (ATTCT).

*, Commercially available.

(Continued)

Chromosome		Mutation	Repeats	Clinical Features
DRPLA More prevalent in Asia	12p13	CAG expansion Atrophin 1 (ATN1)	3–36 49–88	*Early onset:* progressive myoclonic epilepsy (PME); *late onset:* ataxia; onset 20–30 years: HD-like or mixed movement disorder (dystonia, tremor, parkinsonism and dementia).
EA-1*	12p13	**KCNA1** Kv1.1	Dominant negative point mutation	Brief, short lasting (few min) attacks, Interictal myokymia
EA-2*	19p13	**CACNA1A** Cav2.1	Haploinsufficient point mutation	Longer attacks (hours-days), with chronic ataxia developing. There is interictal downbeat nystagmus.

HD, Huntington disease.

For patients with cerebellar ataxia who also have external ophthalmoplegia and sensory peripheral neuropathy, and for whom common SCAs (SCA1, SCA2, and SCA3) and FRDA mutations have been excluded, POLG gene sequencing is indicated.

*Ataxic channelopathies include SCA6, SCA13, SCA15, EA1, EA2, and severe myoclonic epilepsy of infancy (see "Channelopathies in Epilepsy").

EPISODIC ATAXIAS*

Episodic Ataxia Type 1 Voltage-gated K$^+$ channel gene (KCNA1), 12p13	Episodic Ataxia Type 2* Voltage-dependent P/Q type Ca$^+$ channel (CACNA1A), 19p13
Triggered by stress and exertion	
Brief paroxysmal cerebellar ataxic episodes	Long (hours to days) paroxysmal cerebello-vestibular ataxic episodes
Interictal myokymia may be the only interictal finding	Interictal nystagmus (gaze evoked or downbeat) is characteristic
Paroxysmal kinesigenic choreoathetosis may be associated	Mild permanent gait ataxia may be a long-term residual deficit
Responds to phenytoin and acetazolamide	Responds to acetazolamide

*EA-2 is allelic with familial hemiplegic migraine and SCA-6 and has been associated with episodic weakness, migraine, dystonia, epilepsy, and cognitive involvement.

The differential diagnoses of episodic ataxias include:
- Aminoacidurias (Hartnup disease, isovaleric acidemia, neonatal Maple syrup disease)
- Hyperammonemias (ornithine transcarbamylase deficiency and argininosuccinate lyase deficiency)
- Multiple carboxylase deficiency
- **Pyruvate dehydrogenase deficiency**
- Other causes: MS, TIA, basilar migraine, BPPV, carbamyl phosphate synthetase, and paroxysmal dyskinesias

Hereditary Ataxias: Autosomal Recessive Inheritance

Abetalipoproteinemia, A-T, FA, Juvenile GM2, MLD, Marinesco-Sjögren syndrome, Ramsay Hunt syndrome, CACH, xeroderma pigmentosum, and cerebrotendinous xanthomatosis (CTX) usually have childhood onset.

Friedreich Ataxia

Onset of cerebellar ataxia or scoliosis before age 20, along with rapid early progression of areflexia, extensor plantar response, position and vibration loss, skeletal deformities (pes cavus, scoliosis), and absence of ophthalmoplegia and dementia suggest Friedreich ataxia (FRDA). Pes cavus or scoliosis in parents should suggest an autosomal dominant ataxia, such as CMT. An unstable **GAA repeat** within the first **intron** of the **frataxin (*FXN*)** gene on chromosome **9q13** causes FRDA. Affected persons have from **81 to over 1,000 repeats** in both their alleles (homozygous expansion). When the expansion is heterozygous, the other allele must have a point mutation. **Hypertrophic cardiomyopathy and diabetes mellitus** develop when GAA repeats exceed 500. Brain MRI shows **atrophy of the upper cervical cord with nearly normal cerebellum.**

> **Cervical spine (and medullary) atrophy on MRI can also seen in adult-onset Alexander disease.** This disorder is characterized by bulbar dysfunction, ataxia, corticospinal involvement, and palatal tremor and confirmed by GFAP gene analysis.

Vitamin E Deficiency

It is an important and reversible cause of the **FA phenotype** (spinocerebellar degeneration) with or without **retinitis pigmentosa** but without cardiomyopathy or glucose intolerance. Nystagmus, ptosis, or partial **ophthalmoplegia** is seen in half of the patients. **Head titubation** is seen in 28% of patients. Although malabsorption is a common reason, the disorder is often caused by a defect in α-**tocopherol transfer protein (α-TTP, 8q13),** which impairs the incorporation of α-tocopherol into very-low-density lipoprotein. Treatment with 800–900 IU of oral DL-α-tocopherol improves the deficits.

Early-Onset Cerebellar Ataxia with Retained Tendon Reflexes

Clinically indistinguishable from FA with retained reflexes (FARR) or vitamin E deficiency, early-onset cerebellar ataxia with retained tendon reflexes (EOCA-RR) patients have less upper limb ataxia, less proprioceptive loss, and slower progression than FA. Optic atrophy, cardiomyopathy, scoliosis, or diabetes mellitus are rare or completely absent. Some subjects map to chromosome 10 or 13q (as in Charlevoix-Saguenay spastic ataxia).

Early-Onset Cerebellar Ataxia of Holmes Type

This EOCA presents as a progressive ataxia with **hypogonadotrophic hypogonadism and a frontal-dysexecutive syndrome** (like SCA 2). Less common findings are **retinal degeneration, deafness,** distal amyotrophy, choreoathetosis, and dysphagia. Early diagnosis is desirable because **testosterone replacement** may allow normal sexual development. MRI shows **superior vermian** and cerebellar hemisphere atrophy.

Ataxia-telangiectasia (ATM Mutation, 11q)

AT is the most common cause of progressive ataxia of childhood, occurring in 1:40,000 births. **Ataxia, ocular and cutaneous telangiectasias, immunodeficiencies** (IgA deficiency, recurrent sinopulmonary infections), **and endocrinopathies** (stunted growth) are the common presentations in the early childhood (classic) form, whereas **choreoathetosis** and tremor are the hallmarks in young adulthood (variant AT), with ataxia developing later. Peripheral neuropathy develops in both clinical forms. **Oculomotor apraxia and failure to suppress the vestibular ocular reflex** are key findings. Cerebellar atrophy is most prominent at the **vermis.** Patients become wheelchair-bound by 8–12 years in the classic form and 15–21 years in variant AT. **Alpha-fetoprotein (AFP) is elevated** in 90% of patients. AFP is a useful screen test: if positive, the protein truncation test (PTT) will detect 70% of the more than 400 AT-mutated (ATM) mutations. Western blot will show little or no ATM protein kinase in 85% of patients. Routine chromosomal analysis may show **rearrangements of chromosomes 7 and 14. Radiation hypersensitivity** and increased incidence of lymphoma and lymphocytic leukemia should prompt avoidance of diagnostic radiographic procedures and monitoring for malignancies.

Ataxia-ocular Motor Apraxia 1 (*Aprataxin* Mutation, APTX, 9q)

AOA1 is the most frequent cause of pediatric autosomal recessive ataxia in Japan and the second most common in Portugal. AOA1 causes early chorea and ataxia, oculomotor apraxia, and, eventually, cerebellar atrophy but, unlike AT, patients have an **axonal motor and sensory neuropathy** (early **areflexia** and pes cavus) and no mental retardation, telangiectasia, or immunodeficiency. Important serologic findings are **hypoalbuminemia, hypercholesterolemia,** elevated low-density lipoprotein, and low high-density lipoprotein. Optic atrophy may occur.

Ataxia-oculo Motor Apraxia 2 (*Syntaxin* Mutation, 9q)

AOA2, described in Pakistan and Japan (two families), presents with oculomotor apraxia, strabismus, gait ataxia, **areflexia, extensor plantar response,** and choreoathetosis in late childhood. It is a milder form of ataxia with a later onset (around 15 years) and progression to wheelchair dependence (30 years of age). Besides hypercholesterolemia and increased CK levels, it occurs in the setting of **high AFP** (>20 ng/mL), **IgG,** and **IgA.**

Chediak-Higashi Syndrome (*CHS1* Mutation, 1q)

Primarily a disorder of immune (**chronic infections** from neutrophil granule defect) and dermatologic (**oculocutaneous albinism** from melanin granule defect) nature, Chediak-Higashi syndrome can manifest in adults with cerebellar ataxia, **nystagmus,** and **peripheral neuropathy,** with or without **dystonia, parkinsonism,** or **seizures** (children often developed a fatal lymphoproliferative phase). The diagnosis requires examination of a **peripheral blood smear,** which reveals characteristic large granules in the cytoplasm of neutrophils. Bone marrow transplants have been successful in several cases. Aggressive treatment of infections is indicated.

Spastic Ataxia of Charlevoix-Saguenay (*sacsin*, 13q11)

Described first in Quebec and Tunisia but likely underrecognized elsewhere, Spastic ataxia of Charlevoix-Saguenay (ARSACS) causes a combination of spinocerebellar ataxia with slowly progressive **spastic quadriparesis, hypermyelinated retinal nerve fibers** (retinal striation), and **distal amyotrophy** due to **demyelinating neuropathy.** Brain MRI shows **superior cerebellar vermis atrophy** and **pontine linear hypointensities.**

Marinesco-Sjögren Syndrome (*SIL1*, 5q31)

Cerebellar **ataxia,** early-onset or congenital **cataracts,** and mental **retardation** with developmental delay are the triad components of Marinesco-Sjögren syndrome. **Hypotonia, weakness** (due to muscle replacement with fat), short stature, motor and sensory neuropathy, hypergonadotrophic hypogonadism, and skeletal abnormalities (scoliosis), also occur. Electron microscopy of muscle shows autophagic vacuoles, membranous whorls, and electron-dense double-membrane structures associated with nuclei.

Refsum Disease (PAHX, 10p)

Due to a deficiency of phytanoyl-CoA hydroxylase (PAHX), which leads to insufficient **α-oxidation of phytanic acid,** a lipid of exclusive dietary origin, it leads to **cerebellar ataxia, retinitis pigmentosa,** deafness, **ichthyosis,** demyelinating sensory motor **polyneuropathy,** and high CSF protein. **Phytanic acid** is elevated in urine and serum. **Restricting phytanic acid in diet** reverses some of the deficits. **Cardiac arrhythmia** may result in sudden death. Plasma exchange plays a role in acute exacerbations.

Retinitis pigmentosa without ataxia:
- Myotonic dystrophy
- Mucopolysaccharidosis type II (Hunter syndrome)
- Laurence-Moon-Biedl syndrome

Retinitis pigmentosa with ataxia:
- Friedreich ataxia, vitamin E deficiency
- Abetalipoproteinemia
- Refsum disease
- Cockayne syndrome
- Carbohydrate-deficient glycoprotein syndrome type 1aNBIA-1 and HARP
- Aceruloplasminemia
- Kearns-Sayre syndrome
- Neuronal ceroid lipofuscinosis
- Juvenile gangliosidosis GM2 (type III)

Xeroderma Pigmentosum

This disorder consists of **microcephaly, mental retardation,** sensorineural deafness, **hypogonadism,** and erythema, blistering and scarring on **sunlight exposure** due to faulty DNA repair, with vulnerability to skin cancer. Ataxia is due to a combination of **spinocerebellar degeneration** and **peripheral neuropathy** (DeSanctis-Cacchione syndrome of **xerodermic idiocy**).

Cockayne Syndrome

Also resulting from **defective DNA repair** with sensitivity to ultraviolet light, Cockayne syndrome is recognized by early senility, photosensitivity, **cachectic appearance, dwarfism, microcephaly, retinal degeneration,** impaired hearing, **ataxia,** tremor, dysarthria, and **basal ganglia calcifications.** Morphologically, it must be differentiated from **Seckel syndrome** (bird-headed and microcephalic dwarfs from birth), which is not associated with progressive neurologic deterioration.

GM₂ Gangliosidosis (Tay-Sachs Disease) (HEXA Gene, Low Hex A Activity)

This condition is suspected in any child with an apparent spinocerebellar degeneration, especially if there is Ashkenazi Jewish parentage. **Activity of hexosaminidase A (Hex A) is deficient.** The juvenile variant presents with an FA-like spinocerebellar degeneration syndrome with ataxia, tremor, spasticity, dysarthria, optic atrophy, **episodic psychosis,** and dementia. The adult-onset variant manifests as an atypical progressive myoclonic encephalopathy or as a spinal muscular atrophy syndrome. The latter includes **upgaze limitation** from supranuclear gaze palsy, **proximal leg weakness** and wasting (with evidence of chronic denervation by electromyography [EMG]), and hyperreflexia. Prominent macular **cherry-red spot** (from GM₂ ganglioside accumulation; also a feature of sialidosis) is only seen in children who, unlike adults, have no residual Hex A activity.

Childhood ataxia with diffuse central nervous system hypomyelination (CACH, mutations in eIF2B [eukaryotic translation initiation factor 2B] 1–5 genes)

Also known as **leukoencephalopathy with vanishing white matter,** CACH presents with progressive ataxia and diplegia at 2 years with **recurrent coma** following minor head trauma or infections. Cognitive function and ocular motility remain unaffected until motor decline is substantial, even when severe brain abnormalities are seen on imaging studies. Brain MRI shows **cystic-like** periventricular white matter abnormalities without atrophy. No biochemical defects have been identified. Foamy oligodendrocytes are identified on autopsy.

Adult Polyglucosan Body Disease (GSD IV)

It presents with **progressive upper and lower motor neuron signs,** sensory neuropathy, **cerebellar ataxia, dementia,** and **neurogenic bladder,** especially among Ashkenazi Jews. **Spinal cord atrophy** is invariable. Sural nerve biopsy shows periodic acid-Schiff–positive, diastase-resistant focal enlargements of myelinated fibers known as **polyglucosan bodies.**

> These **polyglucosan bodies** are pathologically different from those of **Lafora disease.**They are found in the axon (as opposed to the perikarya and dendrites of Lafora), are due to glycogen branching enzyme deficiency (as opposed to increased glycogen synthase activity as in Lafora), and do not cause progressive myoclonic epilepsy (like Lafora) but an upper and lower motor neuron syndrome.

Cerebrotendinous Xanthomatosis

CTX begins in childhood with **cataracts** and **xanthomata** of tendon sheaths and lungs. Learning difficulties are followed by **dementia, ataxia, spasticity, dysarthria, dysphagia,** and **polyneuropathy. Tongue protrusion** and **seizures** may occur. The basic defect is in bile acid synthesis with accumulation of cholesterol and **cholestanol. Chenodeoxycholic acid,** 750 mg daily, reverses partially or totally the corticospinal, cerebellar, and cognitive deficits.

> **Supranuclear gaze palsy associated with ataxia** suggest Tay Sachs disease, Niemann Pick type C, Gaucher disease, cerebrotendinous xanthomatosis, and spinocerebellar ataxias (SCA3 and SCA7).

Hereditary Ataxias: X-linked Inheritance

Menkes Kinky Hair Disease (Trichopoliodystrophy)

This X-linked recessive disorder is characterized by early growth retardation, peculiar hair (sparse, brittle, twisted), dysmorphic face (full, rosy cheeks, and high-arched palate), changes in the **metaphyses of the long bones,** and cerebral and cerebellar degeneration in boys. Severe neurologic impairment begins at 2–3 months of age and progresses rapidly to decerebration. Brain MRI findings include **hypomyelination, tortuosity of cerebral arteries,** and diffuse atrophy with **ventriculomegaly.** Defective intestinal absorption of copper is due to mutation in the ***ATP7A*** gene coding for an intracellular copper-transporting protein. Low serum copper leads to failure of copper-dependent enzymes, such as cytochrome C oxidase (hypotonia), tyrosine hydroxylase (twisted hair), and dopamine hydroxylase (ptosis and hypoglycemia). If administered early in life, **copper histidinate** increases life expectancy from 3 to 13 years of age. The diagnosis is based on serum (low) and fibroblasts (elevated) copper levels. The incidence of the disease is 1:300,000 births.

COMPARISON BETWEEN THE TWO DISORDERS ARISING FROM DEFECTS IN THE COPPER-TRANSPORTING ADENOSINE TRIPHOSPHATASE (ATPase).

	Wilson Disease	**Menkes Disease**
Defect	ATP7B	ATP7A
Genetics	13q, autosomal recessive	X-linked recessive
Prevalence	1:40,000	1:200,000
Gender	Male:female = 1:1	Always boys
Expression	Liver and brain	Everywhere but liver
Onset	6–60 years	Infants or neonates
Pathophysiology	Copper deposition	Copper deficiency

X-linked Sideroblastic Anemia with Ataxia

Caused by a mutation in adenosine triphosphate (ATP) binding cassette gene (*hABC7, Xq13*) that results in mitochondrial iron accumulation (as with Pearson syndrome and Friedreich ataxia), this condition is suspected when motor delay, **childhood-onset ataxia, and dysarthria,** with or without spasticity, become progressive after the fifth decade. Imaging studies show cerebellar atrophy. The diagnosis rests on the findings of **Pappenheimer bodies on blood smear, ring sideroblasts on bone marrow,** and increased free **erythrocyte *protoporphyrin*** with decreased mean corpuscular volume.

X-linked Adrenoleukodystrophy

X-linked adrenoleukodystrophy is a peroxisomal storage disease whereby abnormal function of peroxisomes leads to the accumulation of very-long-chain fatty acids in the brain and the adrenal glands, leading to a predominantly posterior leukodystrophy and Addison disease. Female carriers may express the myelopathic variant (adrenomyeloneuropathy) of this disorder.

X-linked Intermittent Ataxia with Lactic Acidosis

This thiamine (B1)-dependent episodic but ultimately progressive disorder presents in infancy as **recurrent coma** or in early childhood as **episodic ataxia,** dysarthria, and occasionally lethargy or weakness. When weakness and areflexia develop, **nystagmus** and other oculomotor disturbances are seen. Episodes may be spontaneous or follow periods of stress, infections, or high-carbohydrate meals. It is caused by a **defect in the pyruvate dehydrogenase complex (PDHC), subunit E1,** whose activity can be measured in fibroblasts, leukocytes, or muscle. PDHC deficiency has also been associated with **Leigh syndrome,** mitochondrial myopathies, and lactic acidosis. During attacks, **serum lactate and pyruvate are elevated;** interictally, only serum lactate is mildly elevated. **Thiamine** (100–600 mg/d) and high-fat, low-carbohydrate diet are the cornerstones of management. Daily **acetazolamide** may abort the attacks.

Rett Syndrome

Rett syndrome **(MeCP2),** is lethal to males, and affects 1 in 10,000 females. This X-linked dominant disorder is characterized by **developmental regression** and **autistic behavior in girls** following a period of normal development during the first 16–18 months of life. After this age, head growth decelerates **(acquired microcephaly), hand stereotypies** replace purposeful hand movements, and autistic features appear. Gait apraxia and truncal apraxia and ataxia, tremor, and seizures follow and the patient may oscillate between **hyperventilation and breath-holding spells** (with aerophagia during walking). The phenotypic range has been expanding to include autism, neonatal hypotonia, and learning disability or mental retardation, especially if associated with a subtle movement disorder. Testing for MeCP2 can be extended to girls with gene-negative Angelman syndrome and in boys with bipolar disorder or juvenile-onset schizophrenia and mental retardation. A boy may have the classic Rett syndrome if he has Klinefelter (XXY) syndrome. Rett-like disorders include neuronal ceroid lipofuscinosis and ornithine transcarbamylase deficiency.

COMPARISON BETWEEN RETT SYNDROME AND INFANTILE AUTISM

Rett Syndrome	Infantile Autism
Normal development until 7–18 months	Onset from early infancy
Developmental regression	No loss of previously acquired skills
Profound mental retardation in all functional areas	Differential intellectual function (visual-spatial skills better than verbal skills)
Language always absent but eye contact is present and intense	Peculiar speech patterns with impaired nonverbal communication
Stereotypic hand movements	Stereotypies are complex and varied
Little interest in manipulating objects	Ritualistic and skillful manipulation of objects or sensory stimulation
Hyperventilation with air-swallowing, breath holding, bruxism are common	Hyperventilation, breath holding, and bruxism not common
Chorea and dystonia may be present	Chorea and dystonia not present

Congenital Ataxic Disorders

As the cerebellum has the longest period of embryologic development of any major structure of the brain (32 days of gestation to 1 year postnatally), it is vulnerable to teratogenic insults longer. **Selective vermal hypoplasia** may be associated with other midline forebrain deficits such as holoprosencephaly and callosal agenesis, characteristic of Dandy-Walker, Chiari malformations, and Joubert syndrome. **Global cerebellar hypoplasia** encompasses chromosomal diseases as well as Tay-Sachs disease, Menkes kinky hair disease, some cases of spinal muscular atrophy, and sporadic cases of unknown cause.

> **Congenital metabolic disorders and specific cerebellar abnormalities:**
> **Vermis:** carbohydrate-deficient glycoprotein syndromes (CDGP type 1a)
> **Dentate nucleus:** Leigh syndrome
> **Global cerebellar:** mitochondrial disorders
> **Cerebellar white matter:** CTX
> **Calcification:** Cockayne, CTX (cerebellar white matter)
> **Progressive cerebellar atrophy:** Canavan, Menkes, and mevalonic aciduria

Joubert Syndrome (9q, 11c, 2q [*NPHP1*], and 6q [*AHI1*])

Joubert syndrome is characterized by **episodic hyperpnea,** retinopathy, abnormal eye movements (**oculomotor apraxia** and seesaw nystagmus), hypotonia, rhythmic tongue protrusion, and ataxia associated with **agenesis of the cerebellar vermis.** The associated facial **dysmorphic features** are large head, prominent forehead, high-arched eyebrows, low nasal bridge, epicanthic folds, anteverted nostrils, open mouth, and tented upper lip.

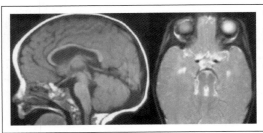

The "**molar tooth sign**" on axial MRI results from **cerebellar vermis hypoplasia**, thick and maloriented superior cerebellar peduncles, and abnormally deep interpeduncular fossa. Corpus callosum is usually thin.

Joubert syndrome is often associated with retinal and renal involvement and is considered part of the cerebello-oculo-renal syndrome (CORS). **The molar tooth sign** helps in distinguishing the Joubert syndrome and related disorders (**JSRD,** see next section) from other hindbrain malformations such as the Dandy-Walker malformation, cerebellar vermis hypoplasia, pontocerebellar hypoplasia, and rhombencephalosynapsis. Funduscopy and electroretinogram are indicated for patients with cerebellar vermis hypoplasia as **Leber congenital amaurosis and colobomas are common.**

Joubert Syndrome-Related Disorders

The Joubert syndrome-related disorders (JSRD) are a group of recessive congenital ataxias consisting of neonatal hypotonia, dysregulated breathing, oculomotor apraxia, and mental retardation. The common denominator is the presence of the **molar tooth sign** on brain MRI.

SPECTRUM OF THE JSRD

Retinopathy, polydactyly, mild or no renal involvement	Hepatic fibrosis and posterior coloboma (retinal or choroidal)	Retinopathy, coloboma, and nephronophthisis (± renal failure)	Notched upper lip, cleft palate, and polydactyly
Joubert syndrome	COACH syndrome	CORS	OFD-VI syndrome

COACH, cerebellar vermis hypoplasia, oligophrenia, congenital ataxia, coloboma, and hepatic fibrocirrhosis. **OFD-VI**, orofacial-digital syndrome type VI; Arima syndrome and Senior-Loken syndrome were previous nomenclatures for CORS. **Meckel-Gruber syndrome** (MKS3) may be part of the JSRD as the molar tooth sign can be seen in addition to encephalocele, polydactyly, cystic dysplastic kidneys, and hepatic fibrosis.

SPECIFIC CONGENITAL CEREBELLAR ATAXIC SYNDROMES WITH MENTAL RETARDATION

Gillespie Syndrome	Paine Syndrome
Inheritance uncertain*	X-linked recessive
Partial aniridia **with unreactive and** dilated pupils in a hypotonic child	**Microcephaly,** spasticity, myoclonus, and seizures

*Mutation of the *PAX6* gene on chromosome 11, responsible for familial and sporadic aniridia, is absent

Congenital Disorders of Glycosylation

Congenital disorders of glycosylation (CDG, previously termed *carbohydrate-deficient glycoprotein syndromes, CDGP)* are a group of hypoglycosylation disorders resulting from defects of *N*-glycosylation (CDG-I, cytoplasm or endoplasmic reticulum [ER]; CDG-II, ER or Golgi) or O-glycosylation (posttranslational in *cis*-Golgi; include two types of muscular dystrophy: **Walker-Warburg** syndrome and muscle-eye-brain disease). **Phosphomannomutase-2 (*PMM2*, 16p)** is the gene for CDG-Ia, the most common subtype. Diagnosis requires isoelectric focusing of transferrin and confirmation of low leukocyte phosphomannomutase activity. The clinical spectrum includes multiple systems, such as:

- **Neurologic: retinitis pigmentosa,** peripheral neuropathy (**hypotonia,** hyporeflexia), and **cerebellar hypoplasia** ("neonatal OPCA [olivopontocerebellar atrophy]")
- **Cutaneous: inverted nipples, lipodystrophic skin,** abnormal distribution of adipose tissue, joint contractures, facial dysmorphism
- **Visceral:** digestive (feeding problems), hepatic **(hepatomegaly),** cardiac **(pericardial effusions),** and renal abnormalities **(nephrotic syndrome)**
- **Hematopoietic system: hypercoagulable syndrome** (low coagulation factors XI, antithrombin III, heparin cofactor II, and proteins C and S are the basis for increased risk for strokes).
- **Endocrine system: hypothyroidism,** hypogonadism, hyperinsulinism, hypoglycemia and osteopenia
- **Immunologic system:** hypogammaglobulinemia

Acquired Ataxias: Selected Disorders

Anti-GQ1b IgG Antibody Syndrome-Related Ataxias

- **Miller-Fisher syndrome** consists of rapid-onset external ophthalmoplegia, cerebellar ataxia, arreflexia, and albuminocytological dissociation. The antecedent infectious agents may be *Campylobacter jejuni,* cytomegalovirus, Epstein-Barr virus, and Streptococcus pyogenes. The IgG autoantibodies (anti-GQ1b) bind to the oculomotor nerves and deep cerebellar nuclei.
- **Bickerstaff's brainstem encephalitis** refers to acute but progressive external ophthalmoplegia, cerebellar ataxia, hyperreflexia, extensor plantar response, and hemihypoesthesia. CSF studies are usually normal. Brain MRI may show asymmetric upper brainstem hyperintensity on T2W sequences with a correspondingly bright lesion on apparent diffusion coefficient sequences (ADC), indicating vasogenic rather than cytotoxic edema.

> The differential of **upper brainstem involvement on brain MRI** includes encephalitis caused by **arboviruses** or *Lysteria* **monocytogenes, Wernicke encephalopathy, paraneoplastic syndromes** (anti-Hu, anti-Ri, and anti-Ma2 antibodies), and **mitochondriopathies.**

Although Miller Fisher syndrome (MFS) and Bickerstaff's brainstem encephalitis (BBE) are proposed to be part of a single autoimmune disease with ophthalmoplegia, ataxia, and drowsiness ("anti-GQ1b IgG antibody syndrome"), MFS is considered a variant of GBS because of peripheral nerve involvement, whereas BBE is defined as a brainstem encephalitis.

Paraneoplastic Cerebellar Degeneration

Paraneoplastic cerebellar degeneration must be entertained in any adult patient with acute or subacute progressive nonfamilial cerebellar syndrome. The underlying malignancies are small cell lung cancer (**anti-Hu** and **anti-CV2**) and breast or ovary (**anti-Yo, anti-Ri** [breast only]). Only **mGluR1** (glutamate receptor type 1) and **anti-VGCC** (voltage-gated calcium channel) antibodies are directed against cell surface antigen and thus have a pathogenic role and may be treated with IVIg or plasmapheresis.

Celiac Disease

Occurring as a malabsorptive syndrome, a neurologic syndrome, or both, celiac disease can present as gait ataxia or peripheral neuropathy or, less commonly, as myopathy, myelopathy, or progressive myoclonic encephalopathy. **Dermatitis herpetiformis** (itchy blistering skin rash) is a rare co-occurrence. **Antigliadin antibodies** (IgG with or without IgA; the latter may be deficient) are the usual screening tools for the diagnosis of celiac disease. **IgG deamidated gliadin peptide antibodies** and **IgA antibodies to transglutaminase TG6** are most specific for cerebellar ataxia even when there is no intestinal involvement. Other autoimmune diseases may coexist. Neuropathology shows striking Purkinje cell loss with cerebellar atrophy. Human lymphocyte antigen (HLA) DQ2 is found in 90% of patients; HLA DQ8 is present in the rest. Gluten sensitivity is the basis for recommending a diet free of wheat, barley, and rye.

Neurodegenerations with Brain Iron Accumulation

Fasting tests for iron metabolism include serum iron concentration (SI), total iron binding capacity (TIBC), percentage of transferrin saturation (*Tsat* = 100 × SI/TIBC), and serum ferritin. **Ferritin** (like copper and melanin) causes high T1W signal and low T2W signal on brain MRI. High ferritin with high *Tsat* indicates hemochromatosis but with low *Tsat*, aceruloplasminemia.

Neurodegeneration with brain iron accumulation 1 (**NBIA-1 or PKAN**, pantothenate kinase-associated neurodegeneration, formerly Hallervorden-Spatz disease) is a progressive disorder of the first two decades of life, characterized by tremor, abnormal tone (rigidity, spasticity, dystonia), hyperreflexia, and **facial dystonia** with contracted platysma and *risus sardonicus*. Nystagmus, **retinitis pigmentosa,** and optic atrophy may occur. The abnormal *PANK2* gene (20p13) has homology to pantothenate kinase, is highly expressed in the brain and essential in CoA biosynthesis, and key in intermediary and fatty acid metabolism. T2W brain MRI shows hyperintensity within a region of hypointensity in the medial GP (**"eye of the tiger"**). Biopsy shows axonal spheroids, **neurofibrillary tangles, but no amyloid plaques.** Hypoprebetalipoproteinemia, acanthocytosis, retinitis pigmentosa, and pallidal degeneration (**HARP**) is part of the NBIA-1 spectrum.

Neuroferritinopathy (**NBIA-2,** ferritin light chain gene, *FTL1*, 19q13) is a progressive autosomal dominant disorder causing limb and/or action-specific facial dystonia (or oromandibular dyskinesia with tongue injury), chorea, or, rarely, parkinsonism. It may cause aphonia, dysphagia, and subcortical/frontal cognitive dysfunction. Serum **ferritin is low.** T2* MRI shows hypointensity within the dentate nuclei, red nuclei, substantia nigra, putamen, globus pallidus, thalami, and the prefrontal cortex. **Cavitation** in pallida and putamen may occur, giving an appearance almost indistinguishable from the eye of the tiger sign.

Aceruloplasminemia causes **diabetes, retinal degeneration,** and neurologic deficits, usually craniofacial (blepharospasm, grimacing, facial/neck dystonia), due to parenchymal iron accumulation from absent ceruloplasmin (Cp). **Ferritin is high** and **iron is low.** Cp is a ferroxidase, essential for mobilizing ferric iron from reticuloendothelial stores into transferrin. **Cp gene** (3q23) mutations raise tissue iron but not copper. T2* MRI shows *uniform* involvement of all basal ganglia and thalami but without cavitation. **Hypoceruloplasminemia** due to heterozygous nonsense mutation in the Cp gene may present with **ataxia,** dysarthria, and hyperreflexia. Plasma iron turnover requires only 5% of normal Cp, explaining the normal iron homeostasis in Wilson disease (WD).

PLA2G6-**associated neurodegeneration** (**PLAN**) may present by 14 months as progressive cerebellar ataxia with cognitive and motor regression, dystonia, axial hypotonia, limb spasticity, **optic atrophy,** and **strabismus (infantile neuroaxonal dystrophy).** Alternatively, it can manifest as early-onset L-dopa-responsive dystonia-parkinsonism with dementia and generalized or frontotemporal atrophy (**PARK14**). Iron deposition, when present, is restricted to the **globus pallidus and substantia nigra** (occasionally in the dentate) as well as cerebellar cortical atrophy and gliosis, a pattern similar to NBIA-1.

Acanthocytosis-Related Neurologic Disorders

Abetalipoproteinemia (Bassen-Kornzweig disease, microsomal triglyceride transfer protein [MTP] mutation, 4q) is associated with fat malabsorption from early childhood leading to hypotriglyceridemia, hypocholesterolemia, and vitamin E deficiency. It causes progressive spinocerebellar ataxia, peripheral neuropathy, dorsal column degeneration, and retinitis pigmentosa.

HARP syndrome is a variant of neurodegeneration with brain iron accumulation (NBAI-1; see "Iron and Neurology"), and consists of **H**ypoprebetalipoproteinemia, **A**canthocytosis, **R**etinitis pigmentosa, and **P**allidal degeneration, with normal vitamin E levels.

Chorea-acanthocytosis or "neuroacanthocytosis" (ChAc, VPS13A gene, chorein protein, 9q) presents with chorea or other movement disorders (including tics, dystonia, and parkinsonism), **orofaciolingual dyskinesias with tongue thrusting and lip biting,** dysarthria, dysphagia, vocalizations, seizures, frontal-dominant dementia, and axonal polyneuropathy with *areflexia.* Tongue and lip biting are part of a "feeding dystonia." Psychiatric features such as depression, anxiety, obsessive-compulsive disorder, and personality disorders are common. CK and liver enzymes are often elevated. **Caudate atrophy,** as in Huntington disease (HD), with high T2W signal in caudate and putamen, is seen in brain MRI. **Chorein** levels can be measured in peripheral blood using a Western blot assay. Genetic testing is not commercially available.

X-linked McLeod syndrome (MLS, *XK* gene, Xp21) is a nonataxic X-linked acanthocytosis affecting pairs of brothers or nephews and uncles but no male-to-male transmission. MLS presents in the fifth decade as myopathy, axonal neuropathy with *areflexia,* increased CK, and dilated cardiomyopathy associated with an abnormal Kell blood group antigen expression. A **Huntington disease–like phenotype** develops in 50% of patients with chorea, subcortical dementia, psychiatric abnormalities, and seizures. **Caudate atrophy** may also be present.

Huntington disease–like 2 (HDL2, *JPH3* gene, encoding *junctophilin 3* protein) is an autosomal dominant disorder only reported in patients of African ancestry.

FAPED, autosomal dominant familial acanthocytosis with paroxysmal exertion-induced dyskinesias and epilepsy, is a rare neuroacanthocytosis syndrome of otherwise normal subjects with paroxysmal phenomena and acanthocytosis. It has been recently traced to a glucose transporter mutation.

Acanthocytes are found when native blood with saline and heparin (10 U/mL) in a 1:1 ratio create >6.3% spiculated cells. Diagnostic tests include CK and liver enzymes (elevated in ChAc, MLS), phenotyping of Kx and Kell erythrocyte antigens (MLS), lipoprotein electrophoresis, and perhaps gene analysis of *XK* (MLS), *VPS13A* (ChAc), *JPH3* (HDL2), and *PANK2* (PKAN).

Dystonia

Sustained muscle contractions of the same group of agonists and antagonists muscles produce abnormal postures or repetitive action-specific movements that are exacerbated by voluntary movements. Younger-onset dystonia (DYT) tends to begin in the arm or leg and generalize, whereas older onset often begins in the face or neck and remains focal.

Classification of Dystonia
Parentheses indicate chromosome localization.

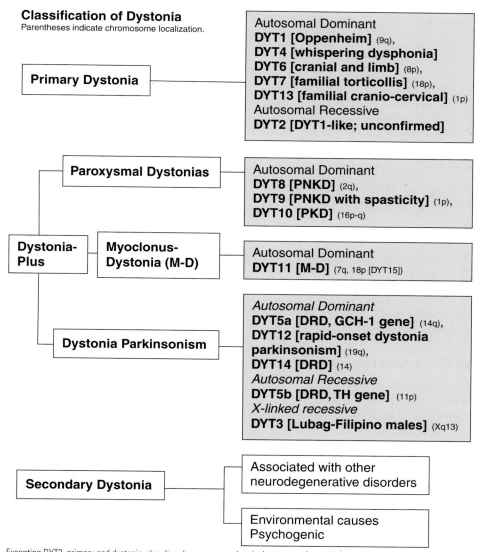

Primary Dystonia

Autosomal Dominant
DYT1 [Oppenheim] (9q),
DYT4 [whispering dysphonia]
DYT6 [cranial and limb] (8p),
DYT7 [familial torticollis] (18p),
DYT13 [familial cranio-cervical] (1p)
Autosomal Recessive
DYT2 [DYT1-like; unconfirmed]

Dystonia-Plus

Paroxysmal Dystonias

Autosomal Dominant
DYT8 [PNKD] (2q),
DYT9 [PNKD with spasticity] (1p),
DYT10 [PKD] (16p-q)

Myoclonus-Dystonia (M-D)

Autosomal Dominant
DYT11 [M-D] (7q, 18p [DYT15])

Dystonia Parkinsonism

Autosomal Dominant
DYT5a [DRD, GCH-1 gene] (14q),
DYT12 [rapid-onset dystonia parkinsonism] (19q),
DYT14 [DRD] (14)
Autosomal Recessive
DYT5b [DRD, TH gene] (11p)
X-linked recessive
DYT3 [Lubag-Filipino males] (Xq13)

Secondary Dystonia

Associated with other neurodegenerative disorders

Environmental causes Psychogenic

Excepting DYT3, primary and dystonia-plus disorders are neurochemical, not neurodegenerative.

Primary Dystonias

DYT1 (Oppenheim's Dystonia, Generalized Primary Torsion Dystonia [PTD])

DYT1 accounts for 90% of early limb-onset dystonia among **Ashkenazi Jews,** in whom **penetrance is 30%,** and in 40%-60% of similar non-Jewish cases. The earlier the age at onset, the greater the likelihood of generalization. The **GAG deletion** (9q34) with glutamic acid loss causes a mutation in **torsinA, a heat-shock, ATP-binding protein** localized in the **nuclear envelope** (as with other "nuclear envelope diseases" such as Emery-Dreifuss muscular dystrophy or LGMD1B, CMT-2, and THAP1) and widely distributed but intensely expressed in nigral compacta (SNpc) neurons. Although brain MRI is normal, fluorodeoxyglucose positron emission tomography (FDG PET) shows increased lenticular and decreased thalamic metabolic activity (from increased direct striatopallidal activity). Because there is only one mutation identified from a single mutation event or founder mutation, routine genetic testing is possible. Mutation testing is recommended for all those with PTD beginning before the age of 26 years, or later if there are relatives with earlier onset of symptoms.

DYT4 (Whispering Dysphonia)

This "non-DYT1 PTD" has been reported in one family with whispering dysphonia, psychiatric symptoms, and focal or generalized dystonia.

DYT6 (Cranial and Limb [Mixed] Type)

This condition frequently starts in craniocervical muscles, in adolescents, and may be associated with severe dysphonia and dysarthria, and progression to the upper body without generalization. It is caused by mutations in the large THAP domain-containing protein 1 (**THAP1,** 8p21-q22), which may disrupt the nuclear localization signal and prevent the protein product from entering the nucleus. DYT6 is more common in Amish-Mennonite and European families.

DYT7 (Familial Focal Dystonia; 18p)

Adult-onset focal dystonia (torticollis, writer's cramp, dysphonia, or blepharospasm) is most prevalent. The unknown mutated gene in 18p may be inherited with low penetrance from a common ancestor in northern Germany.

DYT13 (Familial Cervical-Cranial Predominant)

Mostly of adult onset, DYT13 remains restricted to the craniocervical segmental region or slowly progress to the upper limbs. Mapped in one Italian family to **chromosome 1p,** DYT13 is thought to be allelic to PARK7/*DJ-1* parkinsonism.

DYT2 (Autosomal Recessive PTD)

It is debatable as to whether it exists. It was described in three consanguineous families of Spanish gypsies, with a phenotype resembling DYT1.

Sporadic idiopathic adult-onset dystonia has an uncertain etiology but there are an increased number of polymorphisms in allele 2 of the D5 receptor gene.

Dystonia-Plus

Paroxysmal: DYT8: Paroxysmal nonkinesigenic dyskinesia (PNKD, myofibrillogenesis regulator 1 (*MR-1*) gene, 2q) begins in infancy and early childhood, with attacks of dystonia or choreoathetosis, lasting from 10 minutes to 1 hour, precipitated by caffeine, alcohol, and emotional stress. Response to benzodiazepines is excellent.

Paroxysmal: DYT9: PNKD with episodic ataxia and spasticity (KCNA3, 1p) is phenotypically similar to DYT8 dystonia, with episodic dystonia and paresthesias with additional dysarthria, diplopia, ataxia and spastic paraparesis.

Paroxysmal: DYT10: Paroxysmal kinesigenic dyskinesia (PKD, 16p-q), the most frequent of paroxysmal dyskinesias, occurs in multiple (up to 100/d) and brief (<5 minutes) attacks precipitated by sudden movements or startle, and is relieved by antiepileptics.

DYT11: Myoclonus-Dystonia (ε-sarcoglycan [SGCE] gene, 7q21; 18 p locus) begins in childhood and adolescence with a slowly or nonprogressive course and dramatic response to alcohol. The upper body, especially neck and arms, are involved most often. Depression, alcoholism, obsessive-compulsive disorder, and anxiety cosegregate with the disease gene. Maternal imprinting leads to reduced penetrance if the disease is inherited from the mother.

Dystonia Parkinsonism

DYT3: X-linked dystonia-parkinsonism ("*Lubag:*" *shuffling*; Xq13, TAF1) is a founder-mutation disorder, frequent in males from the island of Panay in the Philippines, has complete penetrance by the end of the fifth decade. Mutations reduce expression of transcription factor TATA-box binding protein associated factor 1 (TAF1), which decreases D2 receptors. Cranial or generalized dystonia, action tremor, and parkinsonism may be combined or in isolation. Heterozygote females may have mild dystonia or chorea. This is the **only primary dystonia with a pathologic correlate:** neuronal loss and astrocytosis ("mosaic gliosis") in the caudate nucleus and lateral putamen.

DYT12: Rapid-onset dystonia-parkinsonism (RDP, 19q13, ATP1A3) consists of rostrocaudally progressing dystonia and tremorless parkinsonism with prominent bulbar findings (dysarthria, grimacing), evolving over hours to weeks, in adolescents and young adults. There is poor response to levodopa. **CSF HVA levels** are low. The causal ***ATP1A3* gene** is linked to the α3 subunit of the Na/K-ATPase. A positive family history is not required to suspect the diagnosis.

DYT16: Young-onset dystonia-parkinsonism (2q31, PRKRA) described in a few families with progressive, generalized, early-onset dystonia with axial muscle involvement, oromandibular (sardonic smile), laryngeal dystonia, and, in some cases, levodopa-unresponsive parkinsonism.

DYT5: Dopa-responsive dystonia-parkinsonism (DRD; Segawa syndrome)

(Also see "Dopamine and Catecholamine Pathways")

DRD starts in childhood and presents as a dystonic gait with diurnal worsening and progression to all four limbs. The phenotype includes juvenile- and adult-onset parkinsonism, adult-onset oromandibular dystonia, spasticity mimicking CP, and exercise-induced limb dystonia. **Hyperreflexia** may occur. There is a dramatic response to low doses of levodopa and, in some, to anticholinergics. **Fluorodopa PET and [123I] beta-CIT SPECT** (single photon emission computed tomography) **scans are normal.** Substantia nigra neurons are hypopigmented but normal.

- **GTP cyclohydrolase I (*GCH1*** mutations [DYT5a, 14q; AD]) affects the rate-limiting enzyme in the biosynthesis of **tetrahydrobiopterin,** BH$_4$, a cofactor for tyrosine hydroxylase (dopamine and norepinephrine), tryptophan hydroxylase (serotonin), and phenylalanine hydroxylase. This DRD is more common in girls and is 30% penetrant. CSF biopterin and neopterin are low. **Hyperphenylalaninemia** ("atypical PKU [phenylketonuria]") and GCH activity assay (<20% of the mean in controls) in blood cells are useful biochemical markers. The tyrosine hydroxylase activity is markedly reduced.
- **Other biopterin metabolism deficiencies** comprise the rare autosomal recessive disorders 6-pyruvoyltetrahydropterin synthase deficiency, dihydropteridine reductase deficiency, and sepiapterin reductase deficiency. These levodopa-responsive disorders may show mental retardation, epileptic seizures, hypotonia, or myoclonus with or without basal ganglia calcification.
- **Aromatic amino acid decarboxylase (AADC) deficiency (7p12; AR)** is suspected when parkinsonism in infants is associated with episodes of oculogyric crisis, dystonia, and limb rigidity with catecholamine-related deficits (hyperhidrosis, miosis, ptosis, nasal congestion, temperature and blood pressure lability, and abnormal sleep). There is reduced metabolism of both 5-hydroxytryptophan (5-HTP) to serotonin (low hydroxyindole acetic acid, HIAA) and L-dopa to dopamine (low homovanillic acid, HVA). In contrast to primary biopterin disorders, the level of 3-O methyldopa (3-O-MD) and 5-HTP is elevated. Patients respond to *dopamine agonists* with pyridoxine and anticholinergics but not to L-dopa.
- **Tyrosine hydroxylase deficiency (mutations in TH [DYT5b, 11p; AR])** should be suspected in infants with severe dystonia, parkinsonism, hypotonia, ptosis, and psychomotor delay.

Nongenetic testing for DRD (necessary, as there is no common mutation):
- **Phenylalanine loading** results in hyperphenylalaninemia without elevation of tyrosine and suggests GCH-1 or biopterin deficiency. The test is normal in DRD associated with tyrosine hydroxylase deficiency.
- **Biopterin level** (decreased), if above is positive, to distinguish it from the hyperphenylalaninemia of phenylketonuria carriers.
- **[11C] Raclopride PET** shows increased D2-receptor binding in symptomatic and asymptomatic gene carriers, suggesting up-regulation of postsynaptic receptors or reduced competition for ligand because of decreased dopamine.

Secondary Dystonias

Causative lesions mostly involve the basal ganglia and, especially, the **putamen.** Thalamus, cortex, cerebellum, brainstem, and spinal cord are less common dystonia-producing regions.

SELECTED CAUSES OF SECONDARY DYSTONIA

Autosomal Dominant	Autosomal Recessive
Huntington disease	Wilson disease [Cu-ATPase gene on 13q] Neuroacanthocytosis
SCA3/MJD	Niemann-Pick type C (cholesterol esterification, 18)
Other SCAs	Gangliosidoses (GM1 and GM2)
DRPLA	Metachromatic leukodystrophy
Neuroferritinopathy (19q13)	Lesch-Nyhan syndrome
X-Linked Recessive	Homocystinuria
Lesch-Nyhan syndrome	Methylmalonic/propionic aciduria
Pelizaeus-Merzbacher	Glutaric aciduria
Deafness-dystonia	Hartnup disease
X-dominant: Rett syndrome	Neuronal ceroid lipofuscinosis
Mitochondrial	Ataxia-telangiectasia
	Familial BG calcifications
MERRF, MELAS	Neurodegeneration with brain iron accumulation-1
Leigh syndrome	Neuronal intranuclear hyaline inclusion disease
LHON	

DRPLA, dentatorubropallidoluysian atrophy; BG, basal ganglia.

Acquired dystonia may arise from encephalitis (including subacute sclerosing panencephalitis, human immunodeficiency virus, and CJD), head trauma, stroke, MS, tumor, pontine myelinolysis, primary antiphospholipid syndrome, hypoparathyroidism, and drug use (levodopa, dopamine D2 receptor blocking drugs [DRBA], ergotism, and anticonvulsants).

Delayed-onset dystonia occurs in symptomatic dystonias resulting from **static brain lesions** (hypoxic, pontine myelinolysis, head trauma, cyanide intoxication). A delayed onset is also seen in postcoma dystonia after the ingestion of mildewed sugar cane whose 3-nitroproprionic acid (3-NP), a complex II mitochondrial toxin, causes striatal necrosis.

Pseudodystonia (mimic torsion dystonia but do not represent true dystonia)
- Sandifer syndrome (see "Paroxysmal Movement Disorders")
- Stiff-person syndrome (see "SPS")
- Isaacs syndrome: continuous muscle activity or neuromyotonia due to motor nerve fiber hyperexcitability
- **Schwartz-Jampel syndrome** (generalized stiffness from myotonia associated with blepharospasm, blepharophimosis, dwarfism, pinched face with low-set ears, joint limitation, contractures, and bone dysplasia)
- **Satoyoshi syndrome** (painful, intermittent muscle spasms, malabsorption, endocrinopathy with amenorrhea, skeletal abnormalities, and alopecia areata)

Other conditions include rotational atlantoaxial subluxation, congenital Klippel-Feil anomaly, Chiari malformation, posterior fossa tumor, syringomyelia, trochlear nerve palsy, and vestibular torticollis.

Tardive Dystonia

As the most frequent form of symptomatic dystonia and the third most common tardive syndrome, tardive dystonia (TD) is a late (*tardive*) and persistent complication of treatment with **dopamine receptor blocking** agents (DRBA) that occur more often in young males. TD presents either focally (oromandibular dystonia) or segmentally with **retrocollis,** extension of the elbows, internal rotation of the shoulders, and flexion of the wrists and may be associated with the more common classic tardive dyskinesia and/or tardive akathisia (feelings of inner restlessness in which moaning is prominent). The required drug withdrawal may be associated with initial symptomatic worsening. **Dopamine depletors** reserpine (0.1 mg/d and increased by 0.1 mg weekly to a maximum of 2 mg/d) and tetrabenazine (12.5 mg tid increased by 12.5 mg weekly to a maximum of 250 mg/d) are the preferred treatment (side effects may include parkinsonism, depression, and orthostatic hypotension) followed by anticholinergics. The addition of baclofen or benzodiazepines may provide further benefit.

> **Non-antipsychotic DRBAs** are used to treat nausea (phenothiazines thiethylperazine [Torecan] and prochlorperazine [Compazine] as well as the substituted benzamides metoclopramide [Reglan], sulpiride, tiapride, and clebopride), depression (tricyclic *amoxapine* [Asendin], *perphenazine/amitriptyline* [Triavil]), cough (*promethazine* [Phenergan]), hypertension (calcium channel blockers *flunarizine* and *cinnarizine*), menopausal flushes (*veralipride*), and Tourette syndrome (*pimozide* [Orap]).

TD may result from **D2 receptor blockade** (the atypical antipsychotics clozapine and quetiapine bind to D4 and $5HT_{2a}$ rather than D2 receptors) and **sensitization of the D1 receptor** (supported by the delayed TD latency, worsening after drug withdrawal, and benefit with bromocriptine, partial D1 antagonist and D2 agonist).

Tardive dyskinesia is more common in older women with a longer, and especially intermittent, exposure to neuroleptics. It has a cumulative incidence of 5% per year. The oral-buccal-lingual region is affected to a greater extent than the limbs and trunks. **Dopaminergic and anticholinergic agents** may increase the severity of the stereotypic abnormal movements. The similar **tardive chorea** occurs in children as part of the **withdrawal emergent syndrome** when DRBA has been discontinued suddenly. It resolves within 6 weeks.

Acute Dystonic Reaction

Acute dystonic reaction (ADR) appears within days from treatment with DRBA or such drugs as amitriptyline, fluoxetine, phenytoin, and dextromethorphan. Ocular (*oculogyric crisis*) and craniocervical muscles (open mouth, tongue protrusion, retrocollis) are most often affected. The treatment requires withdrawal of the offending agent and IV diphenhydramine (Benadryl) 50–100 mg, benztropine (Cogentin) 1–2 mg, or chlorpheniramine, 10–50 mg. Tetrabenazine (but not reserpine) may induce ADR given its D2 dopamine blocking, in addition to depleting, properties. Prophylactic use of anticholinergics with neuroleptic treatment reduces ADR risk.

Treatment Pearls in Dystonia

- **Levodopa** should be given to all patients with childhood or adolescent generalized or segmental dystonia as a trial to address the highly treatable DRD. Doses of <300 mg are usually effective in DRD and this treatment, contrary to what occurs in juvenile Parkinson disease (PD), does not lead in dystonia to levodopa-induced motor fluctuations or dyskinesias.

- **Anticholinergics** (trihexyphenidyl and benztropine) are second-line agents in DRD and other dystonias, as up to 50% respond at least moderately. Peripheral anticholinergic symptoms such as urinary retention and blurry vision can be treated with pyridostigmine (anticholinesterase) and pilocarpine (muscarinic agonist), respectively. Cognitive impairment and hallucinations are potential risks.

- **Baclofen** (GABA$_B$ agonist) is the third-line agent, and fairly dramatic response may occur in children with generalized dystonia, cerebral palsy, and adults with oromandibular dystonia. **Intrathecal baclofen** may be considered for patients with secondary spastic dystonia, dystonia of trunks and legs, and "dystonic storm." Benefits may not be sustained.

- **Dopamine depletors** (tetrabenazine and reserpine) are especially beneficial in tardive dystonia and are preferred over dopamine blockers because they do not cause parkinsonism or tardive dyskinesia. Tetrabenazine, however, may cause acute dystonic reaction.

- **Clonazepam** with or without other benzodiazepines, carbamazepine, and tetrabenazine may be used if above regimens fail.

- **"Marsden cocktail"** includes tetrabenazine, a dopamine blocker, and an anticholinergic, and has been suggested for complicated or difficult-to-treat generalized primary dystonias. Dopamine receptor blocker agents are not recommended because of the tardive side effects.

- **Botulinum toxin** (BTX-A [cleaves SNAP-25, synaptosome-associated protein] and BTX-B [cleaves synaptobrevin/VAMP-2: vesicle-associated membrane protein]) has become the treatment of choice for focal and segmental dystonias. It is also used in generalized dystonia in conjunction with other drugs, for the most disabling or painful muscles.

- **Surgery: Pallidotomy and pallidal stimulation** are used when drugs have failed to improve generalized dystonia. Bilateral pallidal stimulation and unilateral lesion with contralateral chronic stimulation have been shown to provide better outcomes than bilateral pallidotomy.

Although the pathogenesis of primary dystonia is not fully understood, there is evidence of diminished and irregular output from the basal ganglia (GPi/SNr), resulting from **hyperactivity of both the direct (D1) and indirect (D2)** pathways. Because lesioning the medial pallidum can improve symptoms, it has been suggested that it may be the pattern of firing, and not the rate, that is pathogenic in basal ganglia output.

Parkinson Disease

Parkinson disease (PD) is a clinical diagnosis based on the triad of asymmetric L-dopa-responsive tremor, rigidity, and bradykinesia. Several risk factors have been identified:

- **Toxic exposure:** 1-methyl-4-phenyl-1,2,3,6-tetrahydropyridine **(MPTP),** viruses (encephalitis lethargica), herbicides (paraquat), insecticides (rotenone), pesticides, well water, solvents (trichloroethylene).
- **Mitochondrial dysfunction:** MPTP-induced inhibition of complex I of the electron transport chain (40% decrease in complex I activity in substantia nigra pars compacta [SNc])
- **Excitotoxicity:** excessive glutamatergic drive from an overactive subthalamic nucleus (STN), activating NMDA receptors and increasing intracellular levels of calcium
- **Low uric acid:** high urate among PD patients predicts slower decline.
- **Low nicotine:** Cigarette smoking, smokeless tobacco, and passive tobacco exposure are inversely associated with the risk of PD
- **Genetic predisposition:** see "Genetic Considerations in PD."

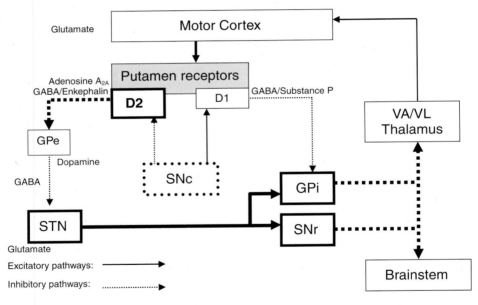

Dopamine deficiency causes overactivity of the indirect pathway, leading to excessive glutamatergic drive to the GPi/SNr, and reduction of the inhibitory GABAergic direct pathway, which combine to greatly suppress the thalamus and motor cortex (explaining akinesia, and to a lesser extent rigidity, and tremor) and brainstem (abnormalities of gait and posture). The model does not explain the reduction in tremor following thalamotomy and the improvement in dyskinesia (without hemiballism) after pallidotomy.

The **ventrolateral SNc and the dorsal putamen** undergo earliest neuronal loss in PD. **Ubiquitin-positive Lewy bodies** are also found in the nucleus basalis of Meynert, locus coeruleus, raphe nuclei, cingulate and entorhinal cortex, olfactory bulb, sympathetic ganglia, and parasympathetic gut neurons.

Genetics of Parkinson Disease

Despite a familial tendency, segregation ratios in PD are low and the disease is believed to be **polygenic** in nature. Twin studies have shown a very high concordance rate in monozygotic twins if the age of onset was below 50 years, **supporting a primarily inherited cause in *early-onset* PD.** Possibly a longer interval to disease onset in a second twin may account for a lower concordance rate among late-onset dizygotic twin PD patients. Considering PD at all ages, longitudinal studies using ^{18}F-dopa PET as a marker of preclinical presynaptic nigrostriatal dopaminergic integrity, found a 75% concordance in monozygotic and 22% in dizygotic twins.

Hypotheses for the genetic pathogenesis of Parkinson disease

- **Ubiquitin-proteasomal system for removal of misfolded or damaged proteins,** which naturally form **defective ribosomal products (DriPs).** Control mechanisms ensure that the DriPs are immediately removed by becoming tagged with **ubiquitin,** a molecule that targets DriPs to the **26S proteasome,** which breaks DriPs into small peptides with the assistance of **ubiquitin C-terminal hydrolase (UCH-L1).** Ubiquitin-activating (E1), ubiquitin-conjugating (E2), and ubiquitin-protein ligase (E3) enzymes are required for tagging any protein with ubiquitin. The ubiquitin-protein ligase **E3** has been recognized in dopaminergic neurons as **parkin.** UCH-L1 is the enzyme involved in the deconjugation of ubiquitin from DriPs.
- **Mitochondrial dysfunction** caused by reduction in mitochondrial complex I activity (pesticide rotenone and MPTP) and increased iron with decreased glutathione in the nigrostriatal system. Oxidative stress also indirectly inhibits the highly ATP-dependent proteasome system, leading to the formation of Lewy body-like inclusions immunoreactive for α-synuclein in rats.

Familial diseases that can mimic Parkinson disease include X-linked dystonia-parkinsonism **(Lubag),** spinocerebellar ataxias 2 and 3 **(SCA 2, SCA3/MJD),** frontotemporal dementia with parkinsonism linked to chromosome 17 **(FTDP-17),** Wilson disease, and Huntington disease.

Parkin and α-synuclein

Disease-causing *parkin* mutations can be homozygous, compound heterozygous (with two mutations on alternate alleles), or single-allele microdeletion or missense mutation with dominant effect. Parkin haploinsufficiency may be sufficient for disease in some cases.

- *Overexpression of α-synuclein,* which is ubiquitous in the human brain, causes oxidative stress, aggregation, and replicates PD features in mice.
- *The common pathway for parkin and α-synuclein* presumably resides in the accumulation of aging and mutant α-synuclein no longer tagged by ubiquitin (especially parkin) in order to be degraded by the 26S proteasome through *synphilin-1.*

Imaging in Parkinson's Disease and Other Parkinsonisms

ABNORMALITIES PER DISEASE ACCORDING TO THREE IMAGING MODALITIES

Diagnosis	(^{123}I) β-CIT SPECT	[^{18}F] F-dopa PET	FDG-PET
ET	Normal uptake	Normal uptake	Th and medulla hypermetabolism
PD	Asymmetric low uptake (Put < Cau)	Asymmetric low uptake (Put < Cau)	Put/Pall and Th hypermetabolism
PSP	Symmetric low uptake (Put = Cau)	Symmetric low uptake (Put = Cau)	Symmetric low uptake (Put = Cau), frontal, midbrain
MSA	Asymmetric low uptake (Put < Cau)	Asymmetric low uptake (Put < Cau)	Asymmetric low metabolism (Put, Cau, cerebellum)
CBD	Asymmetric low uptake (Put = Cau)	Asymmetric low uptake (Put = Cau)	Asymmetric low metabolism (Put, Cau, Th, frontal, inf. parietal)

(^{123}I) β-CIT SPECT, iodine-123 2β-carboxymethoxy-3β-[4-iodophenyl] tropane SPECT (single photon emission computed tomography); F-dopa, fluorodopa; PET, positron emission tomography; FDG, fluorodeoxyglucose; ET, essential tremor; Th, thalamus; Put, putamen; Cau, caudate; Pall, pallidum; PSP, progressive supranuclear palsy; MSA, multiple system atrophy; CBD, corticobasal degeneration.

(^{123}I) β-CIT SPECT assesses the striatal-to-cerebellar ratio uptake of iodine-123 by the **dopamine transporter (DAT),** which is a presynaptic dopaminergic terminal protein that controls dopamine levels by active sodium-chloride-dependent reuptake. DAT is the primary mechanism of dopamine removal from the region of the synaptic cleft and is specific to dopaminergic neurons. Although (^{123}I) β-CIT SPECT does not assess the density of nigrostriatal neurons, it provides *in vivo* information about nigrostriatal degeneration. It differentiates clinically probable PD from healthy subjects and ET with a sensitivity of more than 90%. The SPECT abnormalities diminish with disease progression because of advanced presynaptic nigrostriatal pathology.

[^{18}F]F-DOPA uptake reflects nigrostriatal dopamine-storage capacity and enzymatic decarboxylase activity as a measure of nigrostriatal neuronal integrity. It may detect a nigrostriatal defect several years prior to the onset of clinical manifestations in PD.

FDG-PET assesses the glucose metabolism patterns and is more helpful in the differentiation of parkinsonian syndromes (PD vs. MSA, PSP, and CBD) early in the disease process. The hallmark of glucose metabolism in PD patients is increased metabolism in the putamen and globus pallidus, bilaterally without regard to the affected side. Increased metabolism may also be observed in the ventral thalamus, motor cortex, and cerebellum. This technique has 100% sensitivity and 86% specificity in the identification of early PD patients. A sensitivity of 96% and a specificity of 91% were achieved for PD patients compared with patients with atypical parkinsonism.

Medical Therapy for Parkinson Disease

Treatment-resistant symptoms are dysarthria, freezing of gait (during "on" time), postural instability, dysautonomia, and cognitive dysfunction. For each of these, the response to the treatments listed below tends to be suboptimal.

- **Levodopa** is the most effective treatment for PD. Drug-induced problems are **motor fluctuations** (wearing off and on-off fluctuations due to erratic absorption, especially causing "delayed-on"), **dyskinesias** (peak dose, diphasic, off dystonia), and **psychiatric** (vivid dreams, hallucinations, mania, hypersexuality). Both pre- and postsynaptic degeneration with disease progression shorten therapeutic response.
- **Dopamine agonists** (DA) may be used prior to, or along with, levodopa. Although they do not improve motor disability to the same extent, motor fluctuations and dyskinesias are less frequent. **Pleuropulmonary and retroperitoneal fibrosis** and **erythromelalgia** were complications of ergot-derived dopamine agonists (bromocriptine and pergolide), no longer available. Nonergot agents (ropinirole, pramipexole, rotigotine [transdermal patch]) have greater D3 selectivity. **Ankle edema, hallucinations,** and **somnolence** are more frequent with DA than with levodopa.
- **Selegiline and rasagiline** (selective MAO-B inhibitors) may reduce motor fluctuations. **Serotonin syndrome** may occur if selegiline is administered concurrently with meperidine and other opiates, tricyclic antidepressants, or serotonin reuptake inhibitors.
- **Amantadine** is highly effective against dyskinesias through its NMDA-blocking effect. It may cause ankle edema and livedo reticularis.
- **Catechol O-methyltransferase (COMT) inhibitors** (tolcapone, and entacapone) prolong levodopa half-life and bioavailability, increasing daily "on" time and reducing levodopa need. Diarrhea may require withdrawal in about 3% of cases. Liver insufficiency may develop with tolcapone, which requires periodic monitoring of liver enzymes.
- **Anticholinergics (trihexyphenidyl** and **benztropine)** are used only in early stages and young patients for control of tremor. It has negligible effects on bradykinesia and rigidity. Besides the well-known peripheral side effects, central ones include sedation, memory difficulties, confusion, and hallucinations.
- **Clozapine and quetiapine** are the only atypical neuroleptics that do not worsen parkinsonism. Despite the risk of agranulocytosis, which forces to monitor with weekly blood counts, clozapine also improves other symptoms such as tremor, akathisia, and dyskinesias. Risperidone and olanzapine are capable of worsening parkinsonian deficits.
- **Subcutaneous apomorphine** injections are considered a "rescue" medication in refractory motor fluctuations. Effective doses are between 4 and 6 mg, response latencies between 10 and 15 minutes, and duration of effect around 90 minutes. Blood eosinophilia and red itchy nodules at injection sites have been reported as complications. Continuous subcutaneous infusions (minipump) minimize motor fluctuations and may reduce preexistent dyskinesias but are not available in the United States. Autoimmune hemolytic anemia has been reported with its use.

Surgery for Parkinson Disease

It is indicated in the fluctuating, increasingly intractable patient, in whom motor fluctuations or dyskinesias have become disabling. Bilateral high-frequency chronic deep brain stimulation (DBS) is a safer alternative than ablative procedures in disrupting or inhibiting neuronal activity and does not preclude the use of therapies that depend on the basal ganglia integrity. Stimulation parameters may be tailored postoperatively for best benefit. Both ablation and DBS of the **GPi** and, to a greater extent, the overactive **STN** cause **activation of the premotor and supplementary motor areas** associated with improvement.

DBS imitates the effects of a permanent lesion and matches the best antiparkinsonian effect of levodopa. Possible mechanisms include (1) *"depolarization block"*: constant neuronal depolarization, (2) *"neural jamming"*: disruption of the network by additional impulses generated by the stimulation, (3) *"net inhibition"*: preferential activation of inhibitory neurons when driven at high rates, and/or (4) *"para resonance"*: different nerve thresholds during stimulation at different frequencies generate action potentials or neuronal blockade. Different levels of current in the STN, therefore, may elicit the entire spectrum of motor phenomena of PD. The effects are both **frequency-dependent** (slow rates of Vim stimulation increase tremor whereas fast rates inhibit it) and **polarity-dependent** (negative [cathodic] polarity is more effective than positive polarity). Stimulation has a preferential effect on the speed of motor execution (greater in STN than GPi) rather than reaction time.

- **GPi DBS:** Stimulation of the ventral GPi has the greatest **antidyskinetic** effect with alleviation of rigidity but possibly more akinesia. Stimulation of the dorsal GPi results in greater antiparkinsonian effect but may cause stimulation-induced dyskinesias, possibly as a result of current spread to the GPe, which can be adjusted during programming. GPi DBS may take days or even weeks to reach maximal benefit. **Pallidotomy** is rarely done given the proximity to the internal capsule and optic radiation and the permanent dysphagia, dysarthria, and cognitive impairment associated with bilateral lesions.

- **STN (dorsolateral) DBS:** Reduces **akinesia, rigidity,** and **tremor.** The latter two are reduced within 30 seconds but the beneficial effects on akinesia may take minutes. **It reduces dyskinesias by reducing the need for medications.** There is a 50%–60% reduction in the "off" medication UPDRS score. STN DBS is the procedure of choice and may (neuroprotective hypothesis) halt degeneration of the nigra by limiting the excessive glutamatergic output to the SNc and GPi/SNr.

- **Vim Thalamic DBS:** Reduces contralateral **tremor** as effectively as STN DBS, although it is not as useful to lessen other, potentially more disabling parkinsonian deficits.

Levodopa-induced Dyskinesias

The dyskinesia threshold decreases with progression of disease, whereas the antiparkinsonian threshold remains more constant (and antiparkinsonian efficacy persists unchanged). The early use of dopamine agonists appears to reduce the cumulative exposure to L-dopa and significantly decreases the risk of developing Levodopa-induced dyskinesia (LID), which supports delaying the initiation of L-dopa treatment in PD patients.

Off Dystonia	Monophasic Dyskinesia (Peak-Dose Dyskinesia)	Diphasic Dyskinesia (Onset and End of Dose)
Flexed **dystonic** posture, Foot flexion and inversion Toes clenched or great toe extended	Mainly **choreic** **Upper limbs**, face, trunk Most affected side or **bilateral and axial**	Mainly **ballistic**, dystonic **Lower limbs** Most affected side
"**Off**": Antiparkinsonian medications are worn off⁺	"**On**": Maximal effect of antiparkinsonian drugs	**Transition** between "off" and "on" states
Underactive indirect (D2) striatal output to GPe	**Overactive direct (D1)** striatal output to GPi/SNr	Unclear pathophysiology

⁺Off dystonia disappears after 24 hours have elapsed since the withdrawal of L-dopa and after chronic STN DBS. Low-voltage STN DBS may induce onset-of-dose dyskinesias and higher voltage leads to typical peak-dose dyskinesias.

Necessary elements for the development of LID:
- **Pulsatile (instead of continuous) L-dopa** or selective short-acting D1 or D2 agonist administration. The long half-life of most dopamine agonists may explain their reduced tendency for inducing LID.
- **Nigrostriatal denervation with intact striatal outflow** (MSA, PSP, or any conditions with damage to striatal outflow rarely exhibit LID).

Pathophysiologic underpinnings of LID:
- **Underactive basal ganglia output regions (GPi/SNr)** are due to:
  - **Overactive direct (D1-mediated)** striatal output pathway, possibly driven by **hyperfunction of NMDA receptors.**
  - **Underactive indirect (D2-mediated)** striatal output pathway, possibly driven by **GABA_A receptor upregulation** and causing *GPe overactivity* and subsequent STN underactivity.
- **Striatal increase in preproenkephalin (PPE) and ΔFosB** (chronic Fos-related proteins) are caused by pulsatile treatment with D1 agonists.

Management steps to minimize LID include: (1) Reduction of L-dopa dose or replacement of some of it with a dopamine agonist; (2) add amantadine (NMDA antagonist) or clozapine; (3) try apomorphine subcutaneous pump (not available in the United States); and (4) consider neurosurgical treatments (GPi or STN DBS, or pallidotomy where DBS is not available or practical). Current animal and early human studies are encouraging for the role of glutamate receptor antagonists (reduce D1 output), cannabinoid receptor antagonists, and α2 adrenergic receptor antagonist (inhibits GPe), adenosine A_{2A} receptor antagonist, and 5-HT$_{1A}$-receptor agonists.

Genetic Considerations in Parkinson's Disease

Juvenile parkinsonism, defined as onset of disease before the age of 21 years, has been associated only with *Parkin/PARK2* and *SNCA/PARK1* gene mutations. **Mutations in *Parkin/PARK2, PINK1/PARK6,* and *DJ-1/PARK7*** are considered the classic examples of young-onset parkinsonism with slow disease course. **LRRK2/PARK8-associated parkinsonism** most closely resemble idiopathic PD.

Autosomal recessive Parkinson disease

1. **PARK2** (*parkin* gene [ubiquitin protein ligase]; 6q25) is found in almost 50% of "early-onset" and 80% of patients with onset before age 30. Multiple loss-of-function mutations have been reported. Unequivocal "Parkin disease" is currently made when homozygote or compound heterozygote deletion is found, although heterozygotes are at increased risk for later-onset PD. The classic clinical features are slow progression, dystonic gait at onset, hyperreflexia, **diurnal fluctuation (sleep benefit),** marked response to levodopa with early dyskinesias and psychiatric side effects, and lack of dementia or severe dysautonomia. Pathologically, there is depigmentation of the substantia nigra (SNpc) **without Lewy bodies.** The occasional presence of tau-positive neurofibrillary tangles and neuropil threads with few or no senile plaques is inconsistent with comorbid AD. The parkin gene has 12 exons, of which 3, 4 (earliest onset), and 5 are the most likely to cause PD.
2. **PARK6** (phosphatase and tensin homologue [PTEN-induced putative kinase 1 [*PINK1*] gene; 1p35 [original *Marsala* kindred]) is associated with prominent tremor, **earlier onset (30s), and slower progression** with longer disease duration than idiopathic PD. Early drug-induced dyskinesias are present *without* dystonia or sleep benefit. However, atypical cases have been reported with dystonia at onset, sleep benefit, and even dementia.
3. **PARK7** (*DJ-1* gene; 1p36) causes **early-onset,** asymmetric, slow progressing, levodopa-responsive parkinsonism with **absent rest tremor** and increased likelihood of **focal dystonia** (blepharospasm). It may be allelic to DYT13 (familial craniocervical primary dystonia).
4. **PARK9** (*ATP13A2* gene, also known as **Kufor-Rakeb syndrome)** is phenotypically distinct from PD and presents with levodopa-responsive parkinsonism, pyramidal degeneration, dementia, supranuclear gaze palsy, and facial, faucial, and finger mini-myoclonus.

Gaucher disease gene carrier status is associated with greater prevalence of parkinsonism. **Glucocerebrosidase (GBA) gene mutations** may be up to 5 times more frequent in PD than in controls, not only in Ashkenazi patients, who have a higher mutation frequency. Because the frequency of GBA mutations in the world may be up to 30%, these may be one of the commonest genetic risk factors for PD. The phenotype of GBA mutation carriers ranges from classic L-dopa–responsive PD to DLB. PD patients with GBA mutations develop symptoms about 4 years earlier, are more likely to have a family history, and develop cognitive impairment, compared with PD patients without GBA mutations.

Autosomal Dominant Parkinson Disease

1. **PARK1** (*α-synuclein* **[SNCA]** gene, 4q21), described in Italian [Contursi kindred] and Greek families, is due to the **high-penetrance** α-synuclein gene missense mutations (A53T and A30P), which causes **early onset and rapid course** of asymmetric resting tremor, postural and gait difficulties, dysautonomia, and dementia. SNCA duplications lead to late-onset parkinsonism and dysautonomia, whereas triplications and point mutations are associated with more severe early-onset PD and dementia, which progresses faster to death. Besides Lewy bodies (LBs), there are conspicuous vacuoles in the hippocampus. A PARK1 cohort was mistakenly reported as "PARK4."

2. **PARK3** (2p13), described in northern German families, has **low penetrance** (~40%), suggesting that it might play a role in apparently sporadic cases. The age of onset is in the fifth decade or later and the course is **similar to idiopathic PD.** There is an **increased incidence of dementia** associated with, besides LBs, neurofibrillary tangles and senile plaques.

3. **PARK5** (*ubiquitin C-terminal hydrolase L1 [UCH-L1]* gene; 4p14) has been found in two **late-onset, tremor-predominant** PD patients of a German pedigree. It is unclear whether their *UCH-L1* mutation is causal or incidental.

4. **PARK8 (leucine-rich repeat kinase 2 [LRRK2]/*dardarin* gene; 12p)** can be indistinguishable from idiopathic PD. Its low penetrance suggests that environmental or other genetic influence its expression. The most frequently reported mutation *LRRK2* mutation, G2019S, is found in up to 1% of sporadic and 4% of familial PD cases. Almost 40% of northern African Arab and 20% of Ashkenazi Jewish PD cases carry the mutation. The frequency of *LRRK2* mutations is similar in early-onset and late-onset PD. Although unilateral leg tremor and foot dystonia are common early features in older-onset, early-onset G2019S *LRRK2* carriers more often manifest the "postural instability gait difficulty" phenotype. Unlike those with homozygous or compound heterozygous *Parkin* and *DJ-1* mutation carriers, heterozygous *LRRK2* mutation carriers have anosmia.

Non-PARK classic parkinsonism can also be seen in DYT3 (XDP, Lubag), DYT5 (dopa-responsive dystonia (GCH1), DYT12 (rapid-onset dystonia-parkinsonism), SCA2, SCA3, SCA6, SCA17, and Gaucher disease (GBA mutations). Patients with DYT5/DRD respond well to levodopa but, unlike PD, do not develop motor fluctuations or dyskinesias.

Perry syndrome (*Dynactin* or *DCTN1* mutations) is an autosomal dominant, rapidly progressive levodopa-unresponsive parkinsonism associated with hypoventilation, depression, and severe weight loss. On autopsy, instead of Lewy bodies, there are TDP-43-positive neuronal inclusions, dystrophic neuritis, and axonal spheroids in a predominantly pallidonigral distribution.

Young-onset Dystonia Parkinsonism

The following algorithm, modified from Klein et al., 2009, provides an approach to the diagnostic workup of patients with young-onset dystonia-parkinsonism.

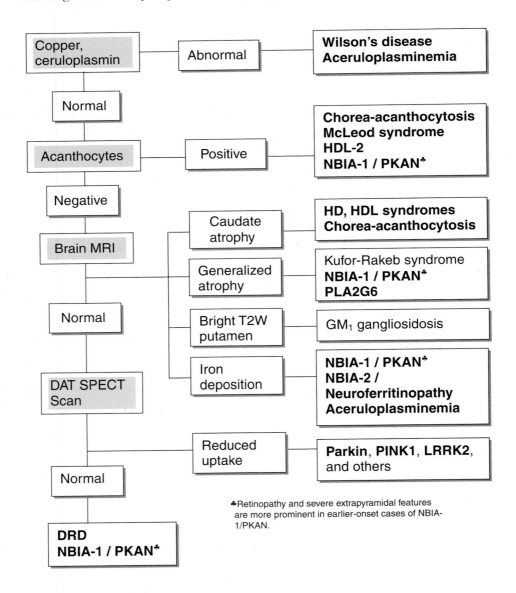

Ethnic background can help steer diagnostic efforts: DYT3 (XDP/Lubag) is seen in Filipinos, from the Island of Panay; SCA2 mostly occur among those of Asian ancestry; HDL-2 in black South Africans; and LRRK2 and Gaucher disease in Ashkenazi Jews.

Tremor in Conditions Other Than PD

Classic essential tremor (ET) refers to a bilateral **4–12-Hz postural and kinetic** flexion-extension tremor (as opposed to the supination-pronation tremor of PD) of the distal upper extremities and potentially also the head, larynx, tongue, face, legs, and occasionally the trunk. It is the commonest movement disorder, with a population prevalence ranging from 0.4% to 6% and a bimodal distribution with peaks in the second and sixth decades. ET appears to result from abnormal intrinsic oscillations originating in the inferior olive and spreading throughout the olivocerebellar network. **Responsiveness to alcohol** occurs in about 50% of the familial cases. ET represents a genetically heterogeneous disorder inherited in an **autosomal dominant** form linked to three loci so far: ETM1 (3q), ETM2 (2p), and one on 6p. The pathologic changes described are loss of Purkinje cells, cerebellar axonal "torpedoes," and brainstem Lewy bodies in the absence of clinical parkinsonism. The only first-line treatments for ET are **primidone** (250–750 mg/d) and **propranolol** (160–320 mg/d). **Botulinum toxin** may be preferred over oral therapy in drug-resistant essential head tremor, vocal tremor, and geniospasm. **Vim thalamic DBS** is the surgical procedure of choice and allows for change in stimulation variables to increase efficacy or reduce side effects.

> **Isolated tremors, especially of the head and voice, may *not* be ET** if they are position-dependent, task-specific, or associated with abnormal posturing, all of which are evidence of underlying dystonia.

Fragile X-associated tremor/ataxia syndrome (FXTAS) is a late-adult–onset neurodegenerative disorder affecting 1:700 men and 1:250 women (largely with premature ovarian failure) due to a premutation expansion of the fragile X mental retardation 1 gene (FMR1) **(55–200 CGG repeats)**. The FXTAS phenotype includes intention tremor, ataxia, parkinsonism, dysautonomia, dysexecutive dementia, and peripheral neuropathy. Brain MRI may show diffuse brain atrophy and increased T2W signal in the middle cerebellar peduncle (the **"MCP sign"**).

> **FXTAS** results from an overexpression of the "toxic" **expanded CGG repeat *FMR1* RNA**, which leads to neural cell dysregulation, **neuronal and astrocytic intranuclear inclusions**, and disruption of the nuclear lamin architecture. Conversely, >200 CGG repeat expansions of *FMR1* RNA (full mutation) causes *FMR1* silencing and absence of *FMR1* RNA and protein (FMRP), the pathogenic basis of the developmental disorder **fragile X syndrome**, the most common form of mental retardation.

Hereditary geniospasm or trembling chin **(8–10 Hz)** is a rare autosomal dominant condition of childhood onset with linkage to chromosome 9q. There is an association with otosclerosis and deafness in some cases. It is precipitated by stress, concentration, and emotion but may cease in adulthood.

Roussy-Lévy syndrome refers to the action tremor of the peripheral neuropathies of hereditary motor and sensory neuropathy (HMSN) type 1, CIDP, and IgM paraproteinemic demyelinating polyneuropathy, and is unrelated to the degree of proprioceptive loss.

Dystonic tremor refers to the combination of tremor and dystonia in the same (writer's cramp, spasmodic dysphonia, generalized dystonia) or different (arm tremor in torticollis) body parts. It occurs in 70% of patients with cervical dystonia and may be distinguished from ET by its irregular and jerky nature, associated abnormal posturing, variable amplitude depending on head or limb position, and responsiveness to sensory tricks. Botulinum toxin is the treatment of choice.

Cerebellar outflow (Holmes tremor) refers to the slow (2–5 Hz) tremor of the head, trunk (titubation), and proximal muscle groups that increases with posture and action. The rest component that distinguishes this tremor from a pure cerebellar tremor results from the involvement of the nigrostriatal system. As such, cerebellar outflow tremor may respond to levodopa. Multiple sclerosis is a common cause of Holmes tremor. Tremor reduction is difficult with conventional drugs and risky with thalamic procedures, although the latter can succeed if a tremor frequency >3 Hz is demonstrated on electrophysiologic studies.

Primary orthostatic tremor (OT) is a fine, occasionally palpable, **14–18 Hz** rippling of weight-bearing limbs and muscles active in sustained isometric contractions, which disappears during walking, sitting, and lying down, and is associated with a subjective feeling of unsteadiness. The latency of the tremor and unsteadiness on standing decreases with age. A single central oscillator (possibly within pontocerebellar circuits) may generate the tremor because the time-locked EMG bursts in all four limbs is only reset by electrical stimulation in the posterior fossa instead of peripherally. OT may respond to clonazepam instead of alcohol and propranolol, as in ET.

Enhanced physiologic tremor is a postural tremor with a frequency of 8–12 Hz better seen in the outstretched hands, which occurs in association with anxiety, stress, exercise, hypoglycemia, pheochromocytoma, thyrotoxicosis, alcohol withdrawal, caffeine intake, or drugs, such as beta-agonists, valproate, lithium, L-thyroxine, prednisone, SSRIs, and tricyclics. Of note, elimination of coffee in lithium-treated patients may worsen tremor: caffeine increases lithium clearance. When managing the underlying etiology is insufficient, low-dose propranolol can be used.

Oculopalatal tremor (formerly, **palatal myoclonus**) refers to two forms of slow (1.5–3 Hz) rhythmic movements of the soft palate:
1. **Symptomatic palatal tremor** results from involvement of the **levator veli palatini** muscles (distal soft palate). The contractions are **synchronous** with other branchial and ocular muscles and persist during sleep. The causal lesion interrupts the **Guillain-Mollaret triangle** (dentato-olivary-rubral pathway) causing **olivary pseudohypertrophic degeneration.**
2. **Essential palatal tremor** results from involvement of the **tensor veli palatini** muscles (proximal soft palate). **Ear clicks,** from the attachment of the eustachian tubes to the tensor veli palatini, are invariably present. No brain lesions or extrapalatal movements are identified.

Progressive Supranuclear Palsy

Described by Steele, Richardson, and Olszewski in 1964, progressive supranuclear palsy (PSP) is about 1/100 as prevalent as PD and just as common as myasthenia gravis and Huntington disease (3–4:1,000,000). PSP is suspected when **poor levodopa response** and **vertical supranuclear gaze restriction** are present in a tremorless and posturally impaired parkinsonian patient who has had **backward falls.**

The cardinal features are slow downward saccades with early normal amplitude, axial-predominant rigidity, and early loss of postural reflexes with **falls within 1 year of disease onset.**

Other features are prominent dysphagia, **facial dystonia** (deep nasolabial folds and furrowed brow), **unblinking stare, apraxia of eyelid opening,** square-wave jerks, **involuntary persistence of ocular fixation,** spastic/ataxic **dysarthria, erect posture with retrocollis,** and **executive dysfunction** with greater decline in set-shifting and categorization skills than PD. **Hypertension** is common.

- **Brain MRI** may show midbrain hyperintensity and atrophy (axial diameter <17 mm) as well as flattened third ventricle from superior colliculi atrophy
- **18F-fluorodopa PET scan** shows decreased uptake in both caudate and putamen (PD exhibits reduction uptake confined to the putamen)
- **18F-deoxyglucose PET scan** reveals an anterior to posterior gradient with greatest hypometabolism in the frontal cortex
- **PET scan with raclopride** (D2 dopamine antagonist) discloses the loss of D2 receptors in the caudate and putamen (which are normal in PD)

Hyperphosphorylated tau-containing **globose neurofibrillary tangles (NFT)** are deposited in the **periaqueductal gray matter,** SN, GPi, GPe, and STN. The **"tufted astrocytes"** and the presence of 15-nm NFT straight tubules rather than 24-nm paired helical filaments (PHF) distinguish PSP from AD. A **four-repeat tau** is the main tau isoform in PSP whereas three-repeat tau is seen in Pick disease (alone) and AD (with four-repeat). PSP and CBD are four-repeat tauopathies, share the same susceptibility genotype (H1/H1 tau), and **lack amyloid deposit** but differ in the topography of tau aggregation (brainstem in PSP, cortex in CBD).

Atypical PSP presentations include "benign" (falls after first year of symptoms), "pure akinesia syndrome," primary progressive freezing of gait, corticobasal syndrome, and frontotemporal dementia (see later discussion). Other entities that need distinction are MSA and nondegenerative diseases such as multi-infarct state, mesencephalic tumors, **Whipple disease,** and **Niemann-Pick disease type C** (vertical supranuclear gaze abnormality, ataxia, and parkinsonism), neurosyphilis, mitochondrial myopathy, and myasthenia gravis. Amantadine and amitriptyline can ameliorate gait and rigidity in PSP. Botulinum toxin injections may be helpful in apraxia of eyelid opening. Cholinergic striatal interneuron loss limits the efficacy of cholinesterase inhibitors.

Pathologic, Clinical, and Genetic Heterogeneity in PSP

Clinical syndromes pathologically diagnosed as PSP ("atypical PSP") may have a more benign prognosis, likely due to more restricted neuropathology. Normal eye movements indicate less damage to omnipause neurons located in the pontine nucleus raphe interpositus.

There is a genetic susceptibility to PSP defined by the tau **H1 haplotype,** which accounts for ~85%–95% of clinically diagnosed PSP haplotypes. Atypical PSP group is less likely to have the PSP susceptibility genotype and more likely to have an AD tau deposition pattern. CSF tau 33 kDa/55 kDa ratio obtained by immunoprecipitation and Western blot analysis is significantly lower in PSP compared to other neurodegenerative disorders, including the other four-repeat tauopathy, CBD. This CSF tau form ratio is a potential biomarker of disease.

Range of PSP phenotypes

- **Classic form (Richardson disease):** gradual onset of postural instability and falls within the first 2 years of disease, vertical supranuclear gaze palsy, a frontal dysexecutive syndrome, and rigidity and bradykinesia unresponsive to levodopa; median disease survival is 6 years.
- **PSP-parkinsonism (PSP-P):** asymmetric limb bradykinesia, positive initial response to levodopa, tremor and limb dystonia in the absence of early falls, eye movement abnormalities, or cognitive dysfunction; it accounts for most parkinsonian cases misidentified as PD early on.
- **Pure akinesia with gait freezing (PAGF):** gradual onset of freezing of gait or speech, absent limb rigidity and tremor, no sustained response to levodopa, and no dementia or ophthalmoplegia within the first 5 years of disease. There is less severe tau accumulation than in the more common Richardson disease. Median survival is 10 years for PSP-P and PAGF.
- **Primary progressive freezing gait (PPFG):** similar to PAGF but with rigidity (pallidonigroluysian degeneration [PNLD] causes "primary" PPFG)
- **Corticobasal syndrome (CBS):** the highly asymmetric parkinsonism of CBS, which run counters with the marked symmetry of PSP, may still represent PSP pathology, and these patients are often confused. The shared pathology of widely differing phenotypes highlights the shared genetics and pathology of these four-repeat tauopathies.
- **Progressive nonfluent aphasia (PNFA),** manifested as severe language deficits within the setting of a tremorless, hypokinetic-rigid syndrome with early falls and oculomotor impairment is a variant of frontotemporal dementia (FTLD), labeled **PSP-PNFA.** However, severe language deficits are currently exclusionary for the diagnosis of PSP.
- **Motor neuron disease (MND)** has also been reported with a PSP-like phenotype (weakness is also currently exclusionary for the diagnosis of PSP). The underlying pathology of these FTLD-MND cases with PSP phenotype is typically TDP-43 proteinopathy without PGRN mutation.
- **Apraxia of speech**

Multiple System Atrophy

Multiple system atrophy (MSA) is an akinetic-rigid syndrome with prominent cerebellar, autonomic, pyramidal, and extrapyramidal involvement occurring at an earlier age than PD and associated with worse prognosis. Two "subgroups" are clinically identifiable: the cerebellar type **(MSA-C)**, previously known as sporadic olivopontocerebellar atrophy (sOPCA), and the parkinsonian type **(MSA-P)**, previously labeled striatonigral degeneration.

Autonomic failure is predominantly central and includes orthostatic hypotension (drop of 20 mm Hg systolic or 10 mm Hg diastolic), urinary incontinence, erectile dysfunction, anhidrosis, and respiratory dysfunction (sleep apnea, snoring, and *inspiratory stridor*). Unlike PD, the dysautonomia is preganglionic (central, see next page) and the peripheral autonomic system is spared. Tremor, often myoclonic, occurs in 10% of patients. Dementia is not a feature of MSA but frontal lobe dysfunction usually develops. **Corticospinal dysfunction** is expressed as extensor plantar response with hyperreflexia. **Cerebellar dysfunction** results in gait or limb ataxia, ataxic dysarthria, and sustained gaze-evoked nystagmus. "Softer" MSA features include **rapid eye movement (REM)behavior disorder,** cold mottled hands **(Raynaud phenomenon), action and stimulus-sensitive myoclonus** of hands and face (correlated with cortical *giant somatosensory-evoked potentials* and EMG discharges [*C-waves*] on electrophysiology), dystonic **anterocollis,** severely hypophonic speech, the "Pisa syndrome," and impaired vestibulo-ocular reflex suppression and optokinetic nystagmus. Response to levodopa can be marked. Dyskinesias or **orofacial dystonia** may complicate levodopa treatment.

- **Brain MRI** shows **T2W hypointensity in the putamen with a lateral hyperintense rim.** "Hot cross bun" sign in the pons may be seen.
- **18F-fluorodopa PET scan** shows reduced putaminal and caudate uptake
- **Proton MR spectroscopy** shows decreased N-acetylaspartate-to-creatine and choline-to-creatine ratios in the putamen and globus pallidus
- **Sphincter EMG** shows abnormal spontaneous activity and long-duration motor unit potentials reflecting denervation from Onuf's nucleus gliosis
- **Tilt table** demonstrates minimal or absent rise in standing norepinephrine levels despite a marked orthostatic drop in blood pressure. In primary autonomic failure (PAF), both standing and supine norepinephrine levels are low.
- **Clonidine** does not increase growth hormone levels like in PAF and PD

Argyrophilic glial cytoplasmic inclusions (GCI) staining for **alpha-synuclein** as in Lewy bodies diseases (PD, DLB, and NBIA-1) are the classic findings. Cell loss can be found in the posterolateral putamen, SN, GP, LC, inferior olives, Purkinje cells, intermediolateral cell column, and Onuf's nucleus. Management of orthostatic hypotension includes liberalizing salt intake, use of elastic stocking, and head elevation at night. **Fludrocortisone** (Florinef, volume expander by decreasing natriuresis, 0.1–0.3 mg/d) and **midodrine** (ProAmatine, peripheral α1-adrenergic receptor agonist, 15–30 mg/d) may be needed. The latter may cause piloerection, scalp pruritus, urinary retention, and supine hypertension.

Dysautonomias

In MSA, the dysautonomia results from central lesions and the sympathetic ganglia are preserved. Basal serum norepinephrine level is normal but the response of serum growth hormone to clonidine, which is dependent on central stimulation of α2-adrenergic receptors, is impaired.

In PD and PAF, the dysautonomia is of peripheral origin: norepinephrine is low, whereas the response of serum growth hormone to clonidine is preserved.

DYSAUTONOMIAS PER TOPOGRAPHY

CNS	Peripheral Autonomic System
Pure autonomic failure (PAF)	**Without peripheral neuropathy**
Multiple system atrophy (MSA)	Pandysautonomia - (AAG, see below)
Parkinson disease (PD)	Cholinergic dysautonomia
	Botulism
Localized*	**With peripheral neuropathy**
Horner syndrome	Diabetes
Holmes-Adie pupil	Amyloidosis
Crocodile tears (Bogorad syndrome)	Guillain-Barré syndrome
Gustatory sweating (Frey syndrome)	Acute intermittent porphyria
Chagas disease (Trypanosoma cruzi)	Familial dysautonomia (Riley-Day syndrome; HMSN III)

*Vasovagal syncope (young) and carotid-sinus hypersensitivity (elderly) are intermittent localized dysautonomias

Autoimmune autonomic ganglionopathy (AAG) is characterized by prominent involvement of the peripheral autonomic nervous system due to ganglionic acetylcholine receptor (AChR) autoantibodies. Patients typically develop generalized autonomic failure including orthostatic hypotension, anhidrosis, and parasympathetic dysfunction. The onset can be acute, subacute, or gradual. Antibody levels correlate with the severity of dysautonomia. Clinical improvement has been reported with the use of immunotherapy including plasma exchange, corticosteroids, and IV immunoglobulin.

CLASSIFICATION OF AUTONOMIC SYSTEM AND CORRESPONDING IMPAIRMENT

	Ganglia and Target	Failure (underactivity)
Parasympathetic	ACh — NA — Glands, smooth muscle, heart	Mydriasis, fixed heart rate, sluggish urinary bladder and bowel, and erectile failure (males)
Sympathetic adrenergic	ACh — NA — Blood vessels, heart	Orthostatic hypotension and ejaculatory failure (males)
Sympathetic cholinergic	ACh — ACh — Sweat glands	Anhidrosis

Autonomic Dysfunction in Neurodegenerative Diseases

Orthostatic hypotension, neurogenic bowel/bladder, and sexual dysfunction may occur in the setting of PD (late), dementia with Lewy bodies (DLB, early or late), MSA (preceding or soon after its onset), and pure autonomic failure (PAF).

Because of the impairment in the brainstem-hypothalamic-pituitary pathways with preservation of postganglionic neurons in MSA, the following tests can be used:

Response to	PD	MSA	PAF
Hypotension	Preserved vasopressin release	**Blunted** vasopressin release	Preserved vasopressin release
Clonidine	Preserved GH secretion	**Blunted** GH secretion	Preserved GH secretion
Supine norepinephrine	Normal	Normal	**Low**
Cardiac SPECT and PET	**Abnormal** cardiac innervation	Normal cardiac innervation	**Abnormal** cardiac innervation

PD, Parkinson disease; MSA, multiple system atrophy; PAF, pure autonomic failure; GH, growth hormone. SPECT (single photon emission computed tomography) and PET (positron emission tomography) imaging use ^{123}I metaiodobenzylguanidine (MIBG) and 6-[^{18}F] fluorodopamine, respectively. In a patient with apparent PAF, normal cardiac innervation should indicate likely development of MSA.

Neuropathology of **MSA shows glial and neuronal cytoplasmic inclusions (GCI)** in the central nervous system *sparing* peripheral postganglionic autonomic. **In PD, PAF, and DLB, different cytoplasmic inclusions (Lewy bodies)** are found in the CNS *and* in peripheral postganglionic autonomic neurons. However, cytoplasmic **accumulation of alpha-synuclein occurs in all four disorders.**

Management of orthostatic hypotension (OH) includes head elevation at night, liberalizing salt intake and caffeine, use of elastic stocking, and avoidance of straining (to prevent Valsalva) and of alcohol or large carbohydrate meals (to prevent splanchnic vasodilation and postprandial hypotension). Dopaminergic agents and sildenafil may worsen hypotension. Pharmacologic interventions include volume expansion with **fludrocortisone** (Florinef, limits natriuresis, 0.1–0.3 mg/d), sympathetic vasoconstriction with **midodrine** (ProAmatine, 15–30 mg/d), and **methylphenidate** (Ritalin, releases presynaptic norepinephrine, 10 mg). Midodrine may cause piloerection, scalp pruritus, urinary retention, and nocturnal supine hypertension. **Pyridostigmine** can improve OH without worsening of supine hypertension. The central sympathomimetic **ephedrine** (15–45 mg tid) is not effective in peripheral dysautonomias such as PAF, PD, and diabetic neuropathy. The antidiuretic vasopressin-2 receptor antagonist **desmopressin** (5–40 µg intranasally or 100–400 mg orally every night) is used when nocturia is prominent. The somatostatin analogue **octreotide** (25–50 µg SQ, 30 minutes before food ingestion) prevents postprandial hypotension without worsening supine nocturnal hypertension. Management of (iatrogenic) supine hypertension requires head-up tilt at night, omission of the evening dose of vasopressor agents, or a prebedtime snack or alcohol.

Corticobasal Degeneration

Corticobasal degeneration (CBD) is a remarkably asymmetric levodopa-resistant, akinetic-rigid syndrome that usually begins after the age of 60 and leads to death within 4–7 years. Loss of dexterity or jerkiness in one *upper* extremity is followed by athetotic posturing and subsequent dystonia. *Lower* limb onset leads to **early postural instability with backward falls** and wheelchair dependence.

> *Major* features are **early postural and gait impairment, asymmetric bradykinesia,** rigidity, **dystonia** (with or without an "alien limb" phenomenon), postural and **kinetic tremor,** and later cortical deficits (progressive **ideomotor apraxia,** aphasia, astereognosis, and agraphesthesia).

Minor criteria are saccadic pursuit, **increased latency but not speed of saccades,** often initiated by head thrusts, dysphagia and dysarthria (slurred and labored), blepharospasm, and hyperreflexia.

Paraclinical investigations for CBD may show the following:
- **Asymmetric frontoparietal cortical atrophy** opposite to the most affected side can be demonstrated on HCT and brain MRI.
- **18F-fluorodopa PET scan** shows decreased uptake in the striatum contralateral to the most affected side
- **18F-deoxyglucose PET scan** reveals hypometabolism in the parietal cortex and thalamus contralateral to the most affected side
- **SPECT scanning** shows reduced postsynaptic striatal D2 receptor binding of [^{123m}I]-iodobenzamide (IBZM)

CBD is a four-repeat tauopathy. The aggregation of microtubule-associated tau forms **neurofibrillary tangles, "astrocytic plaques,"** and neuronal inclusions, mostly in the cerebral cortex (as opposed to PSP, where most pathology is in the brainstem). **Substantia nigra pars compacta (SNc)** is almost universally degenerated. **Ballooned and achromatic neurons** (scant Nissl substance) resembling those of Pick disease are supportive findings.

The **corticobasal syndrome** (CBS) can present as progressive nonfluent aphasia (PNFA or PPA), speech apraxia, frontotemporal dementia (FTD), progressive supranuclear palsy (PSP)-like syndrome, and posterior cortical atrophy syndrome. CBS can result from pathology of CBD, AD, PSP, FTLD-U, and FTLD-tau. CBS due to AD occurs at a younger age than in CBD and is more likely to be associated with myoclonus, and less likely to be associated with tremors. Initial episodic memory complaints tend to predict AD pathology, whereas early frontal behavioral symptoms, nonfluent language disturbance, orobuccal apraxia, and utilization behaviors predict CBD pathology. Apraxia of speech is strongly associated with underlying tau pathology. CBD and PSP share the presence of the four-repeat isoform in tau-positive inclusions (three-repeat in Pick disease), and identical H1 and H1/H1 tau haplotype status.

Machado-Joseph Disease (MJD/SCA 3)

SCA-2, SCA-3, SCA-6, SCA-17, and SCA-21 have been associated with Parkinsonism.

MJD is a multisystem degeneration of the central nervous system and the most common autosomal dominant spinocerebellar degeneration. It results from an **expanded CAG repeat** on chromosome 14q32 (normal, 12–44; SCA-3, 60–84 CAG repeats). The CAG repeat length determines age at disease onset, severity of the clinical phenotype, and rate of progression. Gene-dosage contribution is better appreciated in homozygous patients ("double-dose"), who have more severe disease than heterozygous. The five cardinal features are **cerebellar ataxia, parkinsonism, dystonia, spasticity, and peripheral neuropathy.** Small repeat expansions are associated with ataxia, whereas larger repeats often have worse pyramidal signs and dystonia. Facial fasciculations or myokymia and lid retraction ("bulging eyes") are other helpful clinical clues. **Cognitive impairment is not a feature of MJD.**

Clinically, MJD has been divided into four clinical types:

Type 1: dystonia and spasticity: these patients have an earlier onset, a more severe course with dystonia and spasticity, and severe nuclear (mainly of the abducens nerve) progressive external ophthalmoplegia

Type 2: spasticity and cerebellar ataxia: these patients represent the most common phenotype of MJD/SCA-3

Type 3: cerebellar ataxia and peripheral neuropathy with amyotrophic changes: ophthalmoplegia is supranuclear—rather than nuclear—and may also express with a medial longitudinal fasciculus syndrome, or a limitation in upward gaze and convergence

Type 4: parkinsonism (levodopa-responsive) and peripheral neuropathy: these patients tend to have a later age of onset and a smaller CAG expansion

Intermediate CAG repeat length (53, 54) has been associated with restless leg syndrome and a sensorimotor axonal polyneuropathy in a Dutch family.

Ophthalmologic findings in MJD include square-wave jerks, present in 30%, and gaze-evoked nystagmus in 75% of patients with SCA-3. Impairment of bilateral abduction is common in type 1 SCA-3. Slow saccade is an invariable feature of SCA-2 patients (in whom square-wave jerks and gaze-evoked nystagmus are absent) but occurs, with lesser severity, in only one-third of SCA-3 patients.

The main neuropathologic changes reported are neuronal loss and gliosis in the substantia nigra and dentate nucleus of the cerebellum. The cerebellar cortex is intact. Other changes are seen in the subthalamic nucleus and occasionally in the striatum and pallidum, which may be the reason why parkinsonism is not as common as it could be, predicted on the basis of the primary pathologic involvement of the substantia nigra that occurs in MJD/SCA-3 patients.

Other Parkinsonian Disorders

Vascular parkinsonism is a **"lower half"** parkinsonism (as in normal pressure hydrocephalus [NPH] and senile dementia) distinguished by hesitant, shuffling gait, and postural instability with relatively preserved arm swing and rare or absent resting tremor, hypophonia, and facial masking. **The response to levodopa is usually poor.** Progression tends to be in a step-wise fashion. Pyramidal tract signs and pseudobulbar palsy are common findings.

The categories of associated cerebrovascular disease are multi-infarct disease, **etat crible (multiple dilated perivascular spaces),** Binswanger disease (subcortical arteriosclerotic encephalopathy), and single foci of cerebral infarction or hemorrhage in the midbrain or basal ganglia. Risk factors, such as hypertension, hyperlipidemia, and hypercoagulability should be identified and controlled.

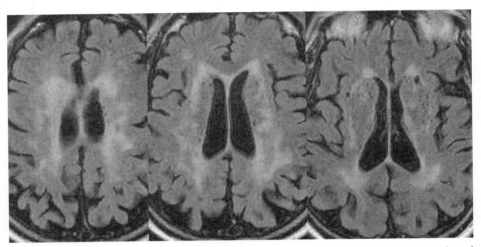

Vascular parkinsonism. Axial brain MRI of a 68-year-old woman with staggering progression of gait and cognitive impairment showing periventricular and deep white matter hyperintensities. These findings suggest microangiopathic disease is the etiology of her lower-body predominant parkinsonism and evolving dementia.

Dementia with Lewy bodies (DLB) applies to the dementia occurring within 1 year from the onset of parkinsonism whereby early **spontaneous hallucinations** and **fluctuating cognition** and alertness are prominent. Extrapyramidal side effects arise from marked **sensitivity to neuroleptic drugs,** whenever these are used. Response to levodopa may be adequate but psychiatric side effects are common. Compared with PD and PD dementia, there is greater cognitive improvement to cholinergic treatment.

Hypoparathyroidism that remains untreated may cause any of the following: **dopa-resistant akinetic-rigid syndrome** or **chorea,** dystonia, myoclonus, paroxysmal choreoathetosis, **tetany,** cerebellar and pyramidal tract signs, **supranuclear vertical gaze palsy,** and epilepsy. **Basal ganglia calcifications** are typical imaging abnormalities.

Normal pressure hydrocephalus (NPH) presents with gait disorder, urinary incontinence, and dementia, usually in that order if all three features are present. The gait is commonly **apraxic** or **"magnetic,"** with inability to lift the feet off the walking surface and turning with normal pivot, and is out of proportion to lesser upper body involvement (the other common form of **"lower half"** or lower-body predominant parkinsonism like vascular parkinsonism). Rest tremor is rare. There is a **higher prevalence of systemic hypertension.** Secondary NPH arises in those with a history of subarachnoid hemorrhage, intracranial surgery or tumors, trauma, meningitis, or subdural hematomas.

Disease-causing hydrocephalus is supported if:

- Head circumference is <59 cm in men or 57.5 cm in women, as greater numbers would indicate congenital hydrocephalus
- **Transependymal flow** (increased periventricular T2W signal) is shown by conventional MRI and **flow void in the cerebral aqueduct** by cine-MRI
- **Modified Evans ratio** (maximum width of the frontal horns divided by a measure of the inner table at the same place) is >3.1
- **Isotope cisternography** shows the radiolabeled isotope stagnant in the ventricles after 72 hours from the lumbar subarachnoid injection with no distribution over the convexities (reliability of this test is poor).

Shunt surgery has a higher likelihood of improving symptoms if:

- Gait dysfunction began before the onset of dementia
- Dementia has been present for <2 years and there is no aphasia or other cortical-based cognitive impairments
- Therapeutic lumbar puncture (CSF removal of 40–50 mL) is associated with transient Improvement, especially in the gait
- There is no history of alcohol abuse
- There is a secondary cause of hydrocephalus
- There is lower frontal-to-posterior ratio of regional cerebral blood flow in 18F-fluorodeoxyglucose PET studies

Drug-induced parkinsonism (DIP) is more likely to be symmetrical, have less resting tremor, and respond better to anticholinergic drugs than PD. A low-frequency, high-amplitude perioral tremor known as the **rabbit syndrome** is highly suggestive. It often appears within the first month after the responsible neuroleptic (including atypical antipsychotics olanzapine and risperidone) has been initiated. Clozapine is safe against the potential for DIP and modestly beneficial for other parkinsonian symptoms such as tremor and dyskinesia. Lack of resolution of DIP within 6 months from discontinuing the offending drug suggests underlying PD unmasked by the neuroleptic drug exposure.

> Parkinsonism can be **rapidly progressive** in motor neuron disease-inclusion body dementia (MND-ID), paraneoplastic limbic encephalitis, Creutzfeldt-Jakob disease (CJD), subacute sclerosing panencephalitis (SSPE), progressive multifocal leukoencephalopathy (PML), and Whipple disease.

Pathology of Tauopathies

Tau is an abnormal cytoskeletal filament that is organized at the ultrastructural level into paired helical filaments that have periodic twists about every 80 nm.

Alzheimer Disease (AD)

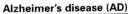

Alzheimer's disease (AD)

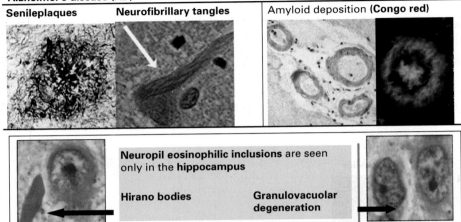

Senileplaques	Neurofibrillary tangles	Amyloid deposition **(Congo red)**

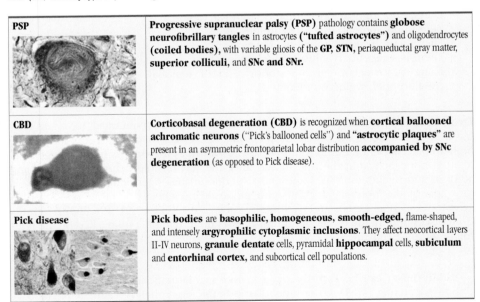

Neuropil eosinophilic inclusions are seen only in the **hippocampus**

Hirano bodies   **Granulovacuolar degeneration**

Marinesco bodies of normal aging (not shown) are **ubiquinated intranuclear eosinophilic inclusion** without a halo (i.e., "Cowdry type B"). Their significance is unclear.

PSP	**Progressive supranuclear palsy (PSP)** pathology contains **globose neurofibrillary tangles** in astrocytes (**"tufted astrocytes"**) and oligodendrocytes **(coiled bodies)**, with variable gliosis of the **GP, STN,** periaqueductal gray matter, **superior colliculi**, and **SNc and SNr.**
CBD	**Corticobasal degeneration (CBD)** is recognized when **cortical ballooned achromatic neurons** ("Pick's ballooned cells") and **"astrocytic plaques"** are present in an asymmetric frontoparietal lobar distribution **accompanied by SNc degeneration** (as opposed to Pick disease).
Pick disease	**Pick bodies** are **basophilic, homogeneous, smooth-edged,** flame-shaped, and intensely **argyrophilic cytoplasmic inclusions**. They affect neocortical layers II–IV neurons, **granule dentate** cells, pyramidal **hippocampal** cells, **subiculum** and **entorhinal cortex,** and subcortical cell populations.

Frontotemporal dementia and parkinsonism linked to chromosome 17 (FTDP-17), recently characterized, results in neuronal loss of the frontal and temporal lobes, substantia nigra, and hippocampus with **"ballooning" and phosphorylated tau (ptau) inclusions** of the remaining neurons.

Pathology of Synucleinopathies

Alpha-synuclein is a synaptic protein, the main component of Lewy bodies, and the **precursor of the non-Aβ component of Alzheimer disease amyloid.** Toxic gain-of-function mutations in alpha-synuclein (A53T and A30P) have been found in Lewy body diseases and MSA.

Parkinson disease 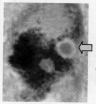 ⇦ **Lewy body:** Cytoplasmic eosinophilic inclusion **H&E** and **ubiquitin** stains	**PD** is characterized by the accumulation of **intracytoplasmic Lewy bodies** in the **substantia nigra, locus coeruleus,** and **nucleus basalis of Meynert.** The inclusions are circular and surrounded by a **clear halo.** The first known genetic cause of PD was the identification of a missense mutation in the α-synuclein gene (*A53T*) in the Contursi kindred
Dementia with Lewy bodies 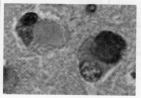	**DLB** is characterized by the accumulation of intracytoplasmic **cortical Lewy bodies.** The areas of greater burden of disease are the **superior temporal cortex, anterior cingulate cortex, parahippocampal cortex,** and **amygdala.** Inclusions may indent the nucleus and *lack a distinct halo.* Identification is aided by using **ubiquitin stain.**
Pure autonomic failure	**PAF** is characterized by the accumulation of intracytoplasmic **Lewy bodies** in peripheral postganglionic autonomic neurons
Multiple system atrophy 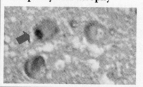	**MSA** is characterized by the appearance of **argyrophilic glial cytoplasmic inclusions (GCIs) containing** α-synuclein tubules present in the substantia nigra, striatum, **locus coeruleus,** pontine nuclei, inferior olives, cerebellum, **intermediolateral columns,** and **Onuf's nucleus** of the spinal cord.

The cytoplasmic inclusions in MSA are found in both *glial* and neuronal cells in the central nervous system *sparing* peripheral postganglionic autonomic neurons. The cytoplasmic inclusions (Lewy bodies) in the Lewy body diseases (PD, PAF, and DLB) are found in the CNS *and* in peripheral postganglionic autonomic neurons; they are lacking in glial cells.

NBIA-1	**Neurodegeneration with brain iron accumulation type 1**
Widespread **axonal spheroids** and large deposits of iron pigment in **globus pallidus** and **substantia nigra pars reticularis** (SNr).	(previously known as Hallervorden-Spatz disease) is recognized by the presence of large numbers of **cortical and brainstem Lewy bodies** strongly staining with α-synuclein.

Chorea

Chorea is an irregular, rapid, flowing, nonstereotyped, random involuntary movement that may be disguised into purposeful activities, and range from distal and writhing (choreoathetosis) to proximal and large amplitude (ballismus).

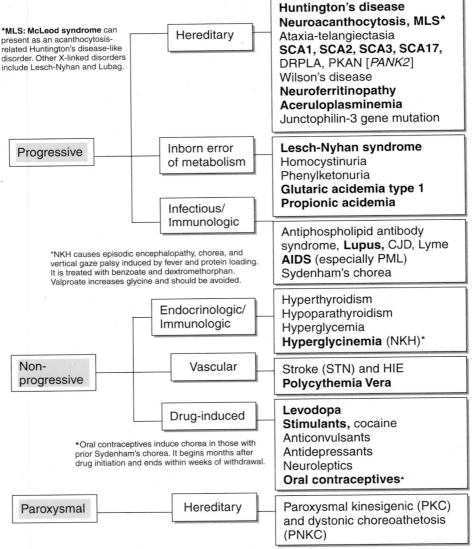

MLS: McLeod syndrome can present as an acanthocytosis-related Huntington's disease-like disorder. Other X-linked disorders include Lesch-Nyhan and Lubag.

Hereditary

Huntington's disease
Neuroacanthocytosis, MLS⁺
Ataxia-telangiectasia
SCA1, SCA2, SCA3, SCA17,
DRPLA, PKAN [*PANK2*]
Wilson's disease
Neuroferritinopathy
Aceruloplasminemia
Junctophilin-3 gene mutation

Progressive

Inborn error of metabolism

Lesch-Nyhan syndrome
Homocystinuria
Phenylketonuria
Glutaric acidemia type 1
Propionic acidemia

Infectious/ Immunologic

*NKH causes episodic encephalopathy, chorea, and vertical gaze palsy induced by fever and protein loading. It is treated with benzoate and dextromethorphan. Valproate increases glycine and should be avoided.

Antiphospholipid antibody syndrome, **Lupus**, CJD, Lyme
AIDS (especially PML)
Sydenham's chorea

Endocrinologic/ Immunologic

Hyperthyroidism
Hypoparathyroidism
Hyperglycemia
Hyperglycinemia (NKH)*

Non-progressive

Vascular

Stroke (STN) and HIE
Polycythemia Vera

Drug-induced

⁺Oral contraceptives induce chorea in those with prior Sydenham's chorea. It begins months after drug initiation and ends within weeks of withdrawal.

Levodopa
Stimulants, cocaine
Anticonvulsants
Antidepressants
Neuroleptics
Oral contraceptives⁺

Paroxysmal

Hereditary

Paroxysmal kinesigenic (PKC) and dystonic choreoathetosis (PNKC)

Benign hereditary chorea (BHC, *TITF-1* gene, 14q) is a nonprogressive autosomal dominant chorea, easily confused with essential myoclonus (which may exhibit dystonia as BHC but does not involve gait or responds to alcohol). Congenital hypothyroidism and respiratory distress are part of the clinical spectrum.

Huntington Disease

Huntington disease (HD) is an autosomal dominant neurodegenerative disease of motor, cognitive, and psychiatric impairment that can begin at any age between 2 and 90 years. It is much more common in Scotland and Venezuela and less common in Finland, China, Japan, and black South Africans. Difficulty with the generation of saccadic eye movements is often the earliest sign. A blink or head thrust may be required to initiate saccadic eye movements **(early oculomotor apraxia).** Clumsiness and fidgetiness evolves into chorea and motor impersistence. HD is caused by a mutation in the *interesting transcript 15 (IT15)* gene. The *IT15* gene contains 67 exons and encodes huntingtin, a cytoplasmic protein necessary for developing and sustaining normal brain function. Exon 1 contains CAG trinucleotide repeats that encode glutamine and proline. In unaffected individuals, there are 10–34 CAG repeats, whereas those affected with HD have >**40 repeats.** In those with 35–39 repeats, the disease is variably penetrant. The age of onset of the disease is inversely proportional to the number of CAG repeats. Individuals with juvenile onset have ≥55 repeats and usually inherit the gene from their father **(paternal inheritance often leads to anticipation:** the child's age of onset is earlier than that of the father's).

The neuropathology shows **caudate and putamen neuronal loss and gliosis** along with more diffuse brain atrophy. Huntingtin forms ubiquitinated aggregates within neurites and nuclei **(neuronal intranuclear inclusions)** in the cortex more than in the striatum. The amount of aggregation is directly dependent on the length of the polyglutamine repeat.

The glutamate antagonist **amantadine** and the dopamine-depleting drug **tetrabenazine** are effective in reducing chorea in patients with HD. Atypical antipsychotics such as olanzapine are helpful and preferable over typical neuroleptics because of the lower risk of tardive dyskinesia with long-term use. Several potentially neuroprotective agents have been tested in clinical trials. **Riluzole and remacemide** improve motor function. Vitamin E, idebenone, and lamotrigine (glutamate antagonist) have shown no benefit.

HD-like 2 (HDL2, CTG repeat expansions in the junctophilin-3 gene, 16q24) affects mainly families of African ancestry with anticipation, caudate atrophy, and cortical intranuclear inclusions as HD. Orolingual dystonia interfering with feeding and variable acanthocytes suggest HDL2 may be a form of neuroacanthocytosis.

Other autosomal dominant HD-like disorders are **HDL4 (SCA-17,** CAA/CAG repeats in the TBP [TATA box-binding protein gene] on 6q27; ataxia is the more common phenotype), **HDL1** (prion protein mutations on 20p12), **DRPLA, neuroferritinopathy,** and benign hereditary chorea. Autosomal recessive HD-like disorders are **HDL3** (4p15, single family from Saudi Arabia, with earlier onset, dementia, and ataxia), **neuroacanthocytosis, NBIA-1,** Friedreich ataxia, and aceruloplasminemia. The X-linked McLeod syndrome is only seen in males.

Sydenham Disease

Sydenham disease (SD) refers to an often self-limited presumably autoimmune chorea that follows, even as late as 6 months, a **group A β-hemolytic streptococcal (GABHS) infection,** largely between ages 5 and 15 years. Girls are affected in a 2:1 ratio to boys. SD can be a late or sole manifestation of rheumatic fever. In such case, other comorbidities ("major" Jones criteria) may be carditis, polyarthritis, erythema marginatum, and subcutaneous nodules. Haloperidol or valproate can be used if chorea requires symptomatic treatment. Secondary antibiotic prophylaxis with penicillin is recommended until age 21 years.

> **SD increases susceptibility to other later-onset choreas,** such as those induced by oral contraceptives, estrogen-containing creams, levodopa, and pregnancy (chorea gravidarum).

Pediatric Autoimmune Neuropsychiatric Disorders Associated with Streptococci (PANDAS) is a controversial disorder with "sawtooth" chronic clinical course, temporally related to a GABHS infection as in SD (although this finding has been challenged recently), in patients between the age of 3 years and the beginning of puberty, expressed as either *obsessive-compulsive disorder* or a *tic disorder* (rather than chorea). It is distinguished from SD by the absence of carditis and polyarthritis, a largely psychiatric presentation with a chronic course, and the failure to respond to antibiotic prophylaxis.

> **GABHS infections** cause the formation of antistreptococcal antibodies that cross-react with neuronal cytoplasmic basal ganglia antigens. **Transient hyperintensity in, and enlargement of, the caudate nucleus and globus pallidus** may occur in Sydenham disease and PANDAS.

Both antistreptolysin O (ASO) *and* anti-DNase B should be used when testing for SD and PANDAS. Titers for anti-DNase B are present for several weeks after ASO titers have normalized and may be the only marker of prior streptococcal exposure when the disorder begins or exacerbates.

Echocardiography is recommended for all suspected cases of SD because silent carditis is often a coexistent condition.

Poststreptococcal acute disseminated encephalomyelitis (PSADEM) is a monophasic postinfectious autoimmune inflammatory disorder associated with GABHS, **abnormal basal ganglia imaging,** and elevated **anti–basal ganglia antibodies** (ABGA). PSADEM is distinguished clinically from SD and PANDAS by the presence of dystonia or rigidity (and, unusually, tremor) rather than chorea or tics, but is also similar to these disorders in the analogous autoimmune pathogenesis and involvement of basal ganglia nuclei. It is also clinically separated from other acute disseminated encephalomyelitis cases by its remarkable extrapyramidal component, which is rare in ADEM cohorts.

Restless Leg Syndrome (Ekbom Syndrome)

Restless leg syndrome (RLS) refers to a distressing need or urge to move the legs (**akathisia**) accompanied by an uncomfortable paresthetic sensation in the legs, worst in the evening, brought on by rest, and relieved with moving or walking. It affects 2.5%–15% of the population, mostly women. Besides a positive family history among first-degree relatives, earlier-onset RLS patients (<40 years) tend to have milder symptoms, slower progression, and less relation between body iron stores and severity of disease. Those with an onset after 50 years are more likely to be idiopathic and have symptoms or signs of neuropathy. Established secondary causes of RLS include **pregnancy, end-stage renal disease, and iron deficiency (with or without anemia)** but **diabetes mellitus, small-fiber neuropathy, and radiculopathy** also increase the risk. Worsening of symptoms has been associated with low magnesium and folate levels. Symptoms resolve with resolution of the condition. Most cases of secondary RLS have a late onset and tend to advance more rapidly.

RLS may be associated (and confused) with brief (1–5 s) and repetitive (every 20–40 s) periodic leg movements during sleep (**PLMS,** formerly termed *nocturnal myoclonus*) or while awake (**PLMW**). Although many patients with insomnia and PLMS do not have RLS, 80% of RLS patients have PLMS. The latter consists of a stereotypic repetitive dorsiflexion movement of the toes, ankle, and knees (resembling a Babinski sign and a triple flexion reflex) during the light **NREM sleep stages 1 and 2.** PLMS can also occur in narcolepsy, sleep apnea syndrome, REM behavior disorder, MSA, or in healthy individuals. PLMW increases with the duration of rest and from morning to night.

The movements of RLS may be of **spinal, possibly propriospinal,** origin. Dysfunction of the diencephalic-spinal dopamine A11 system may explain the efficacy of dopaminergic drugs in relieving RLS symptoms. Iron deficiency may be a predisposing factor by reducing the dopamine transporter.

The best evidence for treatment efficacy in relieving RLS symptoms is for newer dopamine agonists, ropinirole (0.5–6 mg/d) and pramipexole (0.25–1.5 mg/d). **Ropinirole does not undergo renal metabolism and may be more effective in uremic RLS patients.** Ergot-derived dopaminergic agents are rarely used because of their potential for causing valvular cardiopathy and pleuropulmonary fibrosis. Levodopa is effective but may cause more **symptom augmentation** (worsening of RLS symptoms with progressively earlier daily onset, decreased latency to symptoms at rest, and/ or involvement of trunk or upper limbs) than dopamine agonists, presumably from overstimulation of the D_1 compared with D_2 spinal dopamine receptors. Gabapentin, benzodiazepines (clonazepam, temazepam), anticonvulsants, or, if needed, opioids (oxycodone, propoxyphene) may be effective if dopamine agonists fail or intolerable side effects develop. Iron supplementation and opiates can counter augmentation. Iron replacement is most beneficial when ferritin level is <45 μg/L.

Paroxysmal Dyskinesias

Infantile convulsions and chore-oathetosis (16p) is a benign familial infantile seizure (BFIS) syndrome with seizures during infancy, which progresses into, and is now believed to be the same disorder as, PKD.

PKD, mostly sporadic or familial, can also occur in association with MS, PSP, DM, head injury, hyperthyroidism, hypoglycemia, thalamic infarcts, and idiopathic primary hypoparathyroidism.

Paroxysmal kinesigenic dyskinesia (PKD, formerly PKC)	Paroxysmal nonkinesigenic (dystonic) dyskinesia (PNKD)
More common	Less common
Boys > girls 4:1	Boys > girls 3:2
Between 1 and 20 years if no family history	Infancy
Family history in 50% (AD)	Most are AD, some sporadic
DYT10 (16p)	**DYT8 (2q) — myofibrillogenesis regulator 1** **DYT9 (1p): PNKD + spasticity**
Precipitant: **rapid movement** or startle	Precipitants: **alcohol or caffeine**
Duration <1min (never more than 5)	Duration: 10 min to 1 h (up to 4 h)
Frequency: Up to 100/d, decreasing gradually toward adulthood	Frequency: Few episodes a month up to 3 paroxysms daily. It wanes with age
Responsive to PHT and CBZ	**Responsive to benzodiazepines** (clonazepam, diazepam)

Paroxysmal exercise-induced dystonia (PED, intermediate form)◆	Paroxysmal hypnogenic dystonia (truly, frontal lobe epilepsy)
Dystonic spasms of legs (may be presenting sign of young-onset PD)	Brief, occasionally painful dystonic spasms during non-REM sleep
Lasting 1–30 min	Duration is variable
***GLUT1* gene (1p)** in some cases*	***CHRNA4* (20q)** (see following box)
Brought on by sustained exertion	Frontal lobe epilepsy likely cause
Variable benefits to **acetazolamide**	Poor response to anticonvulsants

*Glucose transporter 1 (*GLUT1*) missense mutations (SLC2A1 gene) are found in PED patients with epilepsy and migraine. *GLUT1* deficiency syndrome consists of developmental delay, microcephaly, refractory epilepsy, ataxia, spasticity, *hypoglycorrhachia,* and low RBC glucose uptake.
◆PED can also be the presenting deficit in early-onset Parkinson disease (parkin, LRRK2) and dopa-responsive dystonia.

Paroxysmal dystonia or **tonic spasm** is the most frequent movement disorder in MS. It disappears within weeks spontaneously or after steroid treatment. The lesion may be anywhere within the motor path (midbrain, capsule, cervical cord).

Paroxysmal hypnogenic dystonia is truly a form of familial frontal lobe epilepsy known as autosomal dominant nocturnal frontal lobe epilepsy (**ADNFLE**), due to a mutation in the neuronal **nicotinic** receptor gene *CHRNA4* (**20q**). A novel locus for the same receptor resides on **15q**.

Other Paroxysmal Movement Disorders

The following list excludes paroxysmal ataxias and secondary PKD (multiple sclerosis, cerebrovascular insufficiency, hypo- or hyperglycemia, hypocalcemia, or previous trauma).

- **Sandifer syndrome** (dyspeptic dystonia) refers to the dystonic movements of the head and neck, occasionally with opisthotonos, that occur during feeding in infants with gastroesophageal reflux often associated with hiatal hernia. Symptoms resolve with correction of the underlying gastrointestinal problem.

- **Spasmus nutans** is the combination of horizontal or vertical head tremor or nodding, torticollis, and pendular and asymmetric nystagmus, which appears before the first year of life and resolves spontaneously by 3–4 years. Straightening or fixing the head increases nystagmus, as the head nodding is somewhat compensatory to the oscillatory movements of the eyes. Although spasmus nutans is considered benign and self-limited, there may be an associated **optic nerve glioma** and porencephalic cysts. Cystic tumors of the optic chiasm and third ventricle may show a similar presentation (bobble-head doll syndrome).

- **Bobble-head doll syndrome** is characterized by continuous or episodic involuntary forward-and-backward and side-to-side movements of the head at the frequency of 2–3 Hz. Neuroimaging demonstrates third ventricular lesions, often causing communicating hydrocephalus, such as tumors, suprasellar arachnoid cyst, or aqueductal stenosis. "Yes-yes" head bobbing at this rate may also be part of spasmus nutans, rhombencephalosynapsis (cerebellar malformation), and succinic semialdehyde dehydrogenase deficiency (globus pallidus T2W hyperintensity). Ventriculoperitoneal shunt leads to improvement.

- **Hyperekplexia** (startle disease) results from dominant missense mutations in the **glycine** receptor alpha 1 subunit gene (*GLRA1*), which cause hypertonia in neonates during wakefulness, an exaggerated nonhabituating startle response to any brief stimulation, and hyperactive brainstem reflexes. Tonic spasm and nocturnal myoclonus can be seen. Clonazepam is the drug of choice.

- **Hemifacial spasm** is characterized by tonic and clonic synchronous contractions of the muscles innervated by the ipsilateral facial nerve, which may persist during sleep. Stress, fatigue, anxiety, and voluntary facial movements aggravate symptoms. Vascular compression of the facial nerve root by an ectatic vessel (most commonly, the anterior or posterior cerebellar artery or the vertebral artery) has been shown to be the most common secondary etiology. This compression and the resulting demyelination leads to a "false" synapse with subsequent "axonal talk" between adjacent nerves ("ectopic" or **ephaptic transmission**). It must be distinguished from psychogenic facial spasm (lower lip deviation), facial tic, facial myokymia ("bag of worms"), blepharospasm (dystonic orbicularis oculi overactivity), and tardive dyskinesia. Botulinum toxin injections are the treatment of choice.

Selected Facial Disorders

Ramsay Hunt syndrome (RHS) strictly refers to the onset of peripheral facial nerve palsy accompanied by an erythematous vesicular rash on the ear **(zoster oticus)** or in the mouth due to varicella zoster virus (VZV) infection. CN VIII may be involved causing tinnitus, hearing loss, nausea, vomiting, vertigo, and nystagmus given the proximity of the geniculate ganglion to the vestibulocochlear nerve within the bony facial canal. Patients with RHS often have more severe paralysis at onset and recover less nerve function compared with those suffering from idiopathic facial paralysis (Bell's palsy). Antiviral drugs against VZV or HSV may be given early in the treatment of all patients with RHS. The recommended regimen is a 7–10-day course of famciclovir (500 mg tid) or acyclovir (800 mg, five times daily), as well as oral prednisone (60 mg daily for 3–5 days).

Facial synkinesis is a rare motor overflow phenomena of the face whereby unintentional but synchronous muscle contractions accompany, but are anatomically distinct from, movements of a nonhomologous facial region. Most synkinetic movements are due to postparalytic Bell's palsy from aberrant nerve regeneration or ephaptic transmission. However, some nontraumatic or non–postparalytic facial synkinesis can be distinguished:

- **Marcus Gunn jaw winking** (trigemino-ocular synkinesis) is an autosomal dominant condition with incomplete penetrance in which an infant's eyelid ptosis improves with jaw opening. The stimulation of the trigeminal nerve by contraction of the pterygoid muscles on jaw opening results in the excitation of the branch of the oculomotor nerve that innervates the levator palpebrae superioris ipsilaterally. Marcus Gunn jaw winking is present in approximately 5% of neonates with congenital ptosis. This condition has been associated with amblyopia and strabismus.
- **Inverse Marcus Gunn phenomenon (Marin Amat syndrome)** is a rare facial synkinesis in which eyelids close on jaw opening as the branch of the oculomotor nerve to the levator palpebrae superioris is inhibited.

Idiopathic facial palsy (Bell's palsy) is a common (up to 40/100,000) acute, idiopathic, unilateral paralysis of the facial nerve. Rarely proven, there may be an association with HSV infection. Up to 30% have a poor recovery. Early treatment with prednisolone improves the chances of complete recovery at 3 and 9 months with no additional benefit when acyclovir is given alone or in combination with prednisolone.

Known secondary causes of facial palsy (not Bell's)		
Infection	HSV, HZV **Lyme disease** Leprosy	Tumors	Facial nerve neuromas Other tumors causing facial nerve compression
Sarcoidosis or other granulomatous diseases		**Melkersson-Rosenthal syndrome** Pontine infarcts

Myoclonus

(see also "Myoclonic Encephalopathies")

Sudden, brief, shocklike movements caused by muscle contractions (positive myoclonus) or inhibitions (negative myoclonus) arising from the CNS.

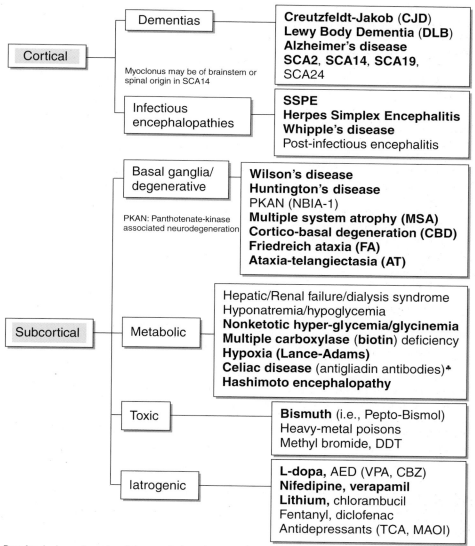

Propriospinal myoclonus is a distinct myoclonic syndrome affecting abdominal wall and lower limb muscles, worsening in the lying position and during the transition into sleep (presleep relaxation phase), associated with premonitory sensation and responsiveness to clonazepam and, anecdotally, to zonisamide. The majority of patients with have their myoclonic generator in the thoracic level of the spinal cord.

*Celiac disease may present with neuropathy, PML, PME, cerebellar ataxia, dementia, myopathy, and bilateral occipital intracerebral calcifications. Transglutaminase antibodies are more specific than the IgG and IgA antigliadin antibodies.

Wilson Disease

Wilson disease (WD) is an autosomal recessive **liver defect in copper excretion** that occurs in 1:40,000 people. Dietary copper is not bound to ceruloplasmin (Cp) for release into the bile and accumulates in the liver, kidney, and brain. The defective **ATP7B** gene (13q) codes for a copper-binding, membrane-bound ATPase homologous to ATP7A, responsible for Menke disease. **Many mutations** and the compound heterozygotes state of most patients make genetic diagnosis unfeasible. Patients present between 10 and 40 years of age with liver, psychiatric, and/or neurologic (particularly, any movement disorder and dysarthria) symptoms. Brain MRI may show **symmetric T2W hyperintensities and T1W hypointensities** in the midbrain ("giant panda sign": high signal in the tegmentum, normal signal in the red nuclei), tectal plate, pons ("panda cub sign" or CPM-like signal changes), caudate, putamen, and thalamus. The diagnosis is established with:

- **Serum Cp (low):** About 90% of neurologic and 75% of hepatic WD have a low Cp. However, 10% of gene carriers (normal heterozygotes) have low Cp levels and 5% of WD patients have normal CP levels. In addition, Cp is an acute-phase reactant: it may "normalize" during infections, neoplasia, inflammation, or pregnancy. Serum copper is not as useful because 90% is bound to Cp, rendering it dependent on the Cp level.
- **24-hour urine copper (high):** always over 100 µg in symptomatic WD but is closer to normal (20–50 µg) in those with prior exposure to penicillamine.
- **Slit-lamp examination for Kayser-Fleischer rings:** copper deposits in the corneal Descemet's membrane are seen in 100% of neurologic WD.
- **Liver biopsy with quantitative copper assay:** diagnostic gold standard; copper level is over 200 µg/g dry weight of liver (normal: 20–50 µg/g).

	Penicillamine	Trientine	Tetrathiomolybdate	Zinc
Action	Chelation and urine excretion of copper. Trientine competes with albumin for binding copper		Forms copper/protein complex, preventing copper absorption	Blockade of copper absorption
Side effects	**Rash** or hives, **bone marrow suppression**, and proteinuria[*]	No rash and less frequent penicillamine toxicities	Copper deficiency is main risk; lack of cellular uptake makes the drug nontoxic[▲]	Abdominal discomfort, increased amylase

[*]Late toxicities include **autoimmune disorders** such as lupus or Goodpasture syndrome, poor immune response, skin disorders such as elastosis perforans serpiginosa, and collagen disorders such as facial wrinkling. In neurologic WD, **further deterioration occurs in about 50%** of such patients with 25% not recovering to prepenicillamine levels.
[▲]Tetrathiomolybdate is the fastest anticopper drug forming a complex that neutralizes endogenous copper and prevents absorption of dietary copper. With doses higher than 120 mg/d, bone marrow copper deficiency and anemia may arise.

Tetrathiomolybdate for 8 weeks is the preferred drug for the initial treatment of neurologic WD, with zinc or trientine used as maintenance therapy. **Trientine** does not mobilize copper from the brain and is therefore not used in the acute neurologic illness. **Penicillamine** use has been discouraged because of the multiple toxicities. Zinc alone is used for presymptomatic and pregnant patients.

Tourette Syndrome

Tourette syndrome (TS) is the most common involuntary movement disorder of childhood (4:1 male-to-female ratio) of **onset before 21 years** and encompasses motor and vocal/phonic tics with coexistent behavioral disorders, especially attention-deficit-hyperactivity disorder **(ADHD)** and obsessive-compulsive disorder **(OCD).** ADHD is usually followed by motor tics, phonic tics, and OCD, with substantial overlap. The diagnosis is made when multiple waxing-and-waning motor and one or more phonic tics have been present for more than 1 year, and the location, number, frequency, type, complexity, and/or severity of tics have changed over time.

Tics are sudden, brief, stereotyped, and semivoluntary (i.e., temporarily **suppressible**) sounds or movements that mimic fragments of normal behavior. They can be **clonic, tonic, dystonic,** and/or **complex** (head shaking, trunk bending, kicking, copropraxia, coprolalia, echopraxia, echolalia, and palilalia among others) and may be preceded by discomfort or premonitory sensations temporarily relieved after the execution of the tics. Tics are also **suggestible** and may exacerbate with stress, heat, excitement, and fatigue.

Increased density of presynaptic dopamine transporter and postsynaptic D2 dopamine receptor (by PET scan) is presumed to be the causal developmental disorder. Streptococcal-induced autoimmune disorder (PANDAS) is a debated etiology. Mutations at or near the ubiquitous *SLITRK1* gene (involved in growth, branching, and interconnection of neurons) cause some cases of TS.

Dopamine blockers used for controlling tics		CNS stimulants used for controlling ADHD	Serotonergic drugs for OCD
Fluphenazine	Ziprasidone	**Methylphenidate**	Fluoxetine
Pimozide	Molindone	Pemoline	Paroxetine
Haloperidol		Dextroamphetamine	Sertraline
Risperidone	**DA depletor**	**α2 agonists**	Fluvoxamine
Thiothixene	Tetrabenazine	Clonidine	Venlafaxine
Trifluoperazine		**Guanfacine**	**Clomipramine**

ADHD, attention-deficit-hyperactivity disorder; OCD, obsessive-compulsive disorder; DA, dopamine agonist.

 Pimozide and clomipramine may prolong the QT interval. Tetrabenazine is the only antidopaminergic that has not been reported to cause tardive complications. The ADHD stimulants methylphenidate, α2 agonists (guanfacine and clonidine), atomoxetine (norepinephrine [NE] reuptake inhibitor), and desipramine (NE/serotonin reuptake inhibitor) do not worsen tic severity, as previously thought. Guanfacine is preferred over clonidine because of less sedation and hypotension and longer half-life.

> **Other inherited tic disorders** besides TS include **Huntington disease,** primary dystonia, **neuroacanthocytosis,** Hallevorden-Spatz disease, tuberous sclerosis, and **Wilson disease**.

Secondary tic disorders include infectious **(CJD, Sydenham disease),** drug-induced or tardive (amphetamines, pemoline, neuroleptics, levodopa, **cocaine,** CBZ, PHT, PB, **LTG**), toxic **(carbon monoxide), head trauma,** encephalitis, stroke, schizophrenia, autism, neurocutaneous and neurodegenerative diseases.

6 | Behavioral Neurology

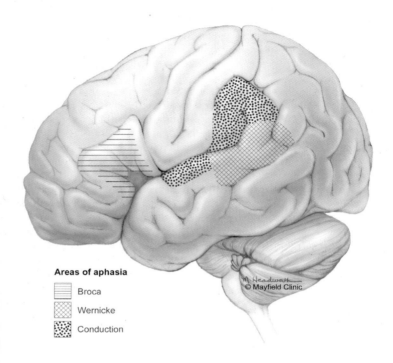

Areas of aphasia

- ▤ Broca
- ▨ Wernicke
- ▩ Conduction

© Mayfield Clinic

The left hemisphere's dominance for language is complemented by the right hemisphere's specialization for visuospatial processing. Studies with split-brain patients have revealed right hemisphere superiority for various tasks involving such components as part-whole relations, spatial relationships, apparent motion detection, and mirror image discrimination, among others. Both hemispheres are equally able to perform many visual tasks provided that they lack a spatial component.

Each disconnected hemisphere may have a separate sense of self. The most intriguing example of self-referential hemispheres is the left hemisphere promptness in detecting a partial self-image, even one that is only slightly reminiscent of the self, whereas the right brain virtually needs a complete picture of the self before it recognizes the image as such. That is to say, the left hemisphere has a linear relationship between the amount of self in a portrait and the probability of detecting self. Conversely, the right hemisphere does not recognize any images as self until they contain more than 80% of self. This chapter will suit the bulk of our left-brain readership, whose left-brain interpreting powers will make the best of the partial information available and make a judgment call on the referencing value of the whole. If the left hemisphere requires less self in an image for self-recognition, it might require fewer pages to grasp and retrieve the body of knowledge that is to follow.

Behavioral Neuroanatomy

Frontal lobe lesions	Left	Right
Frontal operculum	**Broca's aphasia**, defective *verb* retrieval	**"Expressive" aprosodia**
Superior mesial	**Akinetic mutism**	
Inferior or ventromesial: orbitobasal-ventromedial	"Acquired **sociopathy**" *Orbitofrontal* personality	
Inferior mesial: basal forebrain	Anterograde and retrograde **Amnesia and confabulation**	
Dorsolateral prefrontal	Executive dysfunction with **poor working memory**	
	For verbal information	For spatial information

The inferior mesial frontal (IMF) lobe is involved in decision making through an understanding of the current value of stimuli to the individual. Immediate reward may be assessed by medial orbitofrontal cortex (OFC) and medial prefrontal cortex (PFC), whereas delayed reward may be assessed by dorsolateral prefrontal and parietal areas.

Broca's aphasia, from a lesion in the left Brodmann area (BA) **44** and **45,** leads to nonfluent speech, agrammatism, paraphasia, anomia, and poor repetition. Lesions anterior, superior, and deep to, but sparing, Broca's area (ACA-MCA watershed) produce abnormal syntax and grammar but *preserved repetition* and automatic language, as well as uninhibited echolalia, a disorder known as **transcortical motor aphasia. Pseudopsychopathic disorder** is the impairment of social conduct from defects in planning, judgment, emotional reactions, and decision making caused by orbitobasal lesions. Personality changes from orbital damage include impulsiveness, puerility, a jocular attitude, sexual disinhibition, and complete lack of concern for others. Memory disturbances only develop with lesion extension into the septal nucleus of the basal forebrain. Appreciation of verbal humor is most impaired in right frontal polar pathology.

Temporal	Left	Right	Bilateral
Mesial	*Anterograde* amnesia for		**Kluver-Bucy syndrome (KBS)**
	Verbal material	nonverbal material	
Anterior	Impaired retrieval of		Impaired retrieval of concepts and names
	Proper names	concepts/entities	
Inferior	Impaired retrieval of nonunique		Impaired retrieval of concepts and names
	Common nouns	Concepts	
Posterior	**Associative agnosia, optic aphasia**	**Prosopagnosia**	**Visual object agnosia prosopagnosia**

The **hippocampal** complex is responsible for the acquisition of new verbal (left) and nonverbal (right) knowledge. The **amygdala** registers *emotional* information (in facial expressions, for instance) to be used in appropriate social settings. **KBS** is recognized by hyperorality, hypersexuality, *visual agnosia*, and dementia in patients with herpes encephalitis, Pick's disease, Alzheimer's disease, temporal lobe epilepsy, and head trauma. **Retrograde memory** localizes to non-mesial, non-hippocampal, anterior and lateral temporal lobe regions. **Prosopagnosia** stems from bilateral occipitotemporal (fusiform gyri) damage but can reflect isolated right inferomedial (lingual gyrus) temporal lobe injury.

Occipital	Left	Right	Bilateral
Dorsal	**Full or partial Balint syndrome:** simultanagnosia (visual disorientation) ocular apraxia, and optic ataxia		**Balint syndrome,** defective motion perception, **astereopsis**
Ventral	Right - **Hemiachromatopsia** - Left		**Full-field achromatopsia,** visual object agnosia **prosopagnosia**
	Alexia w/o agraphia, upper quadrantanopia	**Apperceptive visual agnosia**	
Occipitotemporal junction	**Associative agnosia, optic aphasia**	**Prosopagnosia** (inability to recognize familiar faces) and **visual object agnosia**	

Balint syndrome, from bi-parieto-occipital lesions corresponding to the posterior superior watershed area (MCA-PCA borderzone territories), is recognized by the combination of **simultanagnosia, ocular apraxia** (psychic gaze paralysis), and **optic ataxia** (disturbance of visually guided reaching behavior). Simultanagnosia alone occurs when occipital cortices are affected without parietal extension. **Astereopsis** (lack of visual depth perception) occurs only in the setting of full Balint syndrome. **Achromatopsia** (black-and-white world) results from bilateral damage to the hue discrimination area, located in the junction of the lingual with the fusiform gyrus. Unilaterally damaged patients (hemiachromatopsia) are usually unaware of the deficit. In **optic aphasia,** qualitatively similar to **associative agnosia,** the lack of visual naming is associated with preserved recognition in which the language centers are disconnected from the visual recognition centers due to a lesion involving both the left optic pathways and the splenium.

Parietal	Left	Right	Bilateral
TP junction	**Wernicke's** aphasia	**Amusia, phonagnosia** poor music recognition, loss of self-agency	**Auditory agnosia**
Inferior	Tactile object agnosia		**Balint syndrome** (parieto-occipital junction)
	Ideomotor apraxia, Conduction **aphasia,**	**Neglect, anosognosia, anosodiaphoria,**	

TP = temporo-parietal; PO = parieto-occipital.
Self-agency is the experience that one is the cause of one's own actions. Self agency is derived from the match between the prediction of the consequences of any voluntary actions (feed-forward signal) and the actual consequences of those actions (sensory feedback), integrated at the right TP junction.

Wernicke's aphasia results from a lesion in BA **22** (posterior part of left superior temporal gyrus), **40,** and **39** (supramarginal and angular gyrus, respectively), known as the *greater Wernicke's area,* and is characterized by fluent, paraphasic speech, impaired repetition, and defective aural comprehension. Lesions anterior, superior, and deep to, but sparing Wernicke's area (PCA-MCA watershed) produce a **transcortical sensory aphasia,** a Wernicke-like aphasia with *preserved repetition.* **Bilateral area 22 lesions** lead to the syndrome of **auditory agnosia,** or inability to identify the meaning of verbal and nonverbal auditory signals, including spoken words and familiar environmental sounds such as a telephone ringing or someone knocking on the door. The left inferior parietal lobe stores the movement representations memories, and damage there will lead to **ideomotor apraxia.** These patients are likely to have **conduction aphasia,** characterized by a disproportionate repetition defect in otherwise mildly paraphasic speech. **Neglect** may present as **anosognosia,** which in turn can lead to excessive lack of concern and minimization of personal deficits, known as **anosodiaphoria.**

Amnesia

Amnestic syndrome is a state in which memory and learning are selectively affected in an otherwise alert and responsive patient.

Korsakoff Syndrome (KS)

KS is an amnestic syndrome of nutritional origin whereby significant retrograde memory loss affects mainly the *temporal sequence* of events extending over years or decades and the *semantic memory*, creating **confabulation.** Thiamine depletion underlies the onset of KS and the often-preceding disorder, **Wernicke encephalopathy** (confusion, ataxia, nystagmus, and ophthalmoplegia). The characteristic neuropathology consists of neuronal loss, microhemorrhages, and gliosis in the paraventricular and **periaqueductal gray** matter as well as the **mammillary bodies.** Persistent memory impairment is associated with involvement of the **dorsomedial nuclei of the thalamus.** Generalized and especially frontal lobe atrophy are also common findings.

Herpes Encephalitis

The encephalitic damage to the medial temporal lobe, including the hippocampi, amygdalae, and the entorhinal and parahippocampal cortices, produces a *retrograde memory loss* with a "flatter" temporal gradient (i.e., less sparing of early memories). Impairments in *semantic memory*, naming, and reading (*surface dyslexia*) result from the involvement of the **left inferolateral temporal lobe.**

Hypoxia

The classic *anterograde amnesia* of anoxic encephalopathy appears to result from severe **loss of pyramidal cells in the CA1 region of the hippocampi** with additional damage to the cerebellum and basal ganglia.

Vascular Disorders

Anterograde amnesia with minimal retrograde amnesia results from **anterior thalamic infarction,** variably supplied by the polar or paramedian arteries, which are, ultimately, branches of the PCA. The anterior and posterior choroidal arteries, branches of the ICA and PCA, respectively, supply the hippocampi. Unilateral damage leads to material-specific memory loss.

Transient Global Amnesia (TGA)

Most commonly occurring in middle-aged or elderly individuals, TGA consists of a period of amnesia and repetitive questioning—without identity loss—lasting 2–12 hours, preceded by headache, stressful events, medical procedures, or vigorous exercise. *Anterograde amnesia* is profound and retrograde amnesia is relatively brief and restricted to recall of episodes instead of facts. TGA is presumed to result from transient dysfunction in limbic-hippocampal circuits. When attacks are brief (<1 hour) and multiple, epilepsy may be the underlying cause **(transient epileptic amnesia).** Interictal memory deficits may be present.

Memory Primer

Anterograde memory depends on the abilities to *encode, consolidate,* and *retrieve* new information. *Encoding* difficulties are thought to be responsible in part for the memory deficits of KS and frontal lobe dysfunction. Encoding is assessed by tasks of *immediate recognition*. Disproportionate deficits in **recall** compared with **recognition** indicate *retrieval* deficits and are observed in patients with frontal lobe and hippocampal lesions:

- **Recall and episodic memory** (based on contextual features of time and spatial location) localizes to the Papez circuit: *hippocampi,* fornices, mammillary bodies, mammillothalamic tract and anterior thalami.
- **Recognition memory** (based on familiarity judgments) depends on the integrity of the *entorhinal and perirhinal cortices.*

Retrograde memory can be dissociated (differential episodic and semantic impairment) and exhibit a temporal gradient (remote memories preserved better than recent ones), as demonstrated in patients with KS, TGA, and anoxia.

Working memory (relatively intact in amnesic patients with KS, HSE, and head injury) is used in the temporary and flexible manipulation of information for such cognitive tasks as reasoning and arithmetic, updated and retrieved within a few seconds but of limited storage capacity and rapidly decayed if not rehearsed. (Testing: serial sevens, digit span backward, Corsi Blocks backward.)

Declarative memory is where information is stored on a permanent or semipermanent basis in medial temporal lobe structures (severely affected in KS and HSE) and is relatively impervious to the effects of decay or interference.

- **Episodic or explicit (long-term)** memory refers to autobiographical or public incidents or events that become part of a *conscious awareness* and are stored in the medial temporal lobe, *hippocampus proper.* (Testing: logical paragraph recall, California Verbal Learning Test, Benton delayed recall.)
- **Semantic** memory refers to the storage of facts, concepts, and language, acquired over time across a variety of different contexts and supported by the *entorhinal and perirhinal cortices* in the anterior temporal lobe. (Testing: category fluency task, pyramids and palm trees test, famous faces test.)

Implicit memory refers to learning of skills that are expressed in the course of task performance without requiring awareness of the basis of this learning. It is relatively preserved in amnesic patients but impaired in certain subcortical dementias such as Parkinson's and Huntington's disease. It includes:

- **Classical conditioning or repetition priming,** which refers to the facilitation in performance that results from previous exposure to task stimuli.
- **Repeated practice or procedural memory,** motor and perceptual skill learning acquired with practice. It has been localized to the motor and prefrontal cortices, basal ganglia, and cerebellum. (Testing: pursuit rotor learning, reverse mirror tracking.)

Agnosias

Agnosia is a recognition failure specific to one sensory channel that cannot be attributed to a primary sensory defect, a generalized cognitive deficit, a language disorder, or a lack of prior knowledge of the stimulus.

Visual agnosias are a group of visual recognition disorders without primary visual defects where tactile and auditory stimuli are correctly identified.

- **Apperceptive visual agnosia** refers to the failure to achieve a structured description of the shape of the object, face, or color. The lesion is located in the **right ventral occipital region.** Denial of blindness and visual confabulation **(Anton syndrome)** are common after bilateral PCA infarcts.
- **Associative visual agnosia** is the inability to attribute meaning to a correctly perceived object (object associative amnesia; good copies of it can be made), face (prosopagnosia), or color (color agnosia). Object and color agnosias arise from damage to the **left occipitotemporal junction,** whereas prosopagnosia relates to the **bilateral occipitotemporal junction** or right medial occipitotemporal regions.

The **callosal syndrome of hemisphere disconnection** consists of left hand tactile agnosia, ideomotor transitive apraxia, and agraphia with constructional apraxia of right hand and intermanual/intentional conflict (also called **diagnostic dyspraxia:** conflict between the desired action and the actually performed act).

Tactile agnosia is a disorder of tactile object recognition by their texture, size, and shape, also called **pure astereognosis,** that occurs in the absence of basic sensorimotor impairment (it could be named *stereoanesthesia*) or other cognitive dysfunction. *Bilateral* involvement results from unilateral damage to **either parietal operculum** (corresponding to the ventrolateral somatosensory association cortex (S2) since lesions in the primary somatosensory cortex (S1) produce impairment in basic and intermediate sensory modalities.

Lesions to the sensory cortex or its thalamocortical projections lead to **cortical sensory loss,** which is translated into lack of **sensory discrimination:** loss of position sense (discrepant with the relative preservation of touch, pain, temperature and vibration sensation), astereognosis, agraphesthesia, and poor two-point discrimination.

Auditory agnosia is the failure to recognize verbal (pure word deafness) or nonverbal (environmental sound agnosia: dog barking or keys jingling) sounds when audiometry is normal. They occur when patients with cortical deafness from bilateral Heschl gyri lesions (which is, by definition, not agnosia since hearing itself is ultimately affected) begin to recover. Patients recovering from Wernicke's aphasia may also go through a state of pure word deafness.

Apraxias

Limb apraxia defines impairment in the ability to perform previously learned or skilled movements in the absence of weakness, deafferentation, or elemental movement disorders. This term may be a misnomer in "apraxia of eyelid opening" (probably focal eyelid dystonia) and "gait apraxia" (locomotion is a repetitive motor pattern that is not consciously learned). Apraxia of speech, due to insular lesions, is distinguished from conduction aphasia, due to midposterior sylvian lesions (angular and supramarginal gyri), by more self-monitored articulatory errors, making speech more halting, effortful, and less prosodic.

Limb-Kinetic Apraxia

These patients are unable to make fine, precise finger movements of the hand contralateral to a frontoparietal cortical lesion. The thesis that limb kinetic apraxia is a *disorder between paresis and apraxia* is supported by the observation that monkeys with corticospinal tract lesions may have clumsiness without weakness.

Ideomotor Apraxia (Patient Knows What to Do but Not How to Do It)

Patients perform movements with *spatial* (positioning, orientation of the limb) or *temporal* (wrist rotation prior to arm extension when using a key) errors. The *body-part-as-tool error* is the most common. It improves on imitation and with use of the actual tool. **Transitive gestures** (demonstrating tool/object use) are typically more impaired than **intransitive gestures** (not involving a tool/object), especially in Alzheimer's disease. Unilateral ideomotor apraxia is an early sign in corticobasal degeneration. Ideomotor apraxia is primarily caused by left **inferior parietal lobe** lesions, which often produce bilateral but asymmetric deficits.

- **Callosal apraxia** consists of severe left-hand transitive apraxia that often results from an infarction of the anterior cerebral artery with involvement of the genu and body of the corpus callosum and sparing of the splenium.
- **Constructional apraxia** (drawing disturbance) is tested by drawing intersecting pentagons and is significantly worse in patients with dementia with Lewy bodies.

Tasks for Transitive Gestures	Tasks for Intransitive Gestures
Use *scissors* to cut a piece of paper, *comb* to fix your hair, *brush* to paint a wall, *screwdriver* to turn a screw, *key* to unlock a door, *razor* to shave your face, etc.	Show me how to *salute*, how to *hitchhike*, wave *goodbye*, go *away*, *come here*, *stop*, *someone is crazy*, *be quiet*, *okay*, *make a fist*

Ideational or Conceptual Apraxia (Patient Does Not Know What to Do)

Patients fail to use tools and objects correctly due to *content errors* or impairment in the *ideation of tool use* (e.g., using a razor as a comb) despite knowing *what* tools are being used (absent agnosia). Ideational apraxia represents a disruption of the praxis *conceptual* system (poor conceptual knowledge of tool use) rather than the praxis *production* system, as in ideomotor apraxia. **Bilateral parieto-occipital damage** is the underlying pathology.

Aphasias

Perisylvian language zones are at the mercy of MCA perfusion. Lesions within the MCA territory produce **nonrepetitive aphasias** (i.e., repetition is impaired):

- **Broca's aphasia** (posterior inferior left frontal cortex, BA 44 and 45) consists of impaired articulation ("apraxia of speech") and simplification of sentence structure (agrammatism)
- **Wernicke's aphasia** (posterior superior left temporal cortex, BA 22) produce a fluent and well structured but meaningless or paraphasic speech and writing. Patients are typically **unaware** of the errors.
- **Conduction aphasia** (arcuate fasciculus, supramarginal gyrus, primary auditory cortex) consists of isolated repetition defect with phonemic paraphasias (e.g., "splant," "plant," "plants," for *pants*)

Lesions outside the perisylvian region are called **transcortical aphasias,** occur in the watershed of vascular territories, and produce **repetitive aphasias:**

- **Transcortical sensory aphasia** (damage to parietal convexity)
- **Transcortical motor aphasia** (damage to cingulate gyrus and supplementary motor area)
- **Mixed transcortical aphasia** is comparable to global aphasia but with preserved repetition. Patients are **echolalic**

	Comprehension	Repetition	Type of Aphasia	Common Causative Lesions
Fluent aphasias	Yes	— yes	Anomic	Nonlocalizing
		— no	Conduction	Strokes in deep parietal white matter
	No	— yes	Transcortical sensory	Occlusion of PCA, watershed MCA-PCA
		— no	**Wernicke**	Left MCA (inf. division)
Nonfluent aphasias	Yes	— yes	Transcortical motor	Occlusion of ACA, watershed ACA-MCA
		— no	**Broca**	Left MCA (sup. division)
	No	— yes	Mixed transcortical	Around BA 44, 45, and 22, but sparing cortex
		— no	Global	Full MCA territory

Generation of a list of words beginning with a specific letter or semantic category (verbal fluency) is considered a **frontal lobe function.** Impaired performance in phonological fluency occurs after right or left superior medial frontal, left dorsolateral, and left posterior lesions. Patients with **left dorsolateral frontal lobe lesions,** who may also have transcortical motor aphasia, exhibit the worst performance in the word list task. For story narrative, left-sided lesions cause perseveration (repetition) and simplification (omission) of sentence elements. Right-sided lesions cause incoherence (wandering from the topic) and irrelevant speech (amplification and over insertion of details). Large right prefrontal lesions may lead to extreme loss of narrative structure and frank confabulation, partly due to a failure of inhibiting distractions.

Acquired Dyslexia and Peripheral Dyslexia

These dyslexias are characterized by a deficit in the processing of visual aspects of the stimulus precluding the matching of words to their stored visual forms.

- **Alexia without agraphia** caused by occlusions of the left PCA was first described by Déjerine (1914) as a *disconnection* syndrome that isolates the "center for the optic images of letters." Pure alexia develops from a left occipital cortex lesion (which causes right homonymous hemianopsia; all visual information is initially processed in the right occipital cortex) and a second lesion in the splenium of the corpus callosum (which prevents visual information to be transferred from the right to the left hemisphere language cortex). Patients cannot read printed words but can recognize words spelled aloud. They may be unable to name visual stimuli but can name them after tactile exploration or verbal description **(optic aphasia).**

- **Neglect dyslexia** reflects an attentional impairment at a higher level of representation in patients who often have left-sided neglect. There is failure to correctly identify the initial portion of a letter string.

Central Dyslexias

These patients have impairments in the "higher" reading functions by which familiar visual word forms mediate access to meaning ("deep" dyslexia) or speech production ("surface" dyslexia) mechanisms.

- **Deep dyslexia** is recognized by the presence of *semantic errors* ("knight" for "castle"), with or without visual ("scale" for "skate") and morphologic ("government" for "governor") errors. There also are greater impairments in reading abstract or "low imaginative" nouns ("destiny") than concrete or "imaginable" nouns ("chair"); and functors (pronouns, prepositions, conjunctions, and interrogatives) and verbs than adjectives and adverbs. Deep dyslexia is largely found in patients with large perisylvian lesions extending into the frontal lobe, who also have global or Broca's aphasia.

- **Phonological dyslexia** is a selective and minor reading deficit that affects the translation of print to sound, relatively preserving the pronunciation of real words, whether orthographically regular ("state") or not ("colonel"), but substantially impairing the oral reading of *nonword letter strings*. Most errors involve the substitution of a visually similar real word ("phone" for *phope*). The dominant superior temporal lobe and especially the angular and supramarginal gyri are usually affected in phonological dyslexics.

- **Surface dyslexia** is another selective reading deficit that affects the print-to-sound translation of *irregularly pronounced words* ("colonel," "borough") preserving the reading of regular words ("state") and nonwords (*blape*). Surface dyslexia is characteristic of semantic dementia and other degenerative dementias such as Alzheimer's disease and frontotemporal dementia. It is rarely observed in patients with focal lesions.

Neglect

Defined as a failure to report, respond, or orient to meaningful or novel stimuli not accounted for by a primary sensorimotor deficit, contralateral to a hemispheric lesion, neglect may range from simple unawareness, to **anosognosia,** to **anosodiaphoria** (lack of concern). Neglect is most commonly associated with lesions that involve the **right inferior parietal lobe** (Brodmann's areas 40 and 39), the convergence site of multiple sensory modalities and perceptual cognitive systems related with the what and where of environmental awareness. Other neglect-inducing lesions are the dorsolateral frontal lobes, the cingulate gyrus, the thalamic and mesencephalic reticular formation, and the basal ganglia.

Distribution of Neglect

- **Spatial neglect** may occur in three dimensions (horizontal, vertical, and radial), can be body centered or environmentally centered, and is tested:
  - Line bisection task: higher yield if line is in contralesional space
  - Target cancellation task: randomly placed targets in a sheet of paper
  - Drawing or copying asymmetric nonsense figures
- **Personal neglect** refers to the failure to groom or even dress one side of the body. A cancellation task may be used for testing personal neglect in which little pieces of sticky paper are applied to different portions of the body and the subject is instructed to remove all the pieces.
- **Representational neglect** occurs when the lesion has directly destroyed the cortical representation of an object (spatial; only scenes ipsilateral to their lesions are recalled) or body part (personal; fail to perform a task in which they are required to imagine a contralesional body part).

Subtypes of Neglect

- **Attentional or sensory neglect.** Sensory neglect is a selective inattention of a given sensory modality (tactile, visual, auditory) in either the hemispatial or personal space. Deafferentation needs to be ruled out before sensory inattention is ascertained.

Initial unawareness of isolated stimuli may recover as *extinction* to **double simultaneous stimulation** becomes apparent during stroke convalescence.

- **Intentional or motor neglect.** Limb akinesia results from failure to prepare for action (intentional system) in the absence of corticospinal damage (pseudohemiparesis). The frontal lobes play a critical role in the intentional systems. Other forms of motor neglect are:
  - Hemispatial neglect (limb moves in ipsilateral but not contralateral space)
  - Directional akinesia (limb moves toward ipsi- but not contralateral space)
  - *Motor extinction* (contralateral limb moves *until* ipsilateral limb moves)
  - Limb, hemispatial, and directional *hypokinesia* (delayed reaction times)
  - Limb, hemispatial, and directional *hypometria* (short reaction amplitude)
  - Limb, hemispatial, and directional *motor impersistence*

Delirium or Acute Confusional State

Delirium (also referred to as toxic-metabolic encephalopathy or acute brain syndrome) consists of a **rapidly developing** and **fluctuating** disturbance of **consciousness** manifested by reduced environmental awareness and a change in cognition or perception that cannot be accounted for by a preexistent or evolving dementia. **Inattention** is the clinical hallmark. The patient may show misinterpretation, illusions, or hallucinations and display diverse and rapidly changing emotions (fear, anxiety, anger, depression, euphoria). A **reversal of the sleep–wake cycle** may be expressed with excessive daytime sleepiness, nocturnal agitation, insomnia, and fragmented or reduced sleep. Psychomotor activity can range from lethargy to restlessness and hyperactivity.

Hypotheses of Causation

1. **The stress-hypercortisolemia hypothesis** postulates that delirium is a manifestation of acute stress mediated by abnormally elevated levels of cortisol, which is known to impair selective attention and information processing. Stroke patients with delirium have significantly higher corticotropin and postdexamethasone cortisol levels in the first hour after onset.
2. **Reduced synthesis of acetylcholine** and epinephrine prompted, at least in part, by a reduction of cerebral oxidative metabolism (reduction of prefrontal cerebral blood flow, for instance). The delirium-prone effects of anticholinergic drugs support this hypothesis.

Search for precipitants may include a search for metabolic derangements (hypo- or hyperglycemia, hypoxemia, uremia, hepatic failure, electrolyte imbalance, thyroid disorders), infections (urinary, respiratory, systemic, or meningeal), subdural hematoma or cerebral contusion, pulmonary emboli, congestive heart failure, excessive bronchial secretions, aspiration, myocardial infarction, toxic exposures (ethanol, sedatives or illicit drugs intoxication or withdrawal), epilepsy, and iatrogenic causes (psychotropic, dopaminergic or anticholinergic drugs, cimetidine, digoxin, and steroids, among others).

> **Stroke can cause delirium** if the infarcts affect the following locations: unilateral or bilateral **PCA territory, dorsomedial and anterior thalamus,** caudate, **anterior cingulate,** lower mesial and **orbital frontal cortex,** right MCA and right ACA territories.

Treatment of delirium hinges on its early detection and the identification and correction of any precipitant(s), along with the use of nonpharmacologic interventions, such as placement in familiar environments, normalization of sleep-night cycles, and reduction or elimination of offending agents (mainly anticholinergic and sedative drugs). Should pharmacologic intervention be needed, atypical neuroleptics (olanzapine and risperidone) are preferred over typical agents such as haloperidol. Benzodiazepines such as lorazepam or diazepam may be helpful in combination with a neuroleptic.

Alzheimer's Disease (AD)

Dementia applies the presence of memory loss (episodic first, semantic later) and a deficit in one other area of cognitive function (language, visuospatial function, attention, orientation, executive functions, motor control, or praxis) associated with social or occupational impairment. AD is the most common neurodegenerative dementia, and it progresses from anomia to agnosia to aphasia to apraxia. From 65 to 85 years of age, the prevalence of AD doubles every 5 years, reaching nearly 50% by age 85. The lifetime risk of developing AD increases with the number of affected relatives, being about 40% with one, 50% with two or more, and 60% in African Americans with any number of affected members.

Accumulation of β-amyloid (Aβ) peptide is central to the AD pathogenesis. Mutations in the **amyloid precursor protein (APP),** the Aβ peptide precursor with more than 700 aminoacid residues, causes early-onset AD. All AD-related mutations increase the production of Aβ. The deposition of Aβ peptide triggers the formation of **neurofibrillary tangles (NFT),** oxidation and lipid peroxidation, glutamatergic excitotoxicity, inflammation, and activation of the cascade of apoptotic cell death.

Autosomal dominant AD may occur in those whose onset occurs under 60 years old (~2%).
- **PS1:** presenilin 1 (chromosome **14** mutation), most common
- **PS2:** presenilin 2 (chromosome **1** mutation)
- **APP:** Amyloid precursor protein (chromosome **21** mutation); Down's syndrome (trisomy **21**) overexpresses APP gene, raising Aβ deposition

Aβ42, forming neuritic plaques or **senile plaques (SP),** is increased in those with each of the above mutations. The enzymes β and γ secretases are responsible for liberating the 42-aminoacid Aβ.

Aβ40, deposited diffusely and **in vessels walls** is increased in those who have the apolipoprotein E ε4 genotype **(ApoE ε4),** believed to be a major risk factor for AD. ApoE ε4 is associated with low rates of glucose metabolism in the posterior cingulated cortex, parietal and temporal lobes, and prefrontal cortex.

Pathological hallmarks of Alzheimer's disease include: (1) **NFT,** which are intraneuronal hyperphosphorylated **microtubule-associated tau** proteins deposited as **paired helical filaments** (PHF), forming a triplet of bands on immunoelectrophoresis. They are formed first in the **entorhinal cortex** and subjacent hippocampus of the medial temporal lobe and **nucleus basalis of Meinert**. NFT-associated dementias include dementia pugilistica, PSP, corticobasal degeneration (CBD), frontotemporal dementia (FTD), adult neuronal ceroid lipofuscinosis (Kufs' disease), and prion disease. (2) Senile plaques (SP) are extracellular aggregates of Aβ peptide formed from the cleavage of membrane-bound APP by β- and γ-secretases. (3) **Lewy bodies** (composed of α-synuclein) are present in 20% of all AD individuals. Conversely, 20% of brains of patients with dementia with Lewy bodies (DLB) contain sufficient density of plaques and tangles to satisfy the pathological diagnosis of AD (AD-DLB).

Sporadic Alzheimer's Disease

The risk factors for AD are advancing age, family history, hypertension, hypercholesterolemia, stroke, head injury with loss of consciousness, less education, smaller head size, low leptin, and apolipoprotein **ApoE ε4 allele** (chromosome 19). **ApoE ε4 allele** raises the density of **β-amyloid protein (Aβ) deposits,** causing nerve cell death by oxidative damage.

- 1 copy of **ApoE ε4** increases the risk of developing AD by 3–5 times
- 2 copies of **ApoE ε4** increases the risk 15 times (50% risk of AD by 60s)
- Homozygosity for **ApoE ε4** is virtually sufficient to cause AD by age 80

Vascular factors that worsen cognition include atherosclerosis, hypertension, diabetes, **cerebral amyloid angiopathy (CAA),** and hyperhomocysteinemia. **CAA** is present in >90% of AD patients and is characterized by the **deposition of Aβ40 in cerebral arterioles,** mostly of the periventricular white matter (while senile plaques in AD predominantly accumulate Aβ42). Plasma Aβ levels are strongly associated with the presence of white matter lesions, especially in patients carrying the ApoE ε4 allele.

Combined Alzheimer's and cerebrovascular disease (mixed dementia) is the most common cause of dementia. There is a synergistic effect between lacunar infarcts and tau deposition. Major vascular risk factors are also risk factors for AD. **Lacunar infarcts** increase the risk of AD 20-fold (Nun study): less AD pathology is needed for clinical dementia if infarcts are present.

> **Cortical cholinergic loss** occurs earlier than other neurotransmitters and correlates well with NFT density. There is decreased **AChE** (presynaptic ↓G4 and ↑G1 forms) and increased **butyrylcholinesterase (BuChE)** activity (↑G1), both of which degrade ACh. BuChE is increased in senile plaques.

Biomarkers of Alzheimer's Disease

- CSF: Low amyloid β-42 and high phosphorylated tau (low aβ-42/p-tau ratio)
- MRI/CT: medial temporal (hippocampi) and parietal lobe atrophy
- PET/SPECT: bilateral *temporo-parietal* hypometabolism/hypoperfusion
- PIB (Pittsburgh Compound B) PET: binds to fibrillar Aβ of senile plaques and blood vessels, revealing widespread increased tracer uptake in neocortical regions, with relative sparing of the occipital and sensory-motor cortices, and minimal uptake in the cerebellar cortex
- FDDNP PET: binds to Aβ of plaques *and* NFT (helpful in early AD or mild cognitive impairment since NFT accumulates earliest in the medial temporal lobe; cognitive function may correlate better with NFT than SP)
- Fluorodeoxyglucose (FDG) PET: low metabolic uptake, which may be best at correlating with cognitive decline over time
- Genetic testing: chromosomal mutations (1, 14, 21), polymorphisms
- Biochemical changes: decreased activity has been found in serotonin and 5-HIAA, somatostatin, noradrenaline, and dopamine β-hydroxylase

Treatment of Alzheimer's Disease

AVAILABLE CHOLINESTERASE INHIBITORS

	Donepezil (Aricept), 1997	Rivastigmine (Exelon), 2000	Galantamine (Razadyne), 2001
Chemical class	Piperidine	Carbamate	Phenanthrene alkaloid
Dosage	5 mg → 10 mg QD	1.5 mg → 3 mg → 4.5 mg → 6 mg bid	4 mg → 8 mg → 12 mg bid
Half-life	70 h	2 h	6 h
Protein binding	96%	40%	18%
Side effects	10% GI, 5% nightmares	30% GI	10% GI, no cramps or sleep disturbances
Metabolism	Liver	Kidney	Liver-½- kidney
Interactions	CYP 2D6, 3A4: PHT, CBZ, DX	None	CYP 2D6, 3A4: PHT, CBZ, DX
Cholinesterase specificity	AchE	Dual **AchE** and **BuChE**	**AchE**; allosteric **nicotinic** modulator

GI, gastrointestinal; PHT, phenytoin; CBZ, carbamazepine; DX, dexamethasone. **Rivastigmine** improves neuropsychiatric symptoms and has become the drug of choice in Lewy body dementia.

Memantine (Namenda) is an N-methyl-D-aspartate (NMDA) antagonist approved by the U.S. Food and Drug Administration (FDA) for the treatment of moderate to severe AD. In pivotal trials, it improved cognition, reduced decline in activities of daily living, and reduced frequency of new behavioral symptoms compared with those receiving placebo when administered to AD patients on stable doses of cholinesterase inhibitors. Memantine interferes with the glutamatergic excitotoxicity or provides symptomatic improvement through effects on the function of hippocampal neurons. The 5-mg initial dose is slowly increased by 5 mg to a target dose of 10 mg bid.

Long-term use of NSAIDs has been found protective against AD in population studies, but prospective evidence is insufficient to support individual treatment with anti-inflammatory agents. NSAIDs suppress microglial activation and deposition of Aβ-amyloid through cyclooxygenase (COX) inhibition. Some NSAIDs (diclofenac, flurbiprofen, ibuprofen, indomethacin, piroxicam, and sulindac, among others) modify γ-secretase cleavage site to reduce formation of the fibrillogenic Aβ42 species. **Tarenflurbil** (R-enantiomer of flurbiprofen), which has no COX- but γ-secretase activity, Aβ vaccination, and bapineuzumab have failed to provide benefits. **Antihypertensive and statin therapies** may reduce the risk of later dementia. Statins enhance α-secretase, which cleaves APP into soluble products, reducing Aβ42 production. **Hormone-replacement is not recommended** for AD prevention. Inhibitors of β and γ secretases, analogues of insulin-degrading enzymes, and metal-binding compounds (such as clioquinol) are under study. Most patients are on a combination therapy with one cholinesterase inhibitor and memantine. Drugs with centrally acting anticholinergic properties such as tricyclic antidepressants, antihistamines, SSRIs (especially paroxetine and sertraline), and digitalis are to be avoided. Strategies that reduce vascular risk (control of blood pressure, statins and angiotensin-receptor blockers, exercise and weight control, moderate red wine consumption) may be beneficial in the long term.

Mild Cognitive Impairment

Mild cognitive impairment (MCI) is a heterogenous intermediary stage between normal cognition and mild dementia, recognized by deficits in isolated cognitive domains that *do not* impair social function or activities of daily living. MCI is subdivided into several subtypes. Amnestic-only MCI is the most common.

Amnestic MCI subtype shows the least reversion to normal and the strongest association with eventual conversion to AD. The rate of conversion to AD is about 15% per year, and up to 80% may develop AD within 6 years of diagnosis. As such, amnestic MCI may represent prodromal AD. Trials of cholinesterase inhibitors in MCI have shown modest benefits possibly due to poorly sensitive measurements, lower-than-anticipated decline rates, and lack of biomarker-enhanced recruitment (which could have been based on hippocampal atrophy, low CSF amyloid-β-42/p-tau ratio, or ApoE ε4, for instance).

MCI in Parkinson's disease (PD) is more commonly executive in nature. These executive impairments can be identified in almost 20% of PD patients at the time of diagnosis using neuropsychological batteries, with the largest deficit in verbal memory (recall of a word list, such as in the California Verbal Learning Test-2) and psychomotor speed (such as tested by the Stroop test). However, the most important cognitive predictors of progression to PD dementia are tasks with a posterior cortical basis: impaired semantic (but not phonemic) fluency, with <20 words in 90 seconds, and inability to copy an intersecting pentagon figure. These factors and age >72 years have an odds ratio of almost 90 for dementia within the first 5 years from diagnosis. The *MAPT* H1/H1 genotype is the most important independent genetic predictor of dementia risk identified to date (odds ratio 12.1).

> **Semantic fluency** is disproportionally impaired in AD and semantic dementia. Phonemic fluency is predominantly impaired in subcortical dementias. Left temporal lobe lesions are sufficient to cause semantic fluency impairment because semantic memory lies within the temporal lobe. Frontal lobe lesions produce comparable semantic and phonemic deficits.

Although the more common cognitive impairments in PD are frontostriatal executive deficits, largely dopaminergic, PD dementia is increased in those with posterior cortical impairment (temporal-parietal, nondopaminergic cortical Lewy body pathology), reflected in deficits in semantic fluency and ability to copy an intersecting pentagons figure. Nontremor dominant or postural instability gait disorder phenotype and late disease onset are additional clinical risk factors for development of dementia. The frontal-executive and posterior-cortical cognitive syndromes in PD are dissociable in terms of both their genetic basis (*COMT* genotype for the former, *MAPT* H1 variant for the latter) and relationship to dementia (strongly associated with the latter).

Vascular Dementia (VaD)

Comprising 20% of all cases of dementia in the United States, VaD is the second most common form of dementia in the United States. Vascular dementia causes an estimated 50% of dementia in Japan. Men are more commonly affected. The prevalence of dementia is nine times higher in patients who have suffered a stroke. *Probable* VaD applies to the onset of dementia within 3 months from cerebrovascular disease. *Definite* VaD requires histopathological evidence of cerebrovascular disease with absent NFT and SP. There are cholinergic deficits in VaD, independent of any concurrent AD pathology.

Two subtypes of VaD have been described: **cortical VaD,** associated with abrupt onset and stepwise progression with cortical features (aphasia, visual agnosia, etc.) and **subcortical VaD,** which is the classic manifestation, with gradual onset and slow progression of subcortical deficits (anxiety, depression, apraxic gait, urinary urgency, and executive dysfunction).

The main distinguishing features between AD and VaD are the presence of focal neurological deficits and vascular risk factors in the latter. **The memory deficit in VaD (as in that of other subcortical dementias) is of *retrieval* whereas in AD is of *encoding*.**

The importance of an accurate and early diagnosis of VaD rests on the effective management of modifiable risk factors: atrial fibrillation, cardiovascular disease, diabetes mellitus, dyslipidemia, hyperhomocysteinemia, hypertension, obesity, sleep apnea, smoking, and strokes (in contrast to the unmodifiable risk factors of age, gender [male], family history, and race [African American]).

Besides monitoring and correction of modifiable risk factors, no pharmacologic agents have been FDA approved for use in VaD. Acethylcholinesterase inhibitors (donepezil 5–10 mg, rivastigmine 6–12 mg/d, and galantamine 24 mg/d) and NMDA inhibitors (memantine 20 mg/d) may slow the progression of VaD, reduce care dependency, and improve function. Lipid-lowering agents can be part of primary and secondary prevention of cardiovascular and cerebrovascular disease. The use of these drugs is also associated with a lower risk for dementia.

Cerebral amyloid angiopathy (CAA), although most commonly recognized as a cause of ICH, may present as an **inflammatory variant** of VaD, with subacute cognitive decline, seizures, headaches, and asymmetric hyperintensities on T2-weighted and fluid-attenuated inversion recovery (FLAIR) brain MRI. There is little or no contrast enhancement. This pattern can be distinguished from the noninflammatory CAA (more symmetric subcortical or periventricular T2 hyperintensities). CAA-related inflammation can be considered a **treatable form of vascular dementia** because most patients improve after anti-inflammatory treatment (IV methylprednisolone). The APOE ε4/ε4 genotype is more common in patients with CAA-related inflammation than in patients with noninflammatory CAA.

Dementia with Lewy Bodies (DLB)

DLB constitutes the third most common cause of dementia (15%–25% of all cases) and is suspected when dementia occurs along with any two of the following (these criteria are highly specific—80%–100%—but poorly sensitive—22%–75%):

- **Recurrent visual hallucinations** and delusions
- **Prominent fluctuations in cognition and attention** (periods of confusion interspersed with periods of lucidity) that must be differentiated from toxic/metabolic encephalopathy and delirium of other causes
- **Dementia occurring within 1 year from onset of parkinsonism** (when dementia symptoms appear more than 1 year after the onset of parkinsonism, patients are classified as having PD dementia [PDD])
- **Hypersensitivity to neuroleptics**, sometimes fatal

REM behavior disorder (loss of muscle atonia during rapid eye movement [REM] sleep) can precede or accompany DLB (as it does in PD and multiple system atrophy [MSA]) in up to 55% of patients.

COGNITIVE FEATURES COMPARING DLB AND AD

DLB is better than AD	DLB as affected as AD	DLB is worse than AD
• Episodic memory (day-to-day events)	• Semantic memory[♣] • Language (verbal fluency)	• Visuospatial orientation • Working memory • Attention

[♣]In *pictorial* semantic memory, DLB fare worse than AD.

Cortical Lewy bodies are found in greatest number in the parahippocampal, entorhinal, and insular cortices as well as in the anterior cingulate region. Neocortical cholinergic activity is more severely depleted, especially in the medial occipital cortex, but postsynaptic muscarinic receptors are better preserved and more functionally intact than in AD (making centrally acting cholinergic drugs the mainstay of treatment). The distribution and severity of cholinergic deficit is shared by DLB and PDD, suggesting that these entities are phenotypic manifestations of the same disease. The **lower density of striatal dopamine D_2 receptors** in DLB may account for both the limited response to levodopa and the increased sensitivity to neuroleptics.

When medications are needed, any cholinesterase inhibitors are appropriate. **Rivastigmine** has shown to improve the psychotic features and cognitive dysfunction in DLB. Neuroleptics should only be used when necessary, given the enhanced sensitivity and worsening of extrapyramidal symptoms. Atypical agents are preferred. **Quetiapine** (Seroquel) may be used first but exhibits low efficacy. **Clozapine** (Clozaril) is the preferred agent, but monitoring for agranulocytosis is needed. Risperidone and olanzapine worsen parkinsonism (and the latter also has anticholinergic properties), making them impractical in DLB. **Levodopa** and dopamine agonists improve parkinsonism in 50% but worsen the hallucinations.

Frontotemporal Lobar Degeneration (FTLD)

FTLD is the second most common form of presenile (younger than 65 years) dementia. It includes the behavioral variant of frontotemporal dementia (bvFTD), primary progressive aphasia (PPA), and semantic dementia (SEMD).

Clinical spectrum of FTLD (location of lesion is determining factor):

*Frontal/**Behavioral***

1. **bvFTD** from **bilateral frontal atrophy** causes relative preservation of memory and language with impairments in abstraction, attention, problem solving, and planning. Echolalia, perseveration, and stereotypical use of words may arise. Parkinsonism and "sweet tooth" are common.
   - **Orbitobasal** ("pseudo-psychopathic"): disinhibition and irritability
   - **Medial frontal (anterior cingulate)**: mutism and apathy
   - **Dorsolateral prefrontal** ("pseudodepression"): apathy, psychomotor retardation and reduced learning and retrieval with decreased problem solving and set shifting (executive dysfunction)

*Temporal/**Language***

2. **PPA or progressive nonfluent aphasia (PNFA),** due to **left inferior frontal, superior temporal gyrus, insular, and inferior parietal atrophy,** causes nonfluent and nonrepetitive speech, word-finding difficulty, and agrammatism ("syntactic" aphasia). Pathology is most commonly tauopathies such as CBD or FTLD-tau but can be the expression of FTLD-U (see below).
3. **SEMD (*fluent* PPA),** due to **left anterolateral temporal atrophy** with relative sparing of hippocampus (right temporal atrophy causes **progressive prosopagnosia),** results in a syntactically fluent but empty speech, semantic paraphasia, and shrinking vocabulary (poor word retrieval). Pathology is most commonly due to FTLD-U.

Neuropathologically, there is atrophy of the frontal and temporal cortices as well as of the basal ganglia and substantia nigra. Neuronal loss is accompanied by **intraneuronal and intraglial microtubule-associated protein tau deposits without extracellular β-amyloid deposits.**

Frontotemporal dementia and parkinsonism linked to chromosome 17 (FTDP-17) is an autosomal dominant form of FTD linked to chromosome 17q21, in patients at or beyond their fifth decade with family histories of alcoholism, psychosis, and suicide, and with tremorless parkinsonism and unspecific behavioral, cognitive, and motor impairments. The forerunner of FTDP-17 was a large family described as "rapidly progressive autosomal-dominant parkinsonism and dementia with pallido-ponto-nigral degeneration (PPND)" by Wszolek et al. in 1992. These families were first described to have the MAPT mutation in chromosome 17. However, a number of families linked to chromosome 17 did not have such tau mutation. More recently, the genetic spectrum of FTDP-17 has been extended to include TDP-43 proteinopathies, with or without PGRN mutation.

Pathology and Genetics of Frontotemporal Lobar Degeneration

The neuropathology of FTLD consists of **tau-positive** filamentous cytoplasmic inclusions in neurons and glia (**FTLD-tau**) or **tau-negative, ubiquitin-positive** intranuclear and cytoplasmic inclusions in neurons only (**FTLD-TDP**). Up to 40% of dominantly inherited **FTLD-tau gain-of-function mutations** are in the *microtubule-associated protein tau gene* (**MAPT**, 17q21). **Loss-of-function FTLD-TDP mutations** have been reported for *valosin-containing protein* or *p97*, an adenosine triphosphatase (ATPase) of the ubiquitin-proteasome system (9p21), *chromatic modifying protein 2B gene* or *CHMP2B*, an endosomal transport protein (3c), and *progranulin* or **GRN**, a growth factor involved in tumorigenesis (1.7 MB centromeric to *MAPT* on 17q21). Ubiquitin-positive lentiform ("cat eye") **intranuclear inclusions** in the neocortex and striatum suggest FTLD-TDP with *PGRN* or *p97* mutations. Mutations in *MAPT* and *GRN* account for 50%–60% of familial FTLD. **FTLD-GRN** is associated with **frontal-temporal-parietal asymmetry,** PNFA, hallucinations and limb apraxia, leading to clinical diagnoses of PNFA, CBD, DLB, or AD. **FTLD-MAPT** is associated with earlier onset of language impairment and may be accompanied by motor neuron disease. The nuclear protein TAR DNA binding protein 43 (TDP-43) is the major protein in FTLD-TDP, FTLD-MND, and *GRN* inclusions. Mutations in the fused in sarcoma/translocation in liposarcoma gene (FUS/TLS) were recently identified as causing about 4% of familial ALS. FUS is, like TDP-43, a nuclear DNA/RNA-binding protein.

SUMMARY OF FTLD-TAU, -TDP, -FUS, AND -UPS MISFOLDED PROTEIN DISEASES

FTLD-Tau (Tauopathies): 3R, 3/4R	FTLD-Tau: 4R
3R: Pick disease (**PiD**)	FTLD with MAPT mutation (**FTDP-17**)
3R: FTLD-MAPT (**FTDP-17**)	Corticobasal degeneration (**CBD**)
3/4R: FTLD-MAPT (**FTDP-17**)	Progressive supranuclear palsy (**PSP**)
3/4R: NFT Dementia	Multiple system tauopathy/dementia (**MSTD**)
(frontal variant of AD)	Argyrophilic grain disease (**AGD**)

FTLD-TDP (Formerly, FTLD-U)	FTLD-FUS
FTLD with ubiquitin inclusions (**FTLD-TDP**)	Neuronal filament inclusion disease (**NIFID**)
FTLD with MND (**FTLD-MND**)	Atypical FTLD-ubiquitin (**aFTLD-U**)
FTLD with PGRN mutation (**FTLD-GRN**)	Basophilic inclusion disease (**BIBD**)
FTLD with TARDBP mutation	FTLD with fused in sarcoma mutation (**FTLD-FUS**)
FTLD with VCP mutation (**FTLD-VCP**)	
FTLD linked to chromosome 9	
FTLD with CHMP2B mutation	

FUS, fused in sarcoma /translocation in liposarcoma gene; 3R, 4R, predominant tau isoform within the inclusion; MAPT, microtubule-associated protein tau mutation; UPS, ubiquitin-proteasome system; VCP, valosin-containing protein.

Frontotemporal dementia with motor neuron disease (FTLD-MND) patients may present with progressive aphasia and personality changes followed within weeks or months by the emergence of bulbar features and mild limb amyotrophy.

Focal Atrophy Syndromes in Dementias

FTLD-MND is associated with more limited atrophy (posterior frontal) compared to FTLD-TDP, which is associated with extensive temporal and frontal atrophy. The restricted distribution of cortical atrophy in FTLD-MND patients may reflect their more rapid progression and early death from neuromuscular problems.

The reliability of a clinical diagnosis as judged by pathology at autopsy depends on the syndrome considered:
- The clinical syndrome of FTD *with* motor neuron disease (FTLD-MND) is often confirmed at autopsy to have ubiquitin-only inclusions.
- The clinical syndrome of FTD *without* MND can be a tauopathy (usually CBD, 42% of cases) or ubiquitinopathy (FTLD-TDP, in 58%).
- The clinical syndrome of progressive nonfluent aphasia (PNFA) is most often (80%) due to a tauopathy, typically CBD and PSP.
- CBD- and PSP-like presentations are highly predictive of tau pathology.

FTLD-U, FTLD-MND, and ALS share ubiquitin pathology, and the protein aggregate in these diseases has recently been found to be the same: TAR DNA binding protein 43 (TDP-43). The following clinical pearls support their common pathology: (1) FTD and MND may afflict a family in separate generations; (2) ubiquitinated neuronal inclusions have been identified in nonmotor cortices of MND cases without clinical evidence of FTD; and (3) ubiquitinated neuronal inclusions have been found in anterior horn cells in MND-ID cases without clinical or pathological evidence of MND. In the absence of MND, the term motor neuron disease inclusion body dementia **(MND-ID)** has been used since the same characteristic histological ubiquitin-positive tau-negative inclusions otherwise present in the anterior horn motor neuron are found in granule cells of the hippocampal dentate gyrus and neocortical neurons.

Posterior Cortical Atrophy Syndrome (PCAt)

PCAt is a dementing syndrome that presents with early impairment of visuospatial skills with less prominent memory loss, associated with atrophy in the parieto-occipital and posterior temporal cortices. Patients exhibit signs of cortical visual dysfunction of the ventral-occipitotemporal ("what") visual processing pathway, such as apperceptive visual agnosia, prosopagnosia, achromatopsia, and alexia, or the dorsal-occipitoparietal ("where") visual pathway: Balint syndrome, transcortical sensory aphasia, apraxia, and some or all of the Gerstmann syndrome elements (agraphia, acalculia, finger agnosia, right-left disorientation). The PCAt syndrome, which mostly affects the dorsal visual pathways, can result from the "visual variant" and "logopenic progressive aphasia" (LPA) variant of Alzheimer's disease (early-onset AD), DLB, corticobasal degeneration (CBD), and Creutzfeldt-Jakob disease. The LPA variant of AD is characterized by slow speech with word-finding pauses and poor repetition associated with left-hemisphere predominant atrophy in posterior temporal and inferior parietal regions.

Frontal Assessment Battery (FAB): Office Assessment of Frontal Function

The FAB (Introduced by Dubois B, et al. *Neurology* 2000;55:1621–1626) is a short bedside cognitive and behavioral battery helpful in assessing whether a dysexecutive syndrome (in such conditions as FTD, PSP, CBD, MSA, and PD) exists. It contains six subtests that explore conceptualization, mental flexibility, motor programming, sensitivity to interference, inhibitory control, and environmental autonomy.

1. **Similarities (conceptualization)**

   "In what way are they alike?"

   A banana and an orange; a table and a chair; a tulip, a rose, and a daisy

   Score only category responses (fruits, furniture, and flowers): 0–3

2. **Lexical fluency (mental flexibility)**

   "Say as many words as you can beginning with the letter 'S,' except surnames or proper nouns."

   Score at 60 seconds: 0 = <3 words; 1 = 3–5 words; 2 = 6–9 words; 3 = >9 words

3. **Motor series (programming)**

   "Look carefully at what I am doing"

   Perform a series of Luria ("fist-edge-palm") three times; "Do it with me now (three times)"; "Now, do it on your own."

   Score consecutive series: 0 = < 3 with examiner; 1 = 3 with examiner; 2 = at least 3 alone; 3 = 6 alone

4. **Conflicting instructions (sensitivity to interference)**

   "Tap twice when I tap once."

   A series of three trials is run (1-1-1) to ensure understanding; "Tap once when I tap twice"—followed by trial (2-2-2)

   Score the series 1-1-2-1-2-2-2-1-1-2: 0 = tapping like examiner at least four consecutive times; 1 = >2 errors; 2 = 1–2 errors; 3 = no errors

5. **Go-no go (inhibitory control)**

   "Tap once when I tap once."

   A series of three trials is run (1-1-1) to ensure understanding; "Do not tap when I tap twice."—followed by trial (2-2-2)

   Score the series 1-1-2-1-2-2-2-1-1-2: 0 = tapping like examiner at least four consecutive times; 1 = >2 errors; 2 = 1–2 errors; 3 = no errors

6. **Prehensive behavior (environmental autonomy)**

   "Do not take my hands."

   Without looking at the patient, the examiner touches the patient's palms to see if he/she will spontaneously take them.

   Score 0 if patient takes the examiner's hand after being told not to do so; 1 = without hesitation; 2 = with hesitation; 3 = hand is not taken

Neuro-ophthalmology and Neuro-otology **7**

It can be said that proper examination of the oculomotor system provides the most localizing and diagnostic "bang for the buck" than that of any other system. Here are some examples of how important this chapter is:

- **Saccadic impairment alone** brings attention to supranuclear eye movement disorders, since nuclear and infranuclear lesions impair saccades, pursuit, and vestibular eye movements equally.
- **Any motility disorder that does not involve the pupil** should include myasthenia gravis and Miller Fisher syndrome in the diagnostic considerations.
- **Any motility disorder, especially if diffuse, that involves the pupil** (mydriasis) should always include botulism in the differential diagnosis.
- **Eye deviated down and out** with impaired elevation, depression, and adduction, ptosis, and mydriasis: internal carotid-posterior communicating artery junction aneurysm causing third nerve palsy until proven otherwise.
- **Same as above but with normal pupil:** suspect microvascular ischemia from diabetes or hypertension.
- **Vertical diplopia,** unlike horizontal diplopia, has a narrow differential: CN IV (trochlear) palsy or skew deviation from a brainstem stroke.

In the presence of CN III (oculomotor) palsy, the method of testing CN IV palsy (superior oblique weakness) by asking the patient to depress the adducted eye cannot be performed. Instead, the patient should be instructed to abduct the eye and then look down; if CN IV is intact, there will be intorsion. Confirming that CN IV is intact in the presence of CN III palsy is important because the combination of an oculomotor and trochlear palsy suggests a lesion in the cavernous sinus.

- **Horizontal gaze palsy** from an abducens nuclear lesion occurs rarely in isolation. Most often, it is accompanied by an ipsilateral facial nerve palsy because the seventh nerve fascicle wraps around the sixth nerve nucleus.
- **When dizziness is central** (brainstem or cerebellar stroke), there is a normal vestibulo-ocular response (as measured by head impulse test [rapid head rotation from lateral to midposition), direction-changing nystagmus, or vertical strabismus on alternating covering of the eyes (skew deviation).
- **When dizziness is peripheral** (acute vestibulopathy) there is an abnormal vestibulo-ocular response, nystagmus beats in the same direction regardless of direction of gaze, or there never is skew deviation.
- **"Peering at the tip of the nose"** from supranuclear gaze palsy with forced downward deviation of the eyes may be due to a thalamic lesion, which can also cause supranuclear thalamic esotropia, probably secondary to excessive convergence tone.
- **Cerebral polyopia** is a form of cortical visual perseveration from parieto-occipital pathology. It refers to two or more visual images persistent with monocular covering and is often accompanied by a homonymous hemianopia.

Transient Monocular Visual Loss (TMVL)

TMVL results from hypoperfusion **(amaurosis fugax)** or disc pressure **(transient visual obscurations).**

Amaurosis fugax (retinal TIA) expresses as a **painless** dark or black shade or "gray-out" that suddenly spreads across the visual field and lasts a few minutes. Positive visual phenomena and **visual worsening with exposure to bright light** also suggest ocular hypoperfusion. It represents the most helpful **localizing sign of carotid occlusive disease.** Funduscopic examination may show multiple mid-peripheral microaneurysms, small-dot-and blot hemorrhages, or nerve fiber layer splinter hemorrhages consistent with **venous stasis retinopathy** (hypotensive retinopathy). The retinopathy is usually due to advanced carotid atherosclerotic or ophthalmic artery disease, and is ipsilateral to the severely obstructed carotid artery.

> **Amaurosis fugax** on exposure to bright light is often associated with severe ipsilateral carotid artery occlusive disease. Patients with amaurosis fugax have a lower risk of subsequent stroke than those with TIAs involving the brain.

The risk of stroke in patients with TMVL and ipsilateral significant carotid stenosis is less than half of those with hemispheric TIAs. The risk of death in patients with TMVL and atheromatous carotid stenosis is approximately 4% per year.

NONVASCULAR TMVL

Ocular Diseases	Optic Nerve Diseases		
Angle closure glaucoma	**Transient Visual Obscurations**		
Dry eyes	Papilledema, optic disc drusen, congenitally anomalous optic disc		
Keratoconus			
Proptosis	**Gaze-evoked:** optic nerve compression		
Retinal detachment			
	Uhthoff's phenomenon		

Painful TMVL suggests giant-cell arteritis, carotid artery dissection, or **angle-closure glaucoma.** The latter is suspected by episodes of unilateral headache or eye pain accompanied by blurred vision and *halos* around lights lasting 30–60 minutes, precipitated by sneezing, pharmacologic mydriasis, and work in dark or dim light environments. Ophthalmic examination shows conjunctival hyperemia, corneal haze, and forward bowing of the iris, with a *mydriatic* and fixed pupil.

Transient visual obscurations are briefer TMVL due to **elevated intracranial pressure** (ICP) from increased pressure at the optic nerve head precipitated by postural changes, such as bending over, and associated with **papilledema.** Unlike other forms of disc edema, visual acuity in papilledema is normal and the visual field deficits are enlargement of the blind spots and visual constriction. Neuroimaging is indicated to explore the causes of raised intracranial pressure (mass lesions, hydrocephalus, or cerebral venous thrombosis). Negative imaging should be followed by a lumbar puncture to confirm the presence of elevated ICP and to analyze the CSF for evidence of meningeal inflammation. Elevated ICP in the presence of normal imaging and CSF studies meet criteria for idiopathic intracranial hypertension.

Migraine may rarely present as TMVL (ocular or retinal migraine). Episodes may last minutes to hours and may be followed by headache or ocular pain in young, healthy people. They build up over time and are associated with scintillations and other positive visual phenomena.

Permanent Monocular Visual Loss (PMVL)

PMVL results from lesions anterior to the chiasm (eye itself or optic nerve).

Acute PMVL (vascular) stems from occlusion of the ophthalmic artery or, more often, either of its two terminal branches (central retinal and posterior ciliary).

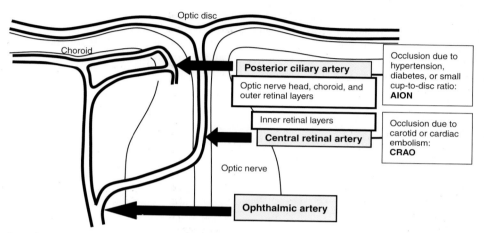

Posterior ischemic optic neuropathy (PION) refers to the rare involvement of the retrobulbar segment of the optic nerve occurring in the setting of severe and prolonged hypotension.

Anterior ischemic optic neuropathy (AION) results from damage to the optic nerve head from **occlusion of branches of the posterior ciliary artery.**

- **Nonarteritic AION** is an acute but **painless altitudinal defect** (often inferior). **Disc edema** may be segmental (often superior). The risk factors are hypertension, diabetes, and **congenitally small optic nerve heads** (no physiologic cupping or "crowded" disc: **small cup-to-disc ratio**).
- **Arteritic AION** is the most common manifestation of **giant-cell arteritis** (GCA) in those older than 60 and may be predated by **episodes of painful diplopia and TMVL.** The fellow eye can deteriorate within days or weeks. Up to 12% of patients with GCA have a normal ESR but high CRP or fibrinogen. High-dose IV steroids may protect the other eye and reverse some of the deficits. A temporal artery biopsy is required for diagnosis.

Central retinal artery occlusion (CRAO) causes diffuse retinal whitening with foveal sparing (choroidal circulation), creating the classic macular **cherry-red spot.** *Painful* CRAO may result from carotid dissection (especially when present with ophthalmoparesis or Horner syndrome) or GCA. Treatments include lowering the Intraocular pressure (acetazolamide), paracentesis, and ocular massage.

Progressive forms of PMVL are unilateral optic neuropathies from infiltrative or compressive mechanisms such as optic nerve gliomas, optic nerve sheath meningiomas, pituitary tumors, or sarcoidosis.

Acute or Subacute MVL in a Younger Patient: Optic Neuritis

Optic neuritis (ON) is recognized by the sudden onset of a **central defect** (rather than altitudinal) that **progresses over days** and is associated with **pain with eye movements.** The earliest findings are relative afferent papillary defects (RAPD), **reduction in color saturation,** and **central scotoma.** The optic disc may be swollen (prebulbar ON) or normal (retrobulbar ON).

> **Relative afferent pupillary defect (RAPD or Marcus Gunn pupil)** is seen in unilateral or asymmetric optic neuropathy. Both pupils constrict less when the affected eye is illuminated and more when the normal eye is shone. Neutral density filters placed over the normal eye can help quantify its severity.

Retrobulbar ON is diagnosed when the above deficits occur in the setting of a normal fundus ("the patient sees nothing and the doctor sees nothing"). Vision recovers over several weeks but optic disc pallor (reflecting degeneration of optic nerve fibers) appears ("the patient sees everything and so does the doctor").

DIFFERENTIAL DIAGNOSIS OF INFLAMMATORY OPTIC NEURITIS

Demyelinating	Infectious
Idiopathic – **multiple sclerosis** and ADEM Devic's disease	*Bacterial:* **Syphilis,** neuroretinitis due to **catscratch disease** (Bartonella henselae), **Lyme disease** (Borrelia burgdorferi), tuberculosis, Whipple's
Inflammatory Disorders	*Viral:* herpes simplex and zoster, HIV, EBV, coxsackie, adenovirus, CMV, hepatitis A and B, measles, mumps, rubeola, and rubella
Sarcoidosis, SLE, polyarteritis nodosa, Wegener granulomatosis	*Parasitic:* toxoplasmosis, cysticercosis, toxocariasis
Other: bee and wasp stings	*Fungal:* cryptococcosis, aspergillosis, mucormycosis, candidiasis, histoplasmosis

Idiopathic ON is the most common acute optic neuropathy in people under the age of 45 with spontaneous visual recovery within 3 weeks in 80% of patients. The risk of MS after ON is 16% at 5 years and as high as 75% at 15 years. **The 10-year risk of MS is 56% in patients with ≥12 MRI T2W lesions,** compared to 22% with a normal baseline MRI (Optic Neuritis Treatment Trial, ONTT, 1995). A very low MS risk comes from the combination of painless ON and normal brain MRI, optic nerve edema, peripapillary hemorrhages, or a macular star. Predictive factors for the development of MS include Caucasian ethnicity, family history, **female gender, retrobulbar ON, pain, and CSF oligoclonal bands.** IV methylprednisolone (250 mg four times daily for 3 days), followed by oral prednisone (1 mg/kg/d) for 11 days (ONTT protocol), hasten the rate of recovery of vision. Oral prednisone is associated with an increased risk of recurrent ON. The **CHAMPS** study (2001) supported the initiation of interferon β-1a treatment at the time of a first episode of ON in patients at high risk for MS based on the presence of subclinical brain MRI lesions. Clinically definite MS was reduced by 44% within 6 months and persisted throughout the study.

Binocular Visual Loss (BVL)

Persistent binocular visual loss (PBVL) results from damage to both optic nerves, the chiasm, or the retrochiasmal visual pathways. Chiasmal and retrochiasmal lesions respect the vertical meridian. Visual acuity is affected (symmetrically) only on bilateral retrochiasmal lesions. Complete blindness of cerebral origin preserves the pupillary light reflex.

	Field Defect	Location
	Bitemporal hemianopia	Chiasm
	Incongruous left homonymous hemianopia	Right optic tract
	Left homonymous **sectoranopia** (lateral choroidal artery)	Right lateral geniculate nucleus
	Left homonymous upper quadrant defect (**"pie in the sky"**)	Right temporal lobe
	Left homonymous defect, denser inferiorly	Right parietal lobe
	Left homonymous lower quadrantanopia (*macular sparing*)	Right occipital lobe (upper bank)
	Left homonymous upper quadrantanopia (macular sparing)	Right occipito-temperol (Meyer's loop)
	Left homonymous hemianopia (*macular sparing*)	Right occipital lobe

The more congruous a partial homonymous visual field defect, the closer the lesion to the occipital lobe. *Macular sparing* occurs only with occipital lobe lesions that spare the most posterior aspect of the occipital lobe which has dual blood supply from the PCA *and* MCA.

Optic neuropathies due to **hereditary** (Leber hereditary optic neuropathy), **toxic** (methanol, ethylene glycol, tobacco, lead, amiodarone, disulfiram, ethambutol), or **nutritional deficiencies** (vitamin B_{12} deficiency) are symmetric and progressive PBVL. The classic visual field defect is a **cecocentral scotoma,** which involves the region between fixation and the physiologic blind spot. The most common bilateral optic neuropathy in the Western world is **primary open-angle glaucoma,** a superior altitudinal visual field loss respecting the horizontal meridian and early on sparing central visual acuity in a patient with elevated intraocular pressure and enlarged cup-to-disc ratio.

Transient binocular visual loss (TBVL) is most commonly part of the visual aura that occurs with **ophthalmic migraine.** An episodic and brief (over minutes) enlarging scotoma in homonymous portions of the visual field is surrounded by jagged, shimmering lights and is followed by contralateral hemicranial throbbing headache. Absence of the latter is more common after the age of 50 (acephalgic migraine or *migraine equivalent*). **TIAs in the basilar or PCA distribution** may cause TBVL, which, unlike migraine, begins suddenly with *concurrent* pain above the contralateral brow and lacks positive phenomena or stereotypical build-up.

Cerebral Visual Loss

Besides the **retinogeniculostriate** (topographic; yielding specific field hemifield defects outlined above) component of visual information, two "higher level" visual streams are described as part of the secondary or association visual cortical areas: the **occipitotemporal** or ventral "what" pathway of object identity, such as form and color, and the **occipitoparietal** or dorsal "where" visual pathway of motion, stereopsis, and spatial location. Diffuse lesions in both occipital lobes or both optic radiations lead to **Anton syndrome,** characterized by cortical blindness with preserved pupillary reactivity, unawareness of blindness, and confabulation.

MAJOR CAUSES OF CEREBRAL VISUAL LOSS

Acute	Progressive
PCA stroke, posterior reversible encephalopathy syndrome (PRES), CVT, and **eclampsia**	Occipital mass (glial tumor, lymphoma), demyelination (MS), dysmyelination (**ADL** and Schilder's disease), **CJD** (Heidenhain variant), **SSPE,** and toxins (chronic **methyl mercury poisoning** – Minamata disease)
Aspergillosis, drugs (**cyclosporine,** tacrolimus), acute intermittent, **porphyria,** hepatic encephalopathy	

CVT, cerebral venous thrombosis; ADL, adrenoleukodystrophy; SSPE, subacute sclerosing panencephalitis.

Occipitotemporal Disorders (Ventral Extrastriate Region): Object Recognition

- **Achromatopsia** from lesions of the contralateral lingual and fusiform gyri; bilateral lesions make patients only see "dirty shades of gray"
- **Object agnosia,** from lesions in both medial temporal lobes, consists of inability to name *and* describe objects until other sensory modality is used
- **Alexia without agraphia** from lesions in the left visual cortex (which causes right homonymous hemianopsia) and splenium of corpus callosum
- **Alexia with agraphia** from lesions in the left angular gyrus and left occipitotemporal cortex
- **Prosopagnosia** or inability to recognize faces, from *bilateral* or right medial temporal lesions
- **Topographagnosia** or geographic disorientation, from right medial occipitotemporal cortex lesions

Occipitoparietal Disorders (Dorsal Extrastriate Region): Object Localization

- **Balint syndrome,** caused by *bilateral* occipitoparietal lesions, consists of **simultanagnosia** (inability to interpret a complex scene with multiple interrelated elements despite accurate "piecemeal" description), **ocular apraxia** (psychic gaze paralysis leading to difficulty initiating saccades), and **optic ataxia** (disturbance of visually guided reaching behavior caused by difficulty in judging the spatial position of objects—visual disorientation)
- **Hemineglect** or a spatially based failure of attention caused by lesions in the right parietal lobe
- **Akinetopsia** or impairment of motion perception leading to misjudgment of speed and direction of moving objects, from bilateral occipitoparietotemporal lesions

Anisocoria

Anisocoria Greater in Dim Light (Smaller Pupil Abnormal)

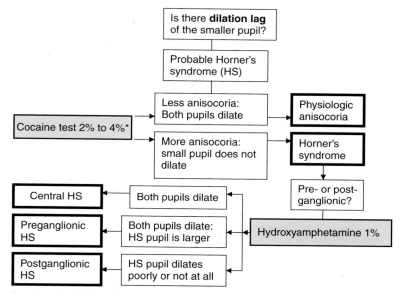

An acute and painful Horner's syndrome should be considered due to an acute carotid dissection until proven otherwise.

*Apraclonidine (0.5% to 1%) is an alternative to cocaine.

Assessment of anisocoria in comatose patients is important. A larger pupil could indicate oculomotor nerve compression by a protruding inferomedial temporal lobe during transtentorial herniation or an aneurysm at the junction of the posterior communicating and internal carotid arteries. A smaller pupil could indicate sympathetic dysfunction due to lateral medullary infarction or an extraparenchimal lesion, such as damage of the superior cervical ganglion by lung cancer (Pancoast syndrome). This myosis may be accompanied by other elements of the Horner's syndrome. Bilateral pinpoint but reactive pupils occur with pontine lesions that transect descending sympathetic pathways. Opioids do not abolish pupillary light reactivity but miosis is severe. Anticholinergic drugs, including amitriptyline, can abolish pupillary light reactivity.

Anisocoria is never caused by retinal or optic damage because pupillary light reflex is consensual. There is reduced but *symmetric* response bilaterally when light is shone at the affected eye (relative afferent pupillary defect). Anisocoria results from abnormalities in the iris or the efferent portion of the pupil pathway.

Anisocoria Greater in Bright Light (Larger Pupil Abnormal)

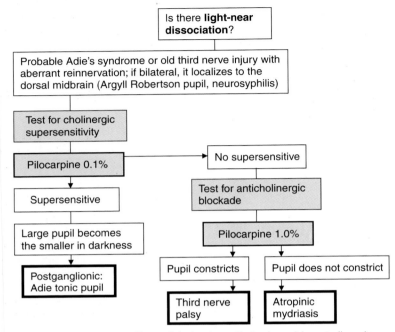

Mechanical anisocoria where pupilloconstriction is subnormal in the abnormal, larger pupil, may be seen in angle-closure glaucoma, trauma, infection, inflammation (prior uveitis), iris tumor or mass (iris melanoma), and laser treatment.

Light-near dissociation most often occur in the following three disorders: (1) Argyll-Robertson pupil (bilateral small pupils, associated with neurosyphilis); (2) Parinaud dorsal midbrain syndrome (bilateral); and (3) Adie tonic pupil (unilateral or bilateral).

Adie tonic pupil is unilateral first. The pupil is large and shows sectoral palsy of the iris sphincter. Constriction to a near stimulus is long lasting and followed by slow redilation. Adie tonic pupils become bilateral at a rate of about 4% per year. **Holmes-Adie syndrome** applies to the association of Adie tonic pupils and hyporeflexia. **Ross syndrome** applies to the above plus segmental anhidrosis.

Acute third nerve palsy with pupillary involvement raises the possibility of compressive pathology (aneurysm, pituitary apoplexy, cavernous sinusitis) and is considered a neurological emergency.

Diplopia

Monocular diplopia is due to ocular refractive problems and resolves with a pinhole. **Binocular diplopia** requires observing the range and speed of gaze with one **(ductions)** and both eyes **(versions)** in the nine positions of gaze.

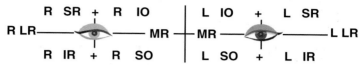

R SR + R IO	L IO + L SR
R LR———⊙——— MR	MR ———⊙———L LR
R IR + R SO	L SO + L IR

The recti muscles are responsible for vertical movements in the abducted position, and the obliques in the adducted position of gaze. IO, inferior oblique; SR, superior rectus; SO, superior oblique; IR, inferior rectus; LR, lateral rectus; MR, medial rectus.

Horizontal misalignment expresses as **esotropia** or inward deviation of the eye, or as **exotropia,** outward deviation. Vertical misalignment is described in relation to the higher eye as **hypertropia,** or lower eye, **hypotropia.** Gaze position affects the degree of eye misalignment in **noncomitant strabismus** (restrictive ocular disorders such as thyroid ophthalmopathy, which typically causes decreased elevation with the eye abducted) but not in **comitant strabismus** (childhood onset), where diplopia is due to decompensation of a long-standing phoria, a *latent* deviation kept in check by fusional mechanisms but expressed when binocularity is interrupted. A *manifest* deviation of the visual axes when both eyes are viewing, not kept in check by fusion, is called **tropia.** When the latter does not cause diplopia, a congenital disorder is suspected.

The cover-uncover test is used to detect tropias and phorias. While fixating on a distant target one eye is covered and any immediate movement of redress of the uncovered eye is observed: inward redress equals exotropia; outward, esotropia. If no tropia is present, our attention is focused to the covered eye to determine if its immediate uncovering would unmask a latent deviation (phoria). **The alternate cover test** can show maximal deviation of any tropia or phoria identified by the cover-uncover test. While fixating on a distant target, the occluder is quickly switched from eye to eye to prevent binocular viewing and break binocular fusion. The movement of the newly uncovered eye indicates a heterotropia or a heterophoria. A secondary deviation (from the nontropic eye) will always be greater than the primary deviation (that of the tropic eye).

Selected Causes of Diplopia According to Cardinal Positions of Gaze

Vertical diplopia—worse when looking up and R **(Right hypertropia)**	Horizontal diplopia—worse when looking to R: Paretic R lateral rectus, or Paretic L medial rectus	Vertical diplopia—worse when looking up and L **(Left hypertropia)**
Either of these pairs may be paretic		Either of these pairs may be paretic

R IR and SO	L IO and SR
(depress R eye)	(elevate L eye)

Horizontal diplopia—worse when looking to L: Paretic L lateral rectus Paretic R medial rectus

R SR and IO	L SO and IR
(elevate R eye)	(depress L eye)

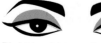

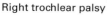

Right trochlear palsy

Left trochlear palsy

Trochlear (fourth nerve) palsy from SO palsy causes **vertical or diagonal diplopia** due to hypertropia with small esotropia, greatest with contralateral gaze and ipsilateral head tilt. A simple test for SO weakness is to hold a pencil horizontally in front of the patient. When slowly lowered, vertical separation of the images forms a V shape whose angle points toward the affected side. **Nuclear trochlear palsy** causes contralateral SO palsy and ipsilateral Horner's syndrome.

There are three steps in diagnosing vertical diplopia due to *left* superior oblique palsy:

(1) Primary position: *left* eye hypertropia (weakness of elevators of right eye, right IO and SR, or depressors of the left eye, left SO and IR);

(2) Gaze to side: deviation is worse on gaze to the *right* (weakness of right SR or left SO);

(3) **Bielschowsky head tilt test:** with the head tilted to the *left*, there is an exaggeration of the left hypertropia (patient's head tend to tilt to the right).

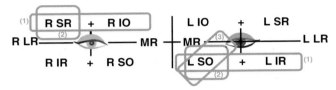

Oculomotor (third nerve) palsy causes exotropia with small hypotropia (eye is "out and down"), upper eyelid ptosis, and a dilated pupil. If there is no intorsion on attempted downgaze, a combined fourth nerve palsy is present (lesion in cavernous sinus is suspected). Since the central caudal nucleus innervates both levator muscles, a **nuclear lesion causes bilateral ptosis.**

Posterior communicating artery aneurysm is the most common etiology.

Superior oblique myokymia patients complain of brief, recurrent episodes of monocular blurring of vision, **vertical or torsional diplopia,** or oscillopsia in one eye usually lasting <10 seconds, but occurring many times per day. The attacks are triggered by looking down and in, which maximally activate the SO muscle. It is often benign and may respond to carbamazepine or baclofen.

Ocular neuromyotonia consists of transient episodes of diplopia precipitated by holding the eyes in eccentric gaze due to potentially painful contraction of one or more muscles innervated by one oculomotor nerve. Vascular compression and radiation therapy to the parasellar region are risk factors. Carbamazepine is an effective treatment. It can be confused with ocular myasthenia, superior oblique myokymia, thyroid ophthalmopathy, and rippling muscle disease.

Duane retraction syndrome consists of congenital aplasia or hypoplasia of the abducens cranial nerve or nucleus (unilateral, rarely bilateral), leading to restricted abduction. In some patients (type III), an attempt at adduction is also limited and associated with eye retraction and **palpebral fissure narrowing** due to anomalous innervation of the medial and lateral rectus muscle by the third cranial nerve. Duane syndrome is more common in women and most often affects the left eye. Thalidomide embryopathy may include Duane features.

Disorders of Saccades

Saccades are voluntary phasic eye movements that redirect the eyes to a new fixation object. Optokinetic and vestibulo-ocular reflexes use saccades as part of an involuntary response.

Saccade synthesis require that *pulse* (phasic muscle *bursts*) and *step* (opposing tonic muscle contraction) are accurately matched to each other.
- Pulses from *burst* neurons in the **pons** paramedian reticular formation (**PPRF**) innervate **horizontally** acting EOM. The PPRF receives "initiation" commands from the *contralateral* frontal eye field and superior colliculus.
- Pulses from *burst* neurons in the **midbrain** rostral interstitial nucleus of the medial longitudinal fasciculus (**riMLF**) innervate **vertically** acting EOM. The riMLF receives supranuclear commands for vertical saccades from *both* frontal eye fields and both superior colliculi.
- **Horizontal and vertical: omni*pause* neurons** in the nucleus raphe interpositus (RIP) inhibit both burst neuron sets (PPRF and riMLF); RIP lesion results in either saccadic oscillations or slow horizontal *and* vertical saccades

Slow saccades are seen in combined PPRF and riMLF lesions, PSP, SCA-2, HD, ataxia-telangiectasia, Whipple disease, Gaucher disease (horizontal saccades), and Niemann-Pick type C (vertical saccades).

Hypometric saccades may result from **dorsal vermis** cerebellar lesions, which also can cause ocular misalignment (esotropia) and impaired smooth pursuit. **Hypermetric saccades** and impaired smooth pursuit may result from **fastigial nucleus** lesions.

Square-wave jerks consist of saccadic intrusions that take the eyes briefly (100–200 ms) off the fixation point, with an intersaccadic interval >1 degree. The jerks are pathologic, and although they have poor localizing value they are commonly associated with cerebellar disease.

Ocular flutter and opsoclonus are saccadic intrusions that, unlike square-wave jerks, lack an intersaccadic interval.

Ocular flutter consists of intermittent brief volleys of rapid horizontal ocular oscillations around fixation. While flutter is horizontal, **opsoclonus** occurs in any direction and is more chaotic and random ("saccadomania") than flutter. Both flutter and opsoclonus can occur from cerebellar disease or postinfectious encephalopathy (specifically, poliomyelitis, salmonella, and coxsackie B3 virus). Opsoclonus plus ataxia and myoclonus is most notably due to paraneoplastic conditions. In children, it is associated with **neuroblastoma** ("dancing eyes, dancing feet" or **Kinsbourne syndrome**) and in adults, with cancer of the breast or ovary (anti-Ri or ANNA-2) or lung (anti-Hu or ANNA-1). Opsoclonus has also been reported with amitriptyline, haloperidol, and lithium use.

Nystagmus

Nystagmus is a rhythmic oscillatory movement of the eyes that may be pendular (slow) or phasic (jerk nystagmus; pursuit-like deviation from fixation and saccadic return to it). Although it is seldom itself symptomatic (the underlying cause may be part of vertigo), a few patients complain of oscillations of the visual field **(oscillopsia).** Jerk nystagmus is named after the direction of the fast component.

VESTIBULAR NYSTAGMUS MAY BE CENTRAL OR PERIPHERAL

Peripheral Nystagmus	Central Nystagmus
Unidirectional (mixed horizontal/torsional♠); fast phase opposite the affected labyrinth	Unidirectional or bidirectional; purely vertical (upbeating or downbeating),♣ torsional,♥ or horizontal♦
Intensity but not direction of nystagmus is more pronounced with gaze toward the side of the fast-beating component (away from a vestibular lesion)	More pronounced toward side of gaze (e.g., left-beating in left gaze, up-beating in upgaze)
Suppressed by visual fixation	**Not suppressed by visual fixation**
Smooth pursuit is intact	Smooth pursuit is broken in ipsilesional direction
Positional nystagmus has latency, adaptability, and **fatigability**	Positional nystagmus has no latency, no adaptability, and **no fatigability**
Tinnitus or deafness may be present	Tinnitus or deafness are absent
Ménière, BPPV, vestibular neuritis, labyrinthitis	Lesions to the vestibulocerebellum (flocculus, nodulus, vermis)

♠ Mixed horizontal/torsional nystagmus is typical for vestibular neuritis but can occur with central lesions.
♣ Pure vertical nystagmus is usually central but can occur with simultaneous lesions of both anterior or both posterior canals.
♥ Pure torsional nystagmus usually indicates a medullary lesion (syringobulbia, lateral medullary infarction) and may be part of the ocular tilt reaction (skew, torsion, and head tilt).
♦ Pure horizontal nystagmus is usually central but can occur with a single horizontal canal lesion.

Downbeat nystagmus is of maximal intensity when the eyes are deviated temporally and slightly inferiorly. Removal of fixation (e.g., by Frenzel goggles) does not influence slow phase velocity to a considerable extent, but the frequency of saccades may diminish. It is seen in disorders of the **craniocervical junction** (e.g., Chiari malformation), **bilateral lesions of the cerebellar flocculus, and medial longitudinal fasciculus,** which carries optokinetic input from the *posterior* semicircular canals to the third nerve nuclei.

Upbeat nystagmus is associated with lesions of the **anterior cerebellar vermis,** in which case the nystagmus increases in intensity with upward gaze, and lesions of the **medulla,** when the nystagmus increases in intensity with downward gaze. It can also occur from lesions of the **ventral tegmental tract or the brachium conjunctivum,** which carry optokinetic input from the *anterior* semicircular canals to the third nerve nuclei. Treatment with the potassium channel blocker 4-aminopyridine has been shown to improve upbeat nystagmus.

Torsional (rotary) nystagmus refers to a rotary movement of the globe about its anteroposterior axis, accentuated on lateral gaze (fast phase away from the side of the lesion), associated with **vestibular lesions of the anterior and posterior semi-circular canals,** such as lateral medullary syndrome. This nystagmus *is affected* by otolithic stimulation: it is accentuated by placing the patient on his or her side with the intact side down.

Seesaw nystagmus is a pendular oscillation that consists of elevation and intorsion of one eye and depression and extorsion of the fellow eye that alternates every half cycle. It may be seen in patients with **chiasmal lesions** (commonly tumors, such as craniopharyngioma), along with **bitemporal hemianopsia,** suggesting loss of the crossed visual inputs from the decussating fibers of the optic nerve at the level of the chiasm. Unlike torsional nystagmus, this type of nystagmus *is not affected* by otolithic stimulation.

Gaze-evoked nystagmus is produced by the attempted maintenance of an extreme eye position when structural lesions impair the neural integrator network, dispersed between the **vestibulocerebellum,** the **medulla** (region of the nucleus prepositus hypoglossi and adjacent medial vestibular nucleus), and the interstitial nucleus of Cajal. Ethanol, anticonvulsants, sedatives, and hypnotics may cause symmetric horizontal gaze-evoked nystagmus. Structural brainstem or cerebellar lesions may cause asymmetric ipsilateral gaze-evoked nystagmus. **Rebound nystagmus** may occur after a period of sustained gaze-evoked nystagmus in patients with cerebellar disease. An unsustained, lower-intensity phenomenon in healthy patients is referred to as **endpoint nystagmus.**

Spasmus nutans is an intermittent, binocular, small-amplitude, high-frequency horizontal pendular nystagmus associated with head nodding and torticollis of onset at age 3–15 months and offset by 3–4 years. It typically resolves by the age of 10 years but may be associated with an anterior visual pathway lesion.

Periodic alternating nystagmus is a conjugate, horizontal jerk nystagmus with the fast phase beating in one direction for a period of ~1–2 minutes, followed by an intervening neutral phase lasting 10–20 seconds. The nystagmus begins to beat in the opposite direction for 1–2 minutes and the process repeats itself. It localizes to the **cerebellar nodulus** and often responds to **baclofen.**

Pendular nystagmus is a rare congenital horizontal nystagmus equal in both eyes and in all directions of gaze, usually associated with poor vision. Albinos and miners who have spent years in dim light may have pendular nystagmus.

Bruns nystagmus, which develops with large cerebellar pontine angle tumors (most often acoustic neurinoma or meningioma), consists of gaze-evoked nystagmus with ipsilesional gaze and peripheral vestibular nystagmus with contralesional gaze.

Selected Cerebellar, Pontine, and Midbrain Oculomotor Syndromes

Impairment in downward saccades are caused by ipsilateral lesions in the **riMLF,** which generates vertical and torsional saccades from the *ipsilateral* CN III and IV (projections to the superior rectus and inferior oblique motoneurons are *bilateral*).

Dorsal midbrain syndrome (Parinaud syndrome) consists of limitation of upward gaze (supranuclear vertical gaze palsy), light-near dissociation, **convergence-retraction nystagmus,** eyelid retraction (Collier's sign), and pseudo-abducens palsy due to a **lesion in the posterior commissure,** which conveys fibers from the interstitial nucleus of Cajal to the contralateral CN III, IV.

Horizontal gaze palsy is caused by lesions in the abducens nucleus, the pontine horizontal conjugate "gaze center." In comatose patients, conjugate deviation of the eyes is due to gaze preference or gaze palsy. The eyes deviate toward the side of the cerebral hemispheric lesion in gaze preference and away from the side of lesion in gaze palsy. Oculocephalic maneuvers do not overcome deviation in gaze palsy. Whereas the slow **horizontal roving eye movements** imply intact brainstem and often toxic-metabolic bilateral hemispheric disease, the faster **ping-pong gaze** of alternating horizontal gaze every few seconds indicates bihemispheric destructive lesions and suggests poor prognosis. **Ocular bobbing** describes rapid conjugate downward eye movements followed by a slow return to primary position, usually accompanied by gaze palsy, reflecting a lesion of the pons. **Ocular dipping,** which refers to a slow downward eye movement followed by a fast return to primary position, lacks localizing and prognostic value but is often seen in the context of hypoxic-ischemic insults.

Internuclear ophthalmoplegia (INO) expresses as ipsilateral adduction paresis (preserved convergence) with contralateral abducting nystagmus due to medial longitudinal fasciculus (MLF) lesions. The MLF is the internuclear pathway by which CN VI neurons conveys conjugate gaze signals to contralateral medial rectus motoneurons to yoke the eyes. **Bilateral INO** lesions result in bilateral adduction weakness, exotropia, and preserved adduction with convergence.

One-and-a-half syndrome results from a combined lesion of CN VI nucleus and adjacent MLF and consists of ipsilateral horizontal gaze palsy and INO, where the only surviving horizontal movement is abduction of the contralateral eye.

Skew deviation is an acquired vertical eye misalignment due to a lesion of the supranuclear pathways connecting the vestibular apparatus to the vertical ocular motor cranial nerve nuclei (most lesions affect the MLF). The higher eye is contralateral to a medullary lesion and ipsilateral to a midpontine lesion (the level at which otolith projections decussate). If accompanied by vertical diplopia, head tilt toward the lower eye, and ocular torsion (incyclotropia of the upper eye; excyclotropia of the upper), it is known as *ocular tilt reaction.*

Giant-Cell Arteritis

As the most common form of *systemic* vasculitis, giant-cell arteritis (GCA) is more often referred to as "temporal arteritis," a topographically insufficient misrepresentation. **Headache** is the most common symptom followed by fever, sweats, **scalp tenderness, jaw claudication,** proximal myalgia, and weight loss. **Visual loss** is the most feared neurologic complication. The highest prevalence occurs in patients of Scandinavian heritage (possibly in association with HLA-DR4) and the lowest among blacks.

The temporal artery may be tender and exhibit decreased pulsation. **ESR** is often markedly elevated (ESR ≥47 mm/h is 92% sensitive for GCA, and an elevated level of CRP is 100% sensitive). If ESR and CRP are considered together, the specificity for the diagnosis of GCA is 97%. Other acute phase changes are reactive **thrombocytosis, anemia,** and **hypoferremia.** Anticardiolipin antibodies, lupus anticoagulant, antiprothrombin antibodies, and antineutrophil cytoplasmic antibody (ANCA) found in these patients are believed to represent an epiphenomenon.

New onset of headache, regardless of location, in any adult over the age of 50 years should suggest the potential presence of giant-cell arteritis. This arteritis selectively affects **extracranial arteries of medium size:**
- **External carotid** artery branches
  Especially the superficial temporal arteries*
- **Ophthalmic and posterior ciliary** arteries
- **Vertebral arteries**

*Systemic vasculitis such as Wegener granulomatosis, the Churg-Strauss syndrome, and Takayasu's arteritis may also involve the temporal artery.

Loss of vision complicates GCA in 15% of cases, usually as the result of **occlusion of the posterior ciliary**—or, less commonly, retinal—artery, which causes an anterior ischemic optic neuropathy **(AION).** Blurring or amaurosis fugax may antedate the onset of blindness. **Polymyalgia rheumatica** is associated with GCA in less than half of the cases. Proximal polyarthralgia and marked morning stiffness characterize this condition.

The definitive diagnosis is made by a long segment (2.5–4.0 cm in length) **temporal artery biopsy,** taking into account the presence of skip lesions. Treatment is with **high-dose daily corticosteroids.** Alternate day corticosteroid therapy is ineffective. When the unilateral specimen does not confirm the diagnosis (about half of all patients) but the clinical index of suspicion remains high, contralateral temporal artery biopsy is diagnostic in up to 14% of cases. The histopathological evidence of arteritis persists for at least 2 weeks after the initiation of corticosteroids. **Takayasu's arteritis,** the other large-vessel vasculitidis, is a disease of young individuals that predominantly affects women. The condition exhibits full-thickness (including intima) *cicatrization* besides giant cells and inflammation on pathology.

Tolosa-Hunt Syndrome

This syndrome of **relapsing painful ophthalmoplegia** encompasses periorbital or hemicranial pain, **ipsilateral ocular motor nerve palsies,** oculosympathetic paralysis, and sensory loss in the distribution of the ophthalmic or, less common, maxillary division of the trigeminal nerve. A **nonspecific inflammatory process** is localized to the region of the **cavernous sinus**/superior orbital fissure. The etiology of this syndrome remains undefined.

Retro- or periorbital pain is boring instead of throbbing, and the ophthalmoplegia may last for days to weeks, remit spontaneously or **within 48 hours after the administration of large doses of systemic corticosteroids,** and recur at intervals of months or years in at least half of the patients. **Loss of visual acuity** is variable and unpredictable, and may, on occasion, be permanent.

Contrast enhanced MRI may show intermediate and enhanced T1W signal abnormalities in the region of the cavernous sinus, especially on coronal sections. The major limitation is the lack of specificity, but **the resolution of imaging abnormalities after a course of systemic steroids** has been suggested to be "diagnostic" of Tolosa-Hunt syndrome.

Lymphomas, vasculitis, and parasellar neoplasms such as chordoma, giant cell tumor, and epidermoid also improve after steroids. Cerebral angiography may disclose "segmental narrowing" of the intracavernous carotid artery

Tolosa-Hunt syndrome is a **diagnosis of exclusion:** trauma, neoplasm, aneurysms, and other forms of inflammation need to be ruled out.

Vascular	Neoplasms	Inflammation	Other
Intracavernous carotid aneurysm	Meningioma Craniopharyngioma	Sarcoidosis	Mucormycosis
		Herpes zoster	Lymphoma
Posterior cerebral aneurysm	Pituitary adenoma Epidermoid	**Giant cell arteritis**	Diabetic ophthalmoplegia
Carotid-cavernous fistula	Cranial tumors: **Chordoma** Chondroma	Wegener granulomatosis	**Ophthalmoplegic migraine***
Carotid-cavernous thrombosis	Giant cell tumor	**Mycobacterium tuberculosis**	Contiguous sinusitis
Basilar aneurysm	Lymphoma	Periostitis	Metastatic tumor

*Ophthalmoplegic migraine is also an exclusionary diagnosis. Relapsing unilateral oculomotor palsy (occasionally, abducens; rarely, trochlear) develops at the height of a headache episode and persists days to weeks after its cessation. A family history of migraine is usually present.

Corticosteroids may not conclusively lessen the degree or duration of the ophthalmoplegia but dramatically reduce the pain. Dosages, duration of treatment, and alternative forms of therapy have not been formally studied.

Dizziness: Vertigo and Lightheadedness

Benign paroxysmal positional vertigo, Ménière's disease, and cerebellar ataxia with bilateral vestibulopathy are covered in the next few pages. Orthostatic hypotension, a major cause of lightheadedness is dealt with in detail in Chapter 9.

Lesions of the labyrinth or CN VIII yield auditory symptoms such as hearing loss, tinnitus, and a sensation of pain, pressure or fullness in the ear. **Lesions in the internal auditory canal** cause associated ipsilateral CN VII palsy. **Lesions in the cerebellopontine angle** result in ipsilateral facial numbness and weakness and ipsilateral limb ataxia.

General Clinical Principles

- Spinning sensation in environment and illusions of movement (oscillopsia) = vestibular; spinning inside but still environment = nonvestibular dizziness.
- Episodic course with events triggered by head movements or positional changes = vestibular dizziness; constant course = nonvestibular dizziness.
- **Unidirectional nystagmus with normal hearing = vestibular neuritis.** Vertigo is sustained and severe, often lasting for days. Other manifestations include nausea, imbalance, and a tendency to fall.
- Unidirectional nystagmus with unilateral hearing loss = viral labyrinthitis, bacterial otomastoiditis, labyrinthine infarct, syphilitic labyrinthitis.
- Direction-changing nystagmus and focal neurological deficits = cerebellar and brainstem lesions (infarcts, hemorrhages, demyelination, etc.).
- Prolonged posttraumatic vertigo with hearing loss = labyrinthine concussion
- Paroxysmal posttraumatic vertigo induced by cough, sneeze = perilymph fistula.

Perilymph fistula causes a "popping" ear sound, sudden-onset hearing loss, and a **positive fistula sign:** rotatory or postural vertigo and nystagmus induced by Valsalva or loud noises and associated with oscillopsia.

Vestibular paroxysmia consists of brief attacks of vertigo, tinnitus, and auditory deficits due to compression of CN VIII by vessels in the posterior fossa, such as the basilar, vertebral, AICA, or PICA. Vestibular paroxysmia may be treated either with carbamazepine, phenytoin, gabapentin, or valproate.

Vasovagal presyncope is recognized by sudden onset of nausea and diaphoresis followed by lightheadedness, dimness of vision, and pallor, most often upon standing. Unlike orthostatic hypotension, the blood pressure does not necessarily drop immediately upon standing. Triggers include hunger, emotional stress, prolonged standing, or exposure to excessive heat, pain, or strong odors. An efferent parasympathetic reflex produces bradycardia and vasodilation of capacitance vessels, particularly in the splanchnic vascular bed.

Hyperventilation may cause lightheadedness, perioral and acral numbness and tingling, and feelings of suffocation and chest pressure. Rapid breathing reduce the pCO_2 to the point of cerebral vasoconstriction.

Benign Paroxysmal Positional Vertigo (BPPV)

BPPV, the most common cause of vertigo, consists of sudden and short-lasting recurrent vertigo elicited by certain rotational movement of the head. It is caused by free-floating debris within the endolymph of the posterior semicircular canal. The debris consists of calcium carbonate crystals **(otoliths)** that dislocate from the utriculus of the vestibular labyrinth and migrate to the more dependent posterior semicircular canal. The otolith movement alters endolymphatic pressure and causes cupular deflection. **Head trauma and labyrinthitis** are uncommon antecedent disorder. BPPV is self-limited but remissions occur unpredictably.

The **10-to-20-second episodes** are induced by certain positions such as rolling over in bed, bending over, or looking upward. **Nausea or vomiting** may precede or accompany the illusory sensation of personal or environmental motion. **Nystagmus** with both **torsional and vertical components** is characteristic. The torsional component is "geotropic" and more prominent during ocular abduction (eye moving toward affected ear) and the vertical component, upward beating, becomes clearer when the eye is adducted (moving away from the affected ear).

Diagnosis requires the **Dix-Hallpike test** (first two steps from Epley maneuver). The rotational nystagmus has a latency of 3–20 seconds and exhibits fatigability with repeated testing. After the patient returns to the seated position, nystagmus of similar magnitude but opposite direction relapses.

RECURRENT VERTIGO (LABYRINTHITIS [VESTIBULAR NEURONITIS] CAUSES *PERSISTENT* VERTIGO)

Otologic	*BPPV*	*Positional*	Seconds	Nausea, vomiting
	Ménière's disease	Spontaneous	Min-hours	Hearing loss, tinnitus
	Labyrinthitis	Spontaneous	1–2 days	Single episode
Neurologic	Migraine	Triggers	Variable	Headache
	Vertebro-basilar	*Positional*	Variable	Diplopia, dysarthria
	Panic disorder	Variable	Variable	No neurologic deficits

Central vertigo resulting from infarcts in the medial branch of the PICA can be positional and show spontaneous ipsilesional beating torsional/horizontal nystagmus in primary position, and *contralesional* truncal lateropulsion and dysmetria. Perceived environmental rotation is toward the lesion (i.e., clockwise in right nodulouvular lesion). Patients prefer to lie with ipsilateral ear down. Additional brainstem signs (Horner''s syndrome, dysarthria, and crossed hypalgesia) with *ipsilesional* lateropulsion suggest Wallenberg syndrome.

Treatment is based on the **Epley maneuver** or other liberatory maneuvers, whose purpose is to relocate free-floating debris from the posterior semicircular canal into the vestibule of the vestibular labyrinth. The maneuver is repeated until the patient is asymptomatic. There is about an 80% success rate after a single treatment. The patient should remain upright for 24 hours to prevent reaccumulation of debris in the posterior semicircular canal. When relapse develops, a second session is necessary. High-grade carotid stenosis and unstable heart disease are contraindications. Side-to-side head movements **(Brandt-Daroff)** are helpful for those who do not have a characteristic response to the Dix-Hallpike test.

Canalith-Repositioning Maneuver (Epley)

(Assuming left posterior semicircular canal affected)

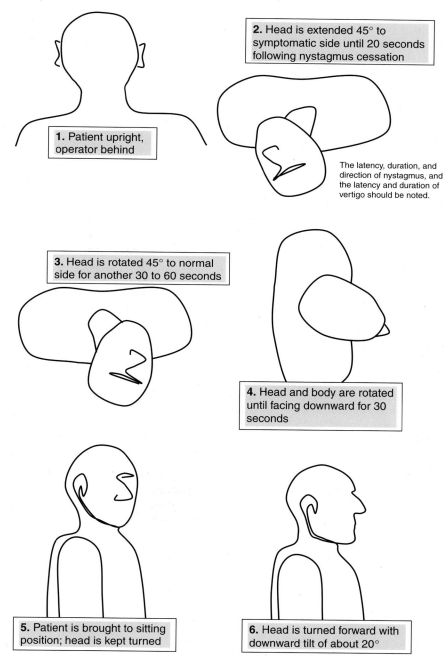

1. Patient upright, operator behind

2. Head is extended 45° to symptomatic side until 20 seconds following nystagmus cessation

The latency, duration, and direction of nystagmus, and the latency and duration of vertigo should be noted.

3. Head is rotated 45° to normal side for another 30 to 60 seconds

4. Head and body are rotated until facing downward for 30 seconds

5. Patient is brought to sitting position; head is kept turned

6. Head is turned forward with downward tilt of about 20°

Ménière's Disease

Ménière's disease is characterized by slowly progressive and **recurrent episodes of vertigo** and hearing loss, tinnitus, nausea, and vomiting, which last from 20 minutes to several hours. **Rotational nystagmus** is the main physical finding. Loud noises may induce transient vertigo **(Tulio's phenomenon).** "Minor attacks" need not be vertiginous and may only be expressed as unsteadiness, especially when turning. Ménière's disease can be difficult to distinguish from vestibular neuritis (where there are not associated auditory symptoms) and vestibular migraine.

> **The fast phase of the nystagmus** is toward the normal ear because the affected ear has decreased function, except very early in an attack.

Endolymphatic hydrops is the pathophysiologic substrate of Ménière's disease and can be documented by electrocochleography. Audiographic assessment usually shows **low-frequency sensory neural hearing loss.** The most specific serial finding is the documentation of **fluctuation of hearing in the low frequencies** (>10 decibels in the low frequencies). Electronystagmography (ENG) and, more recently, videonystagmography measures the slow-phase eye velocity associated with spontaneous and induced peripheral nystagmus. The visually suppressed spontaneous nystagmus of peripheral vestibulopathies can be seen with eyes-closed electronystagmogram (ENG), which may be normal in between attacks. Asymmetric ENG response during caloric testing is also considered significant.

> **Vestibulo-ocular reflex (VOR),** which refers to the smooth compensatory eye movements in the opposite direction of head movement resulting from increased labyrinthine output in the direction of movement, is the physiologic expression of the peripheral vestibular system function. This compensation of eye movements equal to the magnitude of head deviation occurs in the **dark or when the eyes are closed,** but is modified by visual fixation **(visual VOR or VVOR).**

Restriction of caffeine may limit its presumed vasoconstrictive effects in the labyrinthine circulation. **Potassium-sparing diuretics** are preferred to reduce endolymphatic pressure when medications are required. If response is positive in 4–6 weeks, at least 6 months of treatment may be needed, followed by a slow taper. Up to 20% of patients require indefinite treatment. Antihistamine medications such as **meclizine** (12.5–25.0 mg tid or qid), **dimenhydrinate** (50–100 mg daily), and **promethazine** (25 mg tid) block histamine and acetylcholine receptors in the vestibular nuclei. **Betahistine** is often used in Europe. Steroids have not been shown to be effective. The serotonin antagonist **ondansetron** is useful as strong antiemetic, often the main treatment target in the vertiginous patient. Surgical interventions may be required and include intratympanic steroid injections, endolymphatic sac shunt, and destructive procedures such as intratympanic gentamicin injection, vestibular nerve section, and labyrinthectomy.

Cerebellar Ataxia with Bilateral Vestibulopathy (CABV)

This clinical syndrome (Bronstein et al., 1991) is characterized by the **absence of doll's head reflex** in patients with late-onset sporadic ataxia. Oscillopsia (common in those with pure bilateral vestibulopathy) is lacking. On examination, these patients have compensatory saccades while trying to view and earth-fixed target during slow (<1 Hz) horizontal or vertical head oscillations. The electrophysiological correlate is an **impairment of the visually enhanced vestibulo-ocular reflex (VVOR).** Pure cerebellar atrophy without brainstem atrophy or white matter abnormalities has been documented on brain MRI.

The VVOR appears to be the summation of smooth pursuit, optokinetic, fixation, and vestibulo-ocular reflexes:

- **Smooth pursuit (SP)** accurately tracks the target up to a frequency of ~1 Hz and a velocity of ~100°/sec when *target oscillates from side to side.*
- **Optokinetic reflex (OKR)** leads to similar smooth compensatory eye movements when a whole *scene oscillates from side to side.*
- **Vestibulo-ocular reflex (VOR)** produces similar smooth compensatory eye movements at frequencies ranging from <0.1 to >6 Hz when a *head is oscillated from side to side in the dark.* The VOR gain rises from ~0.6 at 0.1 Hz to nearly 1.0 at 0.5 Hz and above.
- **VVOR** is the combination of the above plus fixation, producing similarly smooth compensatory eye movements during activities such as walking or running. It can be activated by *oscillating the head while the patient views a target or a scene.* The VVOR gain is about 1.0 from <0.1 to >6 Hz, thus maintaining retinal slip velocity below 3–5°/sec, the level at which vision starts to degrade.

Measurements of rotatory testing include *gain* = amplitude of eye movement relative to head movement (instantaneous eye velocity divided by instantaneous head velocity); *phase* = lag in eye position relative to head position; and *symmetry* = total slow phase eye movements generated by turning in one direction compared with the other direction.

GENETIC SPINOCEREBELLAR ATAXIAS VERSUS BILATERAL VESTIBULOPATHY

	Genetic SCAs	Bilateral Vestibulopathy
SP and OKR gains	Low	Normal
VOR gain	Normal (except SCA1 and SCA3)	**Low** (by definition)
VVOR	Near normal given a compensatory VOR	Near normal given a compensatory SP and OKR

While SP and OKR impairment is always due to brainstem or cerebellar dysfunction, VOR impairment is generally due to disease affecting vestibular eng-organs or vestibular nerves bilaterally. **The combined impairment of VOR, SP, and OKR suggests a combined lesion of the cerebellum and brainstem,** involving the vestibular nuclei, and this double pathology is suggested by impairment of the VVOR below ~1 Hz.

8 Demyelinating Diseases, Neuro-oncology and Disorders of Neural Tube Closure and Other Congenital Malformations

Multiple sclerosis (MS) introduces the section on neuropathology because of its controversial and continuously redefining place in the field. Not just because we still struggle with the old question of whether the relapsing-remitting form may be a different entity from what is considered its primary progressive counterpart, but because the literature often returns to the theme of MS and acute disseminated encephalomyelopathy (ADEM) as different or, perhaps, neighboring parts of the same pathologic spectrum. And because it seems easier to split what may not be apparently coherent together, the MS body of knowledge has historically suffered from a nomenclatural burst of diseases (Schilder's *encephalitis periaxialis diffusa*, Marburg's fulminant *encephalomyelitis periaxialis scleroticans*, and Balo's *encephalitis periaxialis concentrica*). These, fortunately, have come to terms with their ancestral demyelinating roots by ultimately showing the "sharp-edged plaque" scar that the rest of the MS family carries. The Balo concentric plaques are more often present in persons of Asian descent with a monophasic course that suggests ADEM.

At a basic level, the difference between ADEM and MS is that the former is a clinically isolated syndrome (popularized as *CIS*) and has yet to leave *isolation* and become *recurrent*, or MS. At a deeper level, ADEM is more "gray" (than "white" matter disease) and "confusing" (encephalopathy is rarely present in MS). Further, CIS does not necessarily mean ADEM, a second CIS may not represent MS (but, possibly, *recurrent DEM*, when the deficits are the same or *multiphasic* DEM when the deficits are different), and some CIS may be suspicious enough that a first MS episode is all but established. The latter is the most important of these uncertainties as disease-modifying therapies exercise a greater role when given earlier, as the CIS is yet to recur: the more CISs are treated, the lower the likelihood they will become definite MS.

The latest layer of complexity is the triumph of the "splitters" among MS experts when neuromyelitis optica (NMO) officially departed the MS motherboard and came of age as an autoimmune channelopathy rather than a demyelinating disease. Longitudinally extensive spinal cord lesions and white matter lesions around the spinal canal and third ventricle betrayed NMO's predilection for water channels rather than oligoclonal bands.

As if understanding the pathology of MS and ADEM were not difficult enough, the very title of a review article could have almost said that these disorders "are neither demyelinating nor axonal but the opposite:" *The question 'ADEM: distinct disease or part of the MS spectrum?' can be answered with a resounding no.* Poser CM, Brinar VV. *Clinical Neurology and Neurosurgery* 2004;106:159–171.

Let us review the following pages before considering Alice in Wonderland!

Multiple Sclerosis

MS is a chronic recurrent inflammatory disorder of the CNS resulting in injury to the myelin sheaths, oligodendrocytes, and, eventually, axons. The disease exhibits a north-south gradient, maintained among immigrants younger than 15 years. There are four clinical types: relapsing-remitting (RRMS, 85%), secondary progressive (SPMS), primary progressive, and progressive-relapsing. Clinically definite MS requires two distinct attacks of more than 24 hours, at least 1 month apart, and clinical evidence of two separate lesions (Poser criteria, 1983), or a single attack or "clinically isolated syndrome" if MRI defines dissemination in space and time (McDonald criteria, 2001).

MULTIPLE SCLEROSIS DIAGNOSTIC CRITERIA

Clinical attacks	Objective lesions	Additional requirements to make the diagnosis
≥2	≥2	None
≥2	1	**MRI evidence of dissemination in space (Barkhof)** **or** positive CSF and ≥2 MRI lesions **or** further clinical attack from different site
1	≥2	**MRI evidence of dissemination in time** **or** second clinical attack
1	1	MRI evidence of dissemination in space **or** positive CSF and ≥2 MRI lesions **And** MRI evidence of dissemination in time **or** second clinical attack
0	1	**Positive CSF** **And** MRI evidence of dissemination in space of ≥9 T2 lesions **or** 2 or more spinal cord lesions or 4–8 brain and 1 cord lesion **or** positive VEP with 4–8 MRI lesions **or** positive VEP with less than 4 brain lesions plus 1 cord lesion **And** MRI evidence of dissemination in time **or** continued progression for 1 year

Thompson criteria for PPMS

CSF, cerebrospinal fluid; VEP, visual evoked potential.
Positive CSF: oligoclonal IgG bands (OCB) or elevated IgG index. **Positive VEP:** delayed but preserved waveform. **Barkhof's MRI evidence** of dissemination in space requires three of the following: 9 T2 hyperintense lesions or 1 gadolinium-enhancing lesion; one or more infratentorial lesions; one or more juxtacortical lesions; three or more periventricular lesions (minimal number of lesions required: five [two if gadolinium is used]; one spinal cord lesion can substitute for any one brain lesion; proton density/T2W sequences are most sensitive). (Adapted McDonald, *Ann Neurol* 2001)

MRI evidence of dissemination in time is demonstrated by a gadolinium (Gd)-enhancing lesion in a scan done at least 3 months following a CIS at a site different from that corresponding to the original attack. In its absence, MS can be diagnosed by a follow-up scan after another 3 months showing a Gd lesion or new T2 lesion (Gd use may spare need for second MRI; there is poor correlate between Gd activity and clinical activity; Gd should be used for diagnosis but not for management).

The revised McDonald criteria (2005) permits (1) spinal cord lesions be treated as infratentorial lesions, and (2) any cord lesion may substitute for brain lesions.

Neuroimaging in Multiple Sclerosis

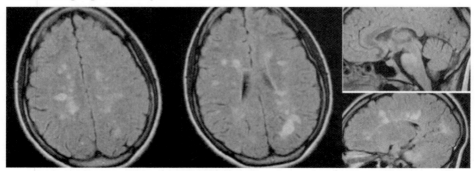

17-year-old woman with facial pain, gait instability, and bilateral leg weakness. CSF showed oligo-clonal bands. FLAIR MRI showed multiple hyperintense lesions in the periventricular and bihemi-spheric deep white matter, with additional involvement of the pons, left cerebral peduncle, bilateral middle cerebellar peduncles, and proximal aspect of the medulla.

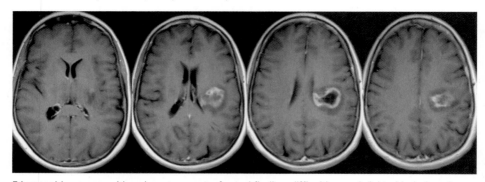

54-year-old woman with subacute onset of word-finding difficulties and right-sided clumsiness. T1W postcontrast MRI shows a thick rim of irregularly enhancing left posterior frontal intra-axial mass, extending to the ependymal surface of the lateral ventricle. The peripheral rim of enhance-ment demonstrated restricted diffusion (not shown). Brain biopsy demonstrated demyelination, perivascular lymphocytic infiltrates, macrophages, and reactive gliosis. These findings are sugges-tive of the **tumefactive form of MS.**

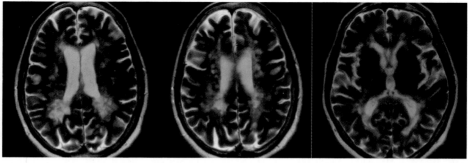

51-year-old woman with a 6-year history of progressive ataxia, parkinsonism, and cognitive impair-ment consistent with PPMS. T2W MRI showed diffuse periventricular and deep white matter signal abnormalities with cystic degeneration of the white matter suggestive of the more severe "cerebral form" of MS. Some of these lesions enhanced after gadolinium.

Pathogenesis of MS

MS is characterized by inflammation, demyelination, and axonal injury. Although the etiology of MS is unknown, the immune system plays a central role in the pathogenesis of the disease, as supported by the effects of immunomodulatory and immunosuppressive therapy on disease activity. Genes also play a role because there is a 30% disease concordance among monozygotic twins compared to 3% among other siblings. The **HLA-DR1501 and HLA-DQ0601** alleles, which encode restriction elements of T cells, are associated a two- to fourfold increased risk of developing MS in white populations. Migration studies and the association between relapses and viral infections support an environmental contribution. The prevalence of **Epstein-Barr virus** (EBV) is substantially high in MS, and antibody responses to EBV nuclear antigen (as opposed to other common virus such as human herpes virus type 6 [HHV-6], CMV, and measles) might predict conversion to MS in patients with CIS.

The MS lesion contains CD4+ and CD8+ T cells, B cells, and macrophages. CD4+ T cells have two subtypes: Th1 and Th2, proinflammatory and anti-inflammatory, respectively. **Th1 cytokines** include interleukin (IL)-2, IL-12, interferon (IFN)-γ, and tumor necrosis factor-α, which activate macrophages for cellular immunity. **The Th2 cytokines** are IL-4, IL-5, and transforming growth factor-β, which activate immunoglobulins-generating B cells for humoral immunity. Blood–brain barrier disruption allows activated T cells to gain access to the CNS. Cell adhesion molecules such as intercellular adhesion molecule-1, vascular cell adhesion molecule-1 and metalloproteinase 9 facilitate entry of T lymphocytes into the brain. Inside the CNS, specific antigenic peptides are shown in major histocompatibility complex (MHC) molecules to T cells. CD8+ T cells recognize them through lass I MHC molecules in neurons and oligodendrocytes; CD4+ T cells, in the perivascular cuff, recognize antigens using class II MHC antigens on dendritic and microglial cells, and release the cytokines that attract macrophages to the lesion. B cells are mostly found in the perivascular space and meninges, where they release IgG antibodies.

Experimental allergic encephalomyelitis (EAE) is the most common animal model of T-cell–mediated inflammatory disease induced by antibodies to myelin oligodendrocyte glycoprotein, causing inflammation, demyelination, oligodendrocyte loss, and axonal damage. Its relevance as a model for MS is questioned because efficacy of some drugs in EAE does not always translate in MS (e.g., IFN-γ, lenercept [tumor necrosis factor-α receptor blocker], anti-CD4 antibodies, and oral myelin) and because EAE neglects the role of B cells in MS pathogenesis.

Three pathologic patterns have been identified in MS. **Pattern 1** shows inflammatory demyelination with prominent macrophages and sharp borders. **Pattern 2,** the most frequent, also has well-defined demyelination and prominent lymphocytic and macrophage infiltration with marked complement deposition (the edges of the lesions correlate with the appearance of Gd enhancement on MRI). **Pattern 3** showed less well-defined borders, far fewer oligodendrocytes, and less remyelination. Patients respond to plasmapheresis in pattern 2 more than in pattern 3, supporting the antibody/complement-mediated nature of the former.

Important Variants of, or Related Entities to, MS

Optic Neuritis and Acute Transverse Myelopathy

The 5-year risk of developing MS after the diagnosis of ON is 16%. The risk increases to 51% if MRI shows two or more T2W lesions. If both MRI and CSF are normal, the likelihood of ON or any other monophasic syndrome to evolve into MS is very low. The risk of MS in ATM, more common among Asians than whites, is **2–8% in complete TM** and up to **80% in incomplete TM.**

Neuromyelitis Optica (Devic Syndrome)

NMO is a distinct inflammatory demyelinating disease characterized by **bilateral or recurrent optic neuritis** with or without **longitudinally extensive spinal cord** lesions (more than three vertebral segments, centrally located). CSF shows neutrophilic **pleocytosis** (>50 white blood cells per cubic millimeter or more than five neutrophils per cubic millimeter) and proteinorrhachia, often **without OCB.** The serum autoantibody **NMO-IgG,** which targets the water channel **aquaporin-4** in astrocytes, is highly specific. NMO-IgG predicts poor visual outcome and recurrence. MRI may show T2W signal abnormalities in the spinal cord (see later discussion) and periependymal region of the third ventricle. Recurrence is higher in **older women.** Children have better prognosis. It is responsive to glucocorticoids, azathioprine, IVIG, and plasma exchange but may worsen with Interferons or glatiramer acetate.

Acute Disseminated Encephalomyelitis

ADEM is a monophasic (within 6 months) **postinfectious encephalopathy,** more common in childhood, which may result from a transient autoimmune response toward myelin induced by molecular mimicry or activation of autoreactive T-cell clones. **Seizures, encephalopathy, basal ganglia/thalamic involvement,** as well as tumor-like brain MRI appearance are more common in ADEM than in MS. The **triggers of ADEM** can be viral, such as **mycoplasma,** measles, varicella zoster (acute cerebellar ataxia), mumps, rubella, influenza, EBV, hepatitis A; and vaccinations against rabies (myelitis and myeloradiculitis), mumps, measles, and diphtheria. CSF shows **pleocytosis with increased intrathecal IgG but typically no OCB. Perivascular demyelination** is seen on pathologic analysis. Up to 20% of patients develop pediatric MS, which has a greater relapse rate (more inflammatory) but slower rate of progression than adult MS. Presence of OCB and a longer steroid taper (>3 weeks) are positive, and seizures and encephalopathy are negative, predictors of progression into MS.

PROGNOSTIC FACTORS IN MS

Better	Worse
Female	**Male**
Relapsing-remitting variant, optic neuritis, sensory involvement	Progressive course, pyramidal and/or cerebellar involvement
Age at onset <30 years	Age at onset >40 years
Low MRI T2 lesion burden	High MRI T2 lesion burden
Infrequent attacks	Frequent attacks

Neuroimaging of Neuromyelitis Optica (Devic Syndrome)

Spine MR images of a patient with spastic tetraparesis with NMO-IgG–positive antibody serology at presentation (upper row) and 4 years later.

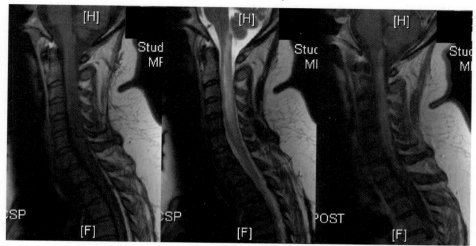

T1W, T2W, and postgadolinium MRI of the cervical spine shows an expansile T2 hyperintense lesion centered in the spinal cord, extending to the dorsal medulla superiorly and to T2-T3 levels inferiorly. The T2 hyperintense signal abnormalities involve most of the spinal cord diameter with some sparing of the periphery of the spinal cord. The spinal cord expansion is most prominent at the C2-C3 levels through the C5-C6 cord levels. There was associated confluent spinal cord enhancement involving primarily the dorsal columns with sparing of the anterior and lateral portions of the spinal cord, extending from the dorsal aspect of the medulla oblongata to the C7-T1 cord levels.

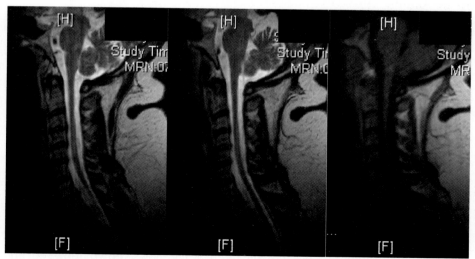

Same patient, 4 years later: T2W and postgadolinium MRI showed decreased interval T2 hyperintense signal within the cervical spinal with no enhancement. The cervical spinal cord shows interval reduction in caliber indicating atrophy.

Important Imitators of MS

X-linked adrenomyeloneuropathy, progressive multifocal leukoencephalopathy, and subacute sclerosing panencephalitis are discussed elsewhere.

CADASIL, MELAS, and CNS lymphoma are dealt with elsewhere in this book.

Infections	Inflammatory disorders	Other conditions
HHV-6	Behçet disease	CADASIL
HTLV-1	Susac syndrome	MELAS
Lyme disease	SLE	CNS lymphoma
Neurosyphilis	Sjögren disease	Spinal stenosis
PML	Other CNS vasculitis	HSP
HIV	Sarcoidosis	Vit B$_{12}$ and E deficiencies

HHV-6, human herpes virus type 6; HTLV-1, human T-lymphotropic virus; HIV, human immunodeficiency virus.

Human herpes virus type 6 (HHV-6), the most neuroinvasive herpes agent, may cause febrile seizures and focal demyelination in immunocompetent and immuno-compromised hosts. Varicella zoster virus may cause leukoencephalitis in the latter.

Tropical spastic paraparesis is caused by human T-cell lymphotropic virus type 1 infection, the first human retrovirus, and mainly affects women between 35 and 45 years of age of Japanese (20%) or Caribbean (5%) ancestry.

Behçet disease is a noninfectious multisystem inflammatory disorder of unknown etiology, common in males of **Mediterranean** countries and **Japan,** characterized by **vasculitic** changes in multiple organs. It consists of a chronic relapsing combination of **oral aphthous ulcerations, genital ulcerations,** and **anterior uveitis.** Attacks of Behçet disease become less frequent and less severe over time. Major morbidity results from ocular, vascular (**venous sinus thrombosis** [VST], increased intracranial pressure, headache, aseptic meningitis), or **brainstem or corticospinal lesions** (neuro-Behçet syndrome). Rare presentations include **intracerebral hemorrhage** from ruptured aneurysms, isolated optic neuritis, and a parkinsonian syndrome. CSF studies may show neutrophilic pleocytosis and proteinorrhachia. Intrathecal IgG production is detected but oligoclonal bands are uncommon and may disappear, whereas in MS remain positive. MRI lesions in 50% of patients are restricted to the **brainstem, diencephalon, and basal ganglia** regions. Onset with headache alone, with, or without papilledema from VST, is predictive of a limited form of disease. Negative prognostic factors are dysarthria, cerebellar and motor symptoms at onset, and a progressive disease pattern.

Susac syndrome applies to a combination of encephalopathy, visual field defects from branch retinal artery occlusions, and hearing loss, occurring in a monophasic, sequential (with stroke-like onset or development), or chronic fashion. Women are more often affected than men (3:1). Headaches, cognitive impairment, behavioral problems, and seizures may occur. Brain MRI typically shows **snowball-like corpus callosum lesions,** with predominant involvement of the central fibers and relative sparing of the callosal periphery (unlike MS and ADEM). CSF shows mild pleocytosis and proteinorrhachia but without intrathecal IgG or OCB (also unlike MS).

Disease-Modifying Therapies for MS

Interferon beta (IFN-β) [IFN-β-1a (Avonex, Rebif) and IFN-β-1b (Betaseron)] has multiple immunomodulatory effects, including a decrease in T-cell trafficking into the CNS and restoration of the Th1-Th2 imbalance. IFN-β **reduces the clinical and MRI relapse rate** in patients with RRMS. The suggested dosages are 30 μg IM per week for Avonex, 44 μg SQ three times weekly (132 μg/wk) for Rebif, and 250 μg SQ every other day for Betaseron. The **PRISMS** (Rebif) study was the first trial of IFN-β in RRMS to show significant reductions in the one-point extended disability status scale (EDSS) and in the T2W disease burden. The **CHAMPS** (Avonex) and **ETOMS** (Rebif) studies showed significant slowing of the rate of conversion to clinically definite MS with IFN-β-1a treatment after the first demyelinating event. The **BENEFIT** (Betaseron) study showed that the risk of developing clinically definite MS at 2 years was reduced by 50% compared with placebo in those treated after a first attack. This study, and head-to-head comparison trials between Avonex and Rebif **(EVIDENCE)** and between Avonex and Betaseron **(INCOMIN),** suggests that **high-dose/high-frequency IFN-β-1b** may be more effective in preventing progression to RRMS than once-weekly low-dose IFN-β-1a (IM or SQ).

Glatiramer acetate (Copaxone) is a synthetic polypeptide composed of the most prevalent amino acids in myelin basic protein believed to reduce proinflammatory cytokines from autoreactive T cells, inhibit monocyte activity, promote Th2 cells, and induce bystander immune suppression in the CNS. The dosage is 20 mg SQ daily. Glatiramer acetate reduces the clinical and MRI attack rate in RRMS by one third. Unlike IFN-β, glatiramer acetate does not cause depression, thyroid disease, liver function abnormalities, or leucopenia but may induce injection site reactions. It provides a similar relapse-free rate than IFN-β-1a 44 μg SQ given three times weekly, although with less suppression of gadolinium-enhancing lesions on MRI but also lower reduction of brain volume (**REGARD,** 2008).

Mitoxantrone (Novantrone) is a chemotherapeutic agent that inhibits topoisomerase II activity providing cytopathic effects on replicating cells. In patients with RRMS and SPMS and incomplete recovery following attacks, mitoxantrone reduced the accumulation of neurologic impairment and number of relapses compared with placebo. Mitoxantrone has **cardiotoxic** properties that limit its total lifetime cumulative dose to 140 mg/m². Mitoxantrone may also cause **acute myelogenous leukemia** in 0.25% of patients. Because of its toxicity, mitoxantrone is regarded as a second-line agent for RRMS and SPMS patients. Strategies to reduce the risk of adverse events include monitoring left ventricular ejection fraction before each dose, short-term treatments, and complete blood cell count monitoring.

Natalizumab (Tysabri) is a monoclonal antibody that binds α-4 integrin on the surface of activated lymphocytes, which in turn binds vascular cell adhesion molecule-1 on the vascular endothelium and prevents the migration of activated proinflammatory T cells into the CNS. Natalizumab conveys a 1:1,000 risk of **progressive multifocal leukoencephalopathy,** especially in combination with Avonex.

Relapse Management and Emerging Therapies in MS

Glucocorticoids are often used in acute MS relapses. Intravenously administered methylprednisolone, 1–2 g/d, or dexamethasone, 2 mg/kg/d administered over 3–5 days, reduces symptoms and shortens the recovery time. Regular pulses may be useful in the long-term management of RRMS patients.

Cyclophosphamide is a cytotoxic alkylating agent that can be added to the treatment regimen of RRMS patients who are experiencing disease progression despite treatment with IFN-β-1a. The recommended dose if 800 mg/m^2 IV every morning, coadministered with methylprednisolone, 1 mg. Adjustments in dosage are based on preinfusion and 10-day postinfusion white blood cell counts.

Azathioprine is a nucleoside analogue of 6-mercaptopurine that impairs DNA and RNA synthesis and appears to reduce the relapse rate in RRMS and SPMS. The recommended dose is 50 mg/day and is titrated to reduce the total white blood cell count to approximately 3,000 cells/mL (usually 2–3 mg/kg/day).

Methotrexate is an inhibitor of dihydrofolate that also augments T-cell suppressor function. Methotrexate can be used also in SPMS at a dose of 7.5 mg/week, with regular liver function monitoring.

Mycophenolate mofetil is an inhibitor of inosine 5'-monophosphate dehydrogenase type II and is a relatively selective immunosuppressant of activated lymphocytes. In patients with persistent disease activity, despite treatment with FDA-approved agents, it has been used with some success at the doses of 500–1,000 mg bid.

Fingolimod, recently approved as the first oral disease-modifying therapy for relapsing remitting MS, acts on the sphingosine-1-phosphate (S1P) receptors, depleting both CD4$^+$ and CD8$^+$ T lymphocytes in blood. Once-daily dose of 0.5 mg reduces relapses by 52% at one year compared with Avonex. Potential side effects include bradycardia, infections, macular edema, and liver problems.

Cladribine is an adenosine deaminase-resistant purine nucleoside that is relatively selective as lymphocyte immunosuppressant. Oral cladribine was recently shown to reduce annualized relapse rates by 58% with the low dose and a 55% reduction with the high dose at 2 years. Cladribine is currently used for the treatment of leukemia, lymphoma, and hairy cell leukemia, but at press time it had not yet received FDA approval for relapsing-remitting MS.

Rituximab is a monoclonal antibody directed against CD20, a cell surface marker present on B lymphocytes. Rituximab was developed for treatment of non-Hodgkin lymphoma and depletes B lymphocytes. Rituximab has shown promise in treatment of primary progressive MS, RRMS, and neuromyelitis optica.

Intravenous immunoglobulin, 0.15–0.20 g/kg every month, appears to reduce the relapse rate in patients with MS but the effects on disability are unknown. **Plasmapheresis** may help resolve acute flares of severe demyelinating disease that are not responsive to glucocorticoids. **HMG-CoA reductase inhibitors** (atorvastatin and simvastatin) are under investigation for MS. They have potent anti-inflammatory properties, are well tolerated, and are administered orally.

Posterior Reversible Encephalopathy Syndrome

PRES may present with confusion, headache or seizures associated with vision loss (ranging from hemianopsia to visual neglect to cortical blindness) with normal optic discs. PRES typically occurs in association with **hypertensive** with cyclosporine, tacrolimus, cisplatin, and immune globulin therapy. PRES is the most common severe neurologic complication in the setting of adult and pediatric hematopoietic stem cell transplantation. **Serious neurotoxicity secondary to calcineurin inhibitors** such as cyclosporine A and tacrolimus occurs in 5% to 6% of patients. Risk factors for the development of neurotoxicity include abnormally high drug levels, intravenous administration, hepatic failure, hypomagnesemia, hypercholesterolemia, significant fluid overload, and concurrent steroid therapy.

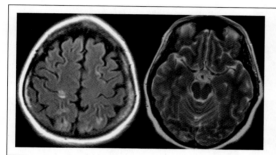

A 39-year-old G1/P1 woman had bilateral visual blurring followed by a generalized tonic-clonic seizure 5 days after delivery. She had been hypertensive during labor. MRI showed multiple patchy areas of increased T2/FLAIR signal abnormalities in bihemispheric cortical and subcortical regions, more pronounced within the parietal and occipital lobes. She was treated with magnesium sulfate.

The characteristic MRI abnormalities are increased signal in both FLAIR and T2W in the occipital lobes, posterior parietal and posterior temporal lobes resulting from **vasogenic edema,** which, unlike the cytotoxic edema of cerebral infarction (which appears bright on DWI with low signal on ADC) causes less brightness on DWI and usually **high signal on ADC.** Despite its name, the brainstem, cerebellum, and anterior hemispheres may also be affected.

Sudden increases in blood pressure exceed the autoregulatory threshold of the capillaries, leading to breakdown of the blood–brain barrier, transudation of fluid, and even petechial hemorrhages. The vertebrobasilar circulation is more vulnerable as it receives **less sympathetic innervation** compared with the anterior circulation arteries.

Blood pressure control and discontinuation of offending agents is the recommended management. IV labetalol and nicardipine are recommended. Nicardipine, in particular, has an advantage of being easily titrated, allowing tight control of blood pressure gradually or rapidly. **Sodium nitroprusside should be avoided** because of the potential for inducing intracranial hypertension as well as cyanide toxicity, which may lead to seizures. IV magnesium may be sufficient in cases of eclampsia. Prompt diagnosis and adequate treatment leads to clinical recovery within 2 weeks, with complete resolution of the MRI signal abnormalities. Most patients do not require lifelong antiepileptic medications.

Brain MRI in PRES

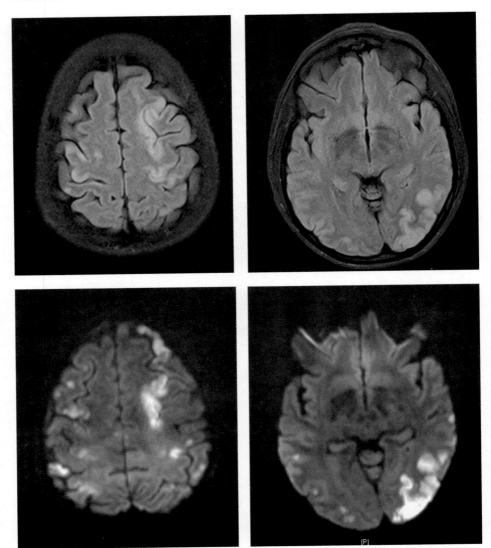

FLAIR (upper row) and diffusion-weighted MR (lower row) brain MRI of a patient with cystic fibrosis, status after bilateral lung transplantation, show scattered foci of cortical and subcortical edema and restricted diffusion involving the cerebral hemispheres bilaterally. The signal abnormalities did not follow a consistent vascular distribution pattern. This is consistent with the diagnosis of PRES.

Autoimmune Channelopathies

Antibodies to acetylcholine receptors (AChRs) are found in 80%–85% of patients with generalized myasthenia gravis. Ganglionic AChR antibodies are implicated in autoimmune autonomic neuropathies. **Antibodies to muscle-specific kinase (MuSK)** are present in a significant proportion of the non-AChR myasthenics with oculobulbar weakness and poor response to treatment. MuSK is a monomeric tyrosine kinase restricted to the NMJ in mature muscle. **The AChR is a postsynaptic pentameric membrane protein** that consists of two α1 subunit and one β1, δ, and ε subunits. Although diagnostic for MG, AChR antibodies can be found in patients with thymoma without myasthenia gravis (MG), after use of D-penicillamine, and in a few women without MG whose babies have arthrogryposis (congenital multiple joint contractures).

Antibodies to AMPA-type glutamate receptor 3 (GluR3) is often present in Rasmussen's encephalitis, a severe form of intractable childhood epilepsy, usually restricted to one hemisphere.

Antibodies to voltage-gated calcium channels (VGCC) are associated with Lambert-Eaton myasthenic syndrome (LEMS) and cerebellar ataxia. LEMS consists of proximal fatigable weakness and areflexia with autonomic symptoms such as dry mouth, constipation, and impotence. About 50% of patients have an associated small cell lung cancer (SCLC), which express VGCCs on their surface. VGCC antibodies thus generated cross-react at the NMJ, making LEMS a prototype paraneoplastic disorder where, uniquely, the antibodies are themselves pathogenic. **The VGCCs are presynaptic multimeric membrane protein** present at the NMJ and autonomic ganglia but not in the CNS, unlike VGKC.

Antibodies to voltage-gated potassium channels (VGKC) are found in **acquired neuromyotonia** (NMT), **Morvan syndrome** (Morvan's fibrillary chorea, MFC), and **limbic encephalitis** (LE). NMT is a peripheral nerve hyperexcitable disorder characterized by muscle twitching, cramps and failure to relax following voluntary contraction due to high-frequency neuromyotonic discharges (pseudomyotonia). MFC is a syndrome that presents with NMT, myokymia, dysautonomia (excessive sweating, hypersalivation, cardiac instability, and constipation), and CNS involvement (insomnia, agitation, and hallucinations). The loss of slow-wave and abnormal REM sleep, and enhanced sympathetic function, has been termed *agrypnia excitata,* a condition shared with fatal-familial insomnia and delirium tremens. MFC may be associated with MG, thymoma, and SCLC. LE with VGKC is most commonly nonparaneoplastic (about 20% have SCLC or thymoma) and, unlike PLE (see later discussion), hyponatremia is frequently found; there is a strong male predominance, and often dramatic response to treatment with a high dose of corticosteroids. Increased T2W and FLAIR hippocampi signal is common. **The VGKCs are ubiquitous presynaptic tetrameric membrane proteins** in the brain.

Autoimmune Encephalopathies

Non-paraneoplastic limbic encephalitis with VGKC antibodies and Morvan syndrome are discussed in the previous section. CJD and inflammatory vasculopathies such as CNS vasculitis, Susac syndrome, Sjögren, and antiphospholipid antibody syndrome are in the differential diagnosis.

Paraneoplastic limbic encephalitis (PLE) consists of anterograde memory impairment, temporal lobe seizures, and psychiatric symptoms. There may be high T2 and FLAIR signal in the mesial temporal lobes. The most common PLE-related tumors are SCLC (associated with ANNA-1 or anti-Hu and CRMP-5 or anti-CV2 antibodies), testicular cancer (anti-Ma2 antibodies), thymoma, and breast cancer. Body imaging with fluorodeoxyglucose positron emission tomography (PET) appears to be more sensitive than computed tomography (CT) alone if cancer is missed on initial screening.

Steroid-responsive encephalopathy associated with autoimmune thyroiditis (SREAT, **Hashimoto encephalopathy**), is diagnosed when high serum levels of **thyroperoxidase** antibody (TPO, also known as antimicrosomal antibody) is present. The nonspecific clinical picture includes fluctuating cognitive impairment, behavioral changes, tremor, myoclonus, transient aphasia, sleep abnormalities, seizures, and gait difficulties. The **presence but not the level of TPO** makes the diagnosis of SREAT, regardless of whether patients are euthyroid or mildly hypothyroid. CSF studies often show elevated protein but may not demonstrate lymphocytic pleocytosis, increased IgG synthesis rate, or oligoclonal bands. The brain MRI in SREAT can be normal or show diffuse white matter signal abnormalities and meningeal enhancement, which may resolve with steroid therapy. Given the presence of **serum TPO in approximately 10% of healthy adults** and the age-related increase in TPO seropositivity, the putative role of thyroid autoimmunity in the pathogenesis of SREAT has been questioned. Thyroid autoantibodies may also be found in paraneoplastic and nonparaneoplastic limbic encephalitis. **Paraneoplastic antibodies,** particularly potassium channel antibodies, should be sought in patients with SREAT to rule out underlying malignancies.

Anti-NMDA-receptor encephalitis, caused by antibodies to NR1/NR2 heteromers of the **NMDA receptor (NMDAR),** is a treatable autoimmune disorder of predominantly young women (ages 15–45 years). It presents with **psychotic symptoms,** seizures, autonomic dysfunction, and rapid progression into a state of **"wakeful unresponsiveness"** with abnormal movements of the trunk and face, particularly **jaw dystonia and buccolingual-facial dyskinesias.** Over one-fourth of all unexplained new-onset epileptic encephalopathies in young women, especially when heralded by psychiatric symptoms, are due to NMDAR antibodies. CSF studies may show lymphocytic pleocytosis. Brain MRI may be normal or show increased T2W and FLAIR signal in the medial temporal lobes. Prompt identification of the characteristic presentation should lead to a search for, and removal of, **ovarian teratoma** as well as initiation of immunomodulation. Autoantibodies against the NMDA receptor originate from neural tissue epitopes expressed within the teratoma. Hypofunctioning of the NMDAR is likely to underlie the psychosis of patients with anti-NMDAR encephalitis because NMDAR agonists ameliorate psychotic symptoms.

Brain Tumors

Intracranial neoplasms is the emerging term, as some tumors do not arise from brain tissue (e.g., meningiomas and lymphomas).

Suggestive symptoms of space-occupying lesions are those of increased intracranial pressure (headache, vomiting, and sixth nerve palsy), morning headache, or seizures. Ionizing radiation is the only established risk factor identified for glial and meningeal neoplasms.

Gliomas

Gliomas are classified according their astrocytic or oligodendroglial origin. The pathologic grading is based on the World Health Organization (WHO) system or the St. Anne-Mayo system, both of which take into account the presence or absence of nuclear atypia, mitosis, microvascular proliferation, and necrosis.

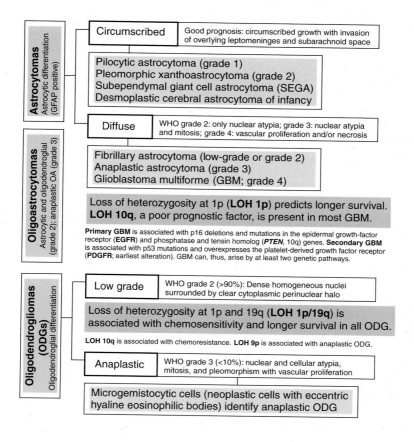

Astrocytomas — Astrocytic differentiation (GFAP positive)

Circumscribed — Good prognosis: circumscribed growth with invasion of overlying leptomeninges and subarachnoid space

Pilocytic astrocytoma (grade 1)
Pleomorphic xanthoastrocytoma (grade 2)
Subependymal giant cell astrocytoma (SEGA)
Desmoplastic cerebral astrocytoma of infancy

Diffuse — WHO grade 2: only nuclear atypia; grade 3: nuclear atypia and mitosis; grade 4: vascular proliferation and/or necrosis

Fibrillary astrocytoma (low-grade or grade 2)
Anaplastic astrocytoma (grade 3)
Glioblastoma multiforme (GBM; grade 4)

Oligoastrocytomas — Astrocytic and oligodendroglial (grade 2); anaplastic OA (grade 3)

Loss of heterozygosity at 1p (**LOH 1p**) predicts longer survival. **LOH 10q**, a poor prognostic factor, is present in most GBM.

Primary GBM is associated with p16 deletions and mutations in the epidermal growth-factor receptor (**EGFR**) and phosphatase and tensin homolog (**PTEN**, 10q) genes. **Secondary GBM** is associated with p53 mutations and overexpresses the platelet-derived growth factor receptor (**PDGFR**; earliest alteration). GBM can, thus, arise by at least two genetic pathways.

Oligodendrogliomas (ODGs) — Oligodendroglial differentiation

Low grade — WHO grade 2 (>90%): Dense homogeneous nuclei surrounded by clear cytoplasmic perinuclear halo

Loss of heterozygosity at 1p and 19q (**LOH 1p/19q**) is associated with chemosensitivity and longer survival in all ODG.

LOH 10q is associated with chemoresistance. **LOH 9p** is associated with anaplastic ODG.

Anaplastic — WHO grade 3 (<10%): nuclear and cellular atypia, mitosis, and pleomorphism with vascular proliferation

Microgemistocytic cells (neoplastic cells with eccentric hyaline eosinophilic bodies) identify anaplastic ODG

Circumscribed Astrocytomas

These are tumors of young adulthood, with a peak incidence in the third to fourth decades of life, typically presenting with a seizure or other focal neurologic deficits. These lesions have no surrounding edema.

Pilocytic astrocytomas represent 5%–10% of all gliomas and 20% of **childhood** brain tumors (making it the second most common pediatric brain tumor after medulloblastomas). These are circumscribed, slow-growing, cystic tumors. The 5-year survival rate is 85%–100%. The **optic chiasm** (in neurofibromatosis type I), hypothalamus and basal ganglia, and the posterior fossa (brainstem and cerebellum) are the most common locations. It may be found around the third and fourth ventricles. Neuroimaging shows a characteristic cyst with **contrast-enhancing mural nodule that may calcify.**

Pleomorphic xanthoastrocytomas represent less than 1% of astrocytomas and usually present with new-onset epilepsy in the **second decade of life.** The tumor is **superficial, partially cystic, and has a mural nodule that may calcify,** and often located in the temporal or parietal lobe.

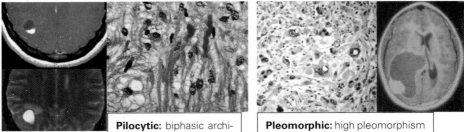

Courtesy: Dr. Mary Gaskill-Shipley

Pilocytic: biphasic architecture, microcysts and **Rosenthal fibers**

Pleomorphic: high pleomorphism with eosinophilic granular bodies

Subependymal giant cell astrocytoma (SEGA) is a **calcified contrast-enhancing** lesion commonly associated with, and occurring in up to 15% of patients with, **tuberous sclerosis.** These intraventricular tumors may evolve from hamartomatous subependymal nodules arising in the *foramen of Monro,* which may lead to intermittent hydrocephalus and intracranial hypertension-related symptoms. Long-term survival is the rule.

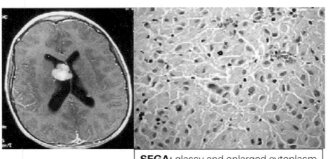

SEGA: glassy and enlarged cytoplasm with eccentric nuclei

Other intraventricular tumors located at the foramen of Monro, besides SEGAs, are subependymoma, central neurocytoma, and intraventricular extension of astrocytomas.

Diffuse Astrocytomas

Fibrillary astrocytoma (WHO grade 2) affects children and young adults and represents 10%–15% of all astrocytomas. The classic MRI appearance is that of T1 hypointensity and T2W/FLAIR hyperintensity **without contrast enhancement or surrounding edema,** frequently affecting the insular cortex. Progression to high-grade malignant gliomas is heralded by the appearance of enhancement on MRI or hypermetabolic areas on PET scans. On pathology, a *gemistocytic* pattern >20% carries a bad prognosis, whereas *microcysts* indicates good prognosis.

Protoplasmic astrocytoma	Gemistocytic astrocytoma
Tumor originates from the cortex and has gelatinlike texture. **Microcysts** and round, small dense nuclei are suspended in a honeycomblike background.	Plump globular or moderately angulated eosinophilic (glassy) cytoplasm with eccentric and pleomorphic nuclei. *p53 mutations* are commonly present.

Anaplastic astrocytoma (grade 3) and glioblastoma multiforme (grade 4, GBM) are the most common glial tumors in the fourth to fifth decades and the sixth to seventh decades, respectively. Brainstem and cerebellar lesions are common locations in children. Most tumors are sporadic but some can occasionally complicate such genetic syndromes as neurofibromatosis 1 and 2, and Li-Fraumeni and Turcot syndromes. Seizures and duration of symptoms greater than 6 months are correlated with better prognosis.

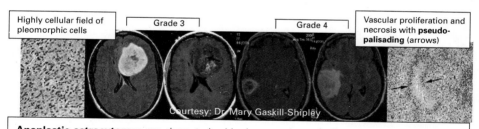

Highly cellular field of pleomorphic cells | Grade 3 | Grade 4 | Vascular proliferation and necrosis with **pseudo-palisading** (arrows)

Courtesy: Dr. Mary Gaskill-Shipley

Anaplastic astrocytomas are characterized by increased mass effect and edema compared to low-grade astrocytomas. Approximately two-thirds of these will demonstrate enhancement. **GBM** shows as thick, irregular enhancement with necrosis. Because of GBM's infiltrative nature, areas of edema surrounding the enhancing lesions typically demonstrate tumor cells.

Surgery or radiation therapy of astrocytomas is deferred in asymptomatic or well-controlled (seizure-free) patients with low-grade tumors, as supported by **PET studies** showing diffuse hypometabolism. If hypermetabolic areas are present, indicating a high-grade tumor, resection should be performed when the lesion is amenable to complete surgical excision. Low-dose focal radiotherapy (45 Gy) is the most effective nonsurgical therapy once progression is clear (early intervention is no better) but may cause disability and may not improve survival. **Bevacizumab,** a humanized monoclonal antibody against vascular endothelial growth factor, is approved for treatment of recurrent glioblastoma.

Oligodendrogliomas

Comprising about 20% of primary brain tumors, oligodendrogliomas (ODGs) are uniquely sensitive to chemotherapy. The preferred locations of these tumors are in the frontal and temporal lobes. The delicate vasculature makes **intracranial hemorrhage** a common neuroimaging presentation. Most patients exhibit seizures, progressive hemiparesis, or cognitive impairment. Overall, ODG fare better (75% 5-year survival for low-grade ODG) than astrocytomas at an equivalent histologic grade.

> **Intracranial hemorrhage** may complicate the primary brain tumors OGD and GBM. Among the metastatic tumors prone to bleeding are **choriocarcinoma, malignant melanoma,** and **renal carcinoma.**

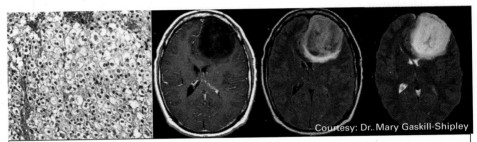

Courtesy: Dr. Mary Gaskill-Shipley

ODG: Perinuclear halos confer the cells a **"fried eggs"** appearance. There are prominent microcysts, **"chicken wire" vessels,** and **calcification.** Brain MRI shows a hemispheric, heterogeneous mass, which often involves cortex and demonstrates variable enhancement. Calcification is shown in head CT as enhancing, irregular cortical hyperintense lesions with cystic components (below).

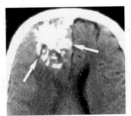

Calcification is present in the primary brain tumors ODG, pilocytic and pleomorphic astrocytomas, SEGA, craniopharyngiomas, choroid plexus papilloma, meningiomas, ependymomas, central neurocytomas, and the metastatic tumors malignant melanoma and renal carcinoma.

Radiographics 2005;25:1669–1688

Treatment of ODG, based on its chemotherapy sensitivity (LOH 1p/19q), consists of a regimen of procarbazine, lomustine [CCNU], and vincristine (PCV), or temozolomide. Sustained remissions with durable clinical improvement, although likely without cure, are documented in low-grade ODG (WHO grade 2). Over 50% of patients with anaplastic ODG (WHO grade 3) recover fully with this regimen, although extensive initial resection is needed. Radiotherapy is reserved for residual tumor only *after* the use of chemotherapy, delaying the potential cognitive dysfunction and reducing the combined toxicity.

The worst prognosis in both primary GBM and anaplastic ODG results from the same genetic profile: *EGFR* amplification, *LOH* 10q, *p16* deletions, *PTEN* mutations without *LOH* 1p or *p53* mutation. MR spectroscopy shows low *N*-acetylaspartate peak and high choline-to-creatinine ratio (>3:1 always suggests malignancy).

Ependymal Tumors

Classic ependymoma is the third most common pediatric brain tumor (8% of all primary brain tumors), mainly intracranial in the first decade of life (**60% infratentorial:** 90% protrude from the fourth ventricle) but **intraspinal in adults** (multiple cord ependymomas are seen in neurofibromatosis type 2 (NF2); astrocytomas predominate in NF1). **Calcification** is common. Poor prognostic factors are age under 2 years, gain of 1q, loss of 9p (including CDKN2A), brainstem invasion, and prior radiation therapy <45 Gy. Degree of histologic malignancy does not predict outcome.

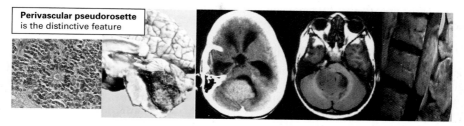

Perivascular pseudorosette is the distinctive feature

Myxopapillary ependymoma is the most common intra-axial tumor of the **conus medullaris and filum terminale** (cervical cord more often harbors *intramedullary* ependymoma). They may present in young individuals (peak age, 28 years) as subarachnoid hemorrhage (vascular tumors) or nocturnal pain upon recumbency.

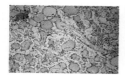

Pseudopapillary architecture with a vascular core embedded in a mucoid matrix is distinctive. Pseudorosettes and rosettes are often seen. It needs to be differentiated from filum terminale paraganglioma

Choroid plexus papilloma is one of the most common primary brain tumors in **children under 2 years,** this cauliflower-looking tumor (resulting from monoepithelial multiple papillae collected around a fibrovascular core) arises in the **trigone of the lateral ventricle (fourth ventricle in adults). Hydrocephalus** occurs both by overproduction of CSF and obstruction to its outflow. It **enhances** and **calcifies** heavily and is **immunopositive for transthyretin** (prealbumin).

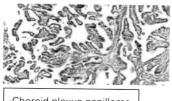

Choroid plexus papilloma

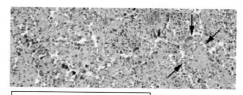

Choroid plexus carcinoma

Choroid plexus carcinoma is difficult to distinguish from choroid plexus papilloma except by its hemorrhagic and invasive nature. Gross surgical resection is associated with favorable prognosis. It is usually negative for transthyretin.

In **adults,** a malignant neoplasm of the choroid plexus is much more likely to be **metastatic carcinoma** than **choroid plexus carcinoma.**

Neuronal Tumors

Well Differentiated (Benign)

Gangliocytoma, dysplastic gangliocytoma, central neurocytoma, and paraganglioma of the filum terminale.

Gangliocytoma

Gangliocytoma is a purely neuronal, quasi-hamartomatous, tumor, which lies on a **dysplastic** brain with malformations such as unilateral **megalencephaly.** Its *cystic nature, with or without a mural nodule,* makes it difficult to differentiate from pilocytic astrocytomas and pleomorphic xanthoastrocytoma. They are the **commonest seizure-associated tumors of the young**.

Dysplastic (Cerebellar) Gangliocytoma (Lhermitte-Duclos)

This tumor is characterized by **progressive hypertrophy of the cerebellar folia** and **granular cell layer** as well as **axonal hypermyelination of the molecular layer. T2W MRI** shows **hyperintense and enlarged folias.** It may represent a true malformation. About 50% of cases have **Cowden syndrome** (multiple hamartomas, autosomal dominant, ***PTEN* gene, 10q**). Other associations are **megalencephaly, polydactyly,** focal gigantism, and heterotopias.

Central Neurocytoma

Intraventricular in location, mostly at the **foramen of Monro,** central neurocytomas develop in young adults. Prognosis is good after total resection. Pathologically, it closely **mimics oligodendrogliomas:** uniform, rounded nuclei with perinuclear halos, branching vascular pattern, and **microcalcifications.**

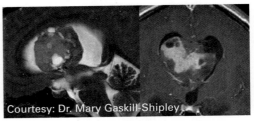

Courtesy: Dr. Mary Gaskill-Shipley

"Intraventricular oligodendroglioma"; mixed hypo-/ isointense intraventricular mass with irregular enhancement.

Oligodendroglioma and central neurocytoma belong to the **clear cell tumors of the CNS** (those with "perinuclear halos"). Other tumors that mimic ODG and central neurocytoma are clear cell ependymoma, clear cell meningioma, dysembryoplastic neuroepithelial tumor (DNET), **metastatic renal cell carcinoma,** and **hemangioblastoma.**

Poorly Differentiated (Malignant)

Ganglioneuroblastoma (gangliocytoma + neuroblastoma) and cerebral neuroblastoma.

Cerebral Neuroblastoma ("Cerebral Medulloblastoma")

It is a poorly differentiated neuronal tumor and a prototypical **supratentorial** primary neuroectodermal tumor (PNET) presenting as a **large, bulky hemispheric mass** with **necrosis, cysts, hemorrhage,** and prominent vessels in the first decade of life (80% are younger than 5 years). It shows heterogeneous density and variable enhancement. Pathologic analysis shows characteristic **perivascular anuclear zones** and **Homer Wright rosettes** (small zones of fibrillarity surrounded by a compact palisading pattern), resembling perivascular pseudorosettes of ependymoma.

Mixed Ganglioneuronal Tumors

Desmoplastic Infantile Ganglioglioma

Desmoplastic infantile ganglioglioma (DIG) is massive and superficial mixed glial-neuronal tumor of infancy (nearly all patients are under 2 years of age), which **enhances** after contrast and is associated with a **cyst.** It is part of the WHO grade 1 tumors and has a good prognosis following gross total resection.

Ganglioglioma

Small, well-circumscribed mass composed by a **cyst with a partially calcified mural nodule,** and show variable enhancement after gadolinium. **Skull erosion** is common if the lesion is superficial. Children and young adults present with seizures. Long-term survival is the rule, even with incomplete resections.

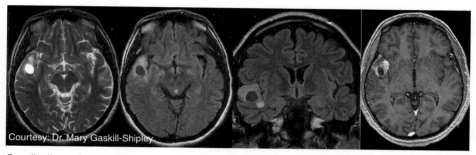

Courtesy: Dr. Mary Gaskill-Shipley

Ganglioglioma: low-grade tumors predominantly affect the temporal lobe, may be calcified, show no overt mass effect or edema, and lead to variable enhancement.

Dysembryoplastic Neuroepithelial Tumor (DNET)

These refer to a **nodular cortical lesion** without edema or mass effect, which may have **megagyric or multicystic appearance** and may be associated with **cortical dysplasia.** The mesial temporal lobe is one of the most common locations. Long history of complex partial epilepsy beginning in childhood is the usual presentation. Occasionally **calcifications** with CT evidence for **calvarial remodeling** may be present. Enhancement is often absent. There is a very small potential for recurrence after gross total resection.

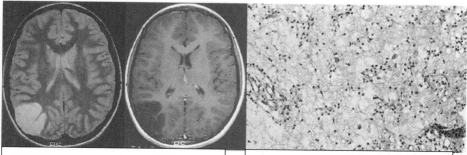

DNET: Homogeneous cortical T2W hyperintensity and T1W hypointensity without enhancement after gadolinium.

DNET as ODG mimicker: prominent ODG-like cells appear "floating" in a mucinous matrix.

Primitive Neuroectodermal Tumors (PNET)

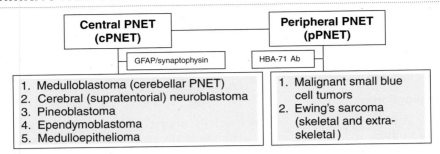

Central PNET (cPNET)	Peripheral PNET (pPNET)
GFAP/synaptophysin	HBA-71 Ab
1. Medulloblastoma (cerebellar PNET) 2. Cerebral (supratentorial) neuroblastoma 3. Pineoblastoma 4. Ependymoblastoma 5. Medulloepithelioma	1. Malignant small blue cell tumors 2. Ewing's sarcoma (skeletal and extra-skeletal)

Medulloblastoma

As the most common primary brain tumor in childhood, medulloblastoma is character-ized as a **spherical** midline (children, 75%) or lateral (adults, 25%) **cerebellar mass, densely cellular** and composed of **small round cells. Early CSF dissemination** occurs in up to 50% at the time of diagnosis, which is best recognized by enhanced MRI or on CSF cytology. It may be associated with basal cell carcinoma **(Gorlin syndrome)** and colon carcinoma **(Turcot syndrome).** Chemotherapy is an effective therapy and contributes to the 50%–60% cure rate after surgical removal and whole neuraxis radiation. Genetic analysis often shows **LOH 17p** (apparently outside the *p53* gene). Amplification of *c-myc* gene (8q) suggests the presence of an aggressive chemoresistant tumor.

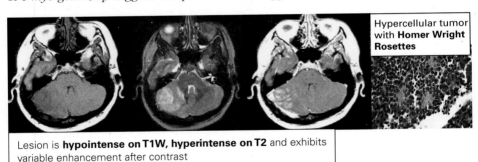

Hypercellular tumor with **Homer Wright Rosettes**

Lesion is **hypointense on T1W, hyperintense on T2** and exhibits variable enhancement after contrast

Medulloblastomas need to be dis-tinguished from atypical teratoid/rhabdoid (AT/RT) tumors (LOH 22q) and **ependymomas** (midline of fourth ventricle, extension into the cerebellopontine angle ("plastic-ity"), and **calcification** on imaging).

Drop metastases or *"subarachnoid invasion"* are seen in the following:
- Medulloblastoma
- Pineoblastoma
- Ependymoma
- Germinoma
- Glioblastoma

Medulloepithelioma

As the **most undifferentiated** tumor among the PNET, medulloepithelioma com-monly presents in very young patients with **increasing head size** due to the **bulky heterogeneous hemispheric mass. Hemorrhage, necrosis,** and **cyst formation** are common.

Meningeal and Mesenchymal Tumors

Meningioma, hemangioblastoma, and hemangiopericytoma.

Meningioma

The most common nonglial primary CNS tumor (20% of all primary tumors), meningioma arises from specialized meningothelial cells called arachnoid "cap" cells mostly in the parasagittal, convexity, sphenoid wing, spinal canal regions and, less commonly, optic nerve sheath and choroid plexus ("intraventricular"). It is most commonly associated with **chromosome 22q loss** (same as **NF2** mutation). **Receptors for estrogen and progesterone** are usually present.

 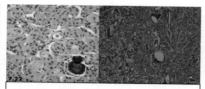 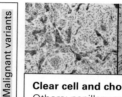

Psammomatous and angiomatous
Microcystic, secretory, metaplastic

Clear cell and chordoid
Others: papillary and Rhabdoid
*Losses of 1p, 9q, 10q, 14q, and 17p
may result in malignant variants*

Hemangioblastoma

Hemangioblastoma (HB) is the most common intra-axial primary neoplasm of the posterior fossa in adults, consisting of a **cystic mass with contrast-enhancing mural nodule** in the cerebellum and, less commonly, medulla and spinal cord. In 25%, HB occurs as part of the **von Hippel-Lindau syndrome** (*VHL* gene, 3p): renal cell carcinoma, pheochromocytoma, and CNS hemangioblastomas including optic nerve and retina. Conversely, 60% of VHL patients develop hemangioblastoma.

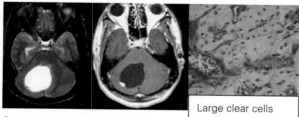

Large clear cells

Courtesy: Dr. Mary Gaskill-Shipley

Cyst with enhancing mural nodule on MRI:
- Pilocytic astrocytoma
- Pleomorphic xanthoastrocytoma
- Ganglioglioma
- Hemangioblastoma
- Craniopharyngioma

Hemangiopericytoma

The origin of hemangiopericytoma from pericytes (contractile cells that surround capillaries) makes these tumors hypervascular and heterogeneous: **low-density cystic or necrotic areas** are common and **enhancement is strong.** There is propensity for both

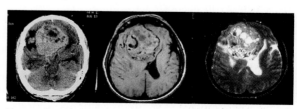

Hemangiopericytoma causing large mass effect in the frontotemporal region.

local **recurrence** and extraneural **metastasis** (especially to lung and bone).

Primary Central Nervous System Lymphoma

Although it represents 1%- 2% of primary brain tumors, the incidence of primary CNS lymphoma (PCNSL) in immunocompromised patients is 3,600 times higher and occurs at a younger age (the peak age is in the sixth to seventh decade in immunocompetent persons), presumably resulting from reactivation of EBV) infection. The tumor is often multifocal and subcortical (periventricular), which explains its low propensity for seizure development. Diffuse microscopic spread accounts for its ability to produce distant disease and local recurrences. Dramatic but transient **response to corticosteroids** leads to its reputation as a **"ghost tumor."** Prognosis is poor and median survival is only 3–5 months in untreated patients.

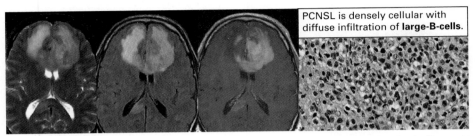

PCNSL is densely cellular with diffuse infiltration of **large-B-cells.**

Lesions may be isointense to hypointense on T2W MRI because of high cell density (unlike most other pathologies, which are hypodense on CT and hyperintense on T2W MRI because of increased water content). In this case, there is transhemispheric extension and secondary involvement of the callosal splenium.

In the presence of ring enhancement, other etiologies are suspected:

Infections	Demyelination	Vascular lesions
Pyogenic brain abscess	**Multiple sclerosis**	**Resolving infarction**
Toxoplasmosis	**Other**	Hematoma
Cysticercosis	Postoperative changes	Thrombosed giant aneurysm
Necrotic fungal infection	Radiation necrosis	

MRI is highly diagnostic in abscesses: it will show a central core of restricted diffusion.(hyperintensity) on diffusion-weighted sequences and a thin rim of low signal on T2W sequences.

Stereotactic biopsy is the diagnostic procedure of choice but can be avoided when lymphomatous cells are discovered in the CSF (18% of patients) or in a vitreous-body biopsy (**uveitis, 10%–20% of patients,** some asymptomatic). The initial required investigations in suspected PCNSL are HIV testing, chest radiograph, CSF analysis, and slit-lamp examination, even though systemic involvement is rare at onset (<5%). Surgery is restricted to brain biopsy because of the multifocality of the tumor. Chemotherapy with high-dose **methotrexate** is associated with response rates of up to 80%, with better overall survival in those whose tumor express the protein **Bcl-6.** When methotrexate is used in combination with radiotherapy, the median survival is increased to at least 40 months, with 25% surviving 5 years or longer. Because this regimen is complicated by **delayed neurotoxicity** (progressive leukoencephalopathy and cognitive dysfunction), especially in those over age 60 years, some advocate postponing radiotherapy in methotrexate responders. Combination chemotherapy regimes are ineffective.

Pineal Tumors and Keratin-Containing Masses

Mainly germinoma and craniopharyngioma, respectively.

Germinoma

This is the **most common germ cell tumor** (followed by teratomas) and the **most common pineal tumor,** occurring predominantly in **young males.** The thalamus and basal ganglia are atypical locations. Germinoma is **hyperdense** on CT but isointense on MRI. There is **strong contrast enhancement,** which also allows for the assessment of **ependymal and subarachnoid spread.**

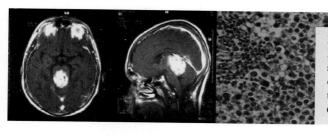

Biphasic cell population: **large** neoplastic cells with **small** reactive lymphocytes, staining for placental alkaline phosphatase (PLAP)

Germ cell tumors—also highly responsive to radiotherapy–, ODG and medulloblastomas are the most **chemosensitive tumors.**

The uncommon pineal germ cell tumors **choriocarcinoma** and **yolk sac tumor** result in high CSF titers of β-human chorionic gonadotropin and α-fetoprotein, respectively.

Craniopharyngioma

This suprasellar tumor arises from the remnants of the hypophyseal Rathke's cleft as a well-defined **cyst with mural nodule.** It may result in growth failure, diabetes insipidus, visual field defects (bitemporal hemianopsia or bitemporal lower quadrantanopsia), and obstructive hydrocephalus. It is the most common supratentorial brain tumor in children. A second peak occurs between the fifth and sixth decades. CT shows foci of hypercalcemia (below, right upper). Brain MRI shows hyperintense strong nodular or rim enhancement (below, right lower). Treatment consists of resection with radiotherapy.

Adamantinomatous (classic)	Papillary
Palisading, "wet" keratin, calcification, "machinery oil" fluid	Well-differentiated squamous epithelium with little keratin, palisading, or calcification
Children and adults	**Adults** only
More infiltrative	Less infiltrative

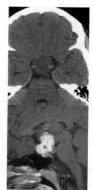

Dr. Mary Gaskill-Shipley

Pituitary Adenoma

These are mostly benign epithelial neoplasms that result from clonal expansion of single adenohypophyseal parenchymal cells. They may reach up to 15% of all intracranial neoplasms. Three-quarters secrete are functioning (i.e., secrete inappropriate amounts of hormones. **Prolactinomas** may rapidly expand during pregnancy and cause hyperprolactinemia (amenorrhea, galactorrhea). Other adenomas secrete **growth hormone, corticotropin,** and rarely gonadotrophin and thyrotropin. Local pressure on the optic chiasm classically causes **bitemporal hemianopsia.**

Lipoma

Lipomas results from abnormal **persistence of the *meninx primitiva*,** a mesenchymal neural crest derivative. Common locations are the corpus callosum, quadrigeminal plate, and cerebellopontine angle. Brain MRI shows fat as **hyperintensity on T1W and hypointensity on T2W sequences.**

> **The corpus callosum may be preferentially affected** in primary CNS lymphoma, intracranial lipoma, glioblastoma multiforme (GBM), Marchiafava-Bignami disease, and agenesis of the corpus callosum.

Arachnoid Cyst

Resulting from meningeal maldevelopment, arachnoid cysts appear by imaging as an extraaxial mass that resembles CSF.

Rathke Cleft Cyst

Rathke cleft cyst develops from the remnants of the closure of the proximal **Rathke's pouch,** which is the embryologic precursor of the anterior lobe, pars intermedia, and pars tuberalis of the pituitary gland. It is **hyperintense on T1W** MRI.

Colloid Cyst

Derived from **neuroectodermal** cells, the colloid cyst is located at the **foramen of Monro** potentially creating symptoms of intermittent hydrocephalus. It is **hyperintense on T2W** MRI. Both Rathke cleft and colloid cysts exhibit a **layer of columnar or cuboidal cells** with a brush border called **goblet cells.**

Metastatic Brain Lesions

The most common metastases derive from lung, breast, malignant melanoma, renal carcinoma, and gastrointestinal tract. The most frequent site for metastatic tumors in the brain is the gray-white matter junction, especially in the distribution of the middle cerebral artery. Leptomeningeal metastases most often complicate breast cancer, leukemia and lymphoma, melanoma, and SCLC. Common systemic tumors that rarely metastasize to the brain are prostate, cervical, ovarian, uterine, squamous cell carcinoma, and sarcomas in general.

> **Hemorrhagic metastases are mostly seen in renal carcinoma, malignant melanoma, and choriocarcinoma.** GBM and ODG are the primary brain tumors with greater bleeding tendency.

Paraneoplastic Syndromes of the CNS

Autoantibodies	Tumors	Clinical syndrome
Anti-Hu (ANNA-1)	SCLC	Limbic encephalitis (anti-CV2/CRMP-5)
		Multifocal encephalomyelitis
		Cerebellar degeneration (anti-CV2)
		Opsoclonus myoclonus
Anti-Ri	Breast	Cerebellar degeneration
	Breast, ovary	Opsoclonus myoclonus
Anti-Yo	Breast, ovary	Cerebellar degeneration
Anti-recoverin	SCLC	Cancer-associated retinopathy (CAR)

Paraneoplastic encephalomyelitis due to **anti-Hu** antibodies, which occur mainly in SCLC, show early and prominent sensory symptoms ("PEM/SSN") and no response to PLEX. There may be high T2W and FLAIR signal in the mesial temporal lobes **(anti-Hu)** or bilateral striatum **(CRMP-5)**. **Anti-Ma2** has been identified in serum and CSF of patients with **testicular cancer.**

Non-paraneoplastic encephalomyelitis, responsive to PLEX or IVIG, results from immune responses against neuronal cell-surface neuronal receptors rather than to intracytoplasmic targets of paraneoplastic disorders. These have been identified in the setting of antibodies to **VGKC** (thymoma; may cause oscillopsia and saccadic paresis), **GluR1/2 AMPA receptor** (primary hippocampus involvement; rapidly progressive abnormal behavior and psychosis), **GABA$_B$ receptor** (early and prominent seizures), and **anti-NMDA receptor** (ovarian teratoma; see "Autoimmune Encephalopathies").

Paraneoplastic cerebellar degeneration (PCD) is suspected in any adults with acutely or subacutely progressive nonfamilial pancerebellar deficit. In decreasing order, the commonest PCDs derive from SCLC (anti-Hu, most are progressive), adenocarcinomas of breast and ovary (anti-Ri, anti Yo), and Hodgkin's lymphoma **(anti-Tr,** only in CSF). Rapid Purkinje cell loss limits treatment response.

Opsoclonus-myoclonus occurs in 2%–3% of children with neuroblastoma (NB), of neural crest origin, mainly of the chest. NB may spontaneously remit (regressive type), mature into a ganglioneuroma (maturative type), or resist to treatment (progressive type). After acute lymphoblastic leukemia, NB is the second most frequent malignancy in childhood. Prognosis of NB is better in the paraneoplastic form. Corticotropin or oral corticosteroids produce rapid and dramatic neurologic improvement in at least two-thirds of children. Other presentations for NB include hypertension (catecholamine metabolites), watery diarrhea (secretion of vasoactive intestinal peptide), or cord compression (dumbbell infiltration at the neural foramen). When ataxia and opsoclonus accompany **gynecologic cancer,** serum and CSF **anti-Ri antibodies** should be sought.

Rhombencephalitis (brainstem encephalitis) may present with gaze palsy, diplopia, or central sleep apnea with acute respiratory failure. It has been associated with anti-Hu, anti-Ri, and anti-Ma2 antibodies.

Paraneoplastic Syndromes of the PNS

Autoantibodies	Tumors	Clinical syndrome
Anti-Hu Anti-amphiphysin	SCLC	Subacute sensory neuronopathy
Anti-VGKC	Thymoma	Neuromyotonia
Anti-VGCC	SCLC	Lambert-Eaton syndrome

Subacute sensory neuronopathy results from the effect of antibodies against the **dorsal root ganglia. Sensory deficits of the upper body are asymmetric** and lead to ataxia and pseudoathetosis. More than 90% of patients have SCLC. It accompanies PEM in 75% of cases. In patients with known cancer, a sensory neuropathy may develop from therapy (cisplatin, paclitaxel, and docetaxel neuropathies), nutritional deficits (B_{12} deficiency), or metastasis.

Neuromyotonia (Isaac syndrome) leads to diffuse muscle stiffness, cramps, and myokymia ("continuous muscle fiber activity") in patients with thymoma, SCLC, Hodgkin's lymphoma, or plasmacytoma. Some patients with **thymoma** have antibodies against **voltage-gated potassium channels** (VGKC), which cause prolonged motor neuron depolarization. About 50% of thymoma patients have myasthenia gravis; conversely, about 15% of MG patients have a thymoma.

Lambert-Eaton myasthenic syndrome (LEMS) results from an autoimmune attack against the **presynaptic voltage-gated P/Q calcium channels** (anti-VGCC) on motor neurons. SCLC is present in 50% of LEMS patients and LEMS develops in about 3% of SCLC patients. Antiglial nuclear antibody (AGNA) antibodies against SOX1, a protein implicated in neural development and expressed in SCLC, are found in 40% of patients. Symptoms include proximal leg weakness, **areflexia, dry mouth with metallic taste,** and dysautonomia (impotence or postural hypotension). LEMS may be precipitated by paralysis from neuromuscular blocking agents or use of **aminoglycosides, magnesium, calcium-channel blockers,** and **iodinated IV contrast agents.** Anti-VGCC levels do not correlate with disease severity but SCLC prognosis is better in its presence. NCV shows small CMAP (<10% of normal). Low-frequency repetitive stimulation (3 Hz) leads to further CMAP fall, but exercise or **high-frequency stimulation (20–50 Hz) causes facilitation** (>200% is diagnostic). Treatment with methylprednisolone, azathioprine, plasmapheresis, or IVIG (2 g/kg over 5 days) produces improvement in many patients but oncologic therapy, if SCLC is present, is the definitive intervention. Cholinesterase inhibitors (especially pyridostigmine) may dramatically relieve weakness or dry mouth in some patients. **Aminopyridines (3,4-DAP,** which blocks potassium channels) and **guanidine** improve strength and autonomic function in most patients.

Motor neuron syndrome and cancer may be associated with anti-Hu (paraneoplastic, ongoing neurologic involvement), no antibodies (women with breast cancer showing a primary lateral sclerosislike picture), or be coincidental (more typical amyotrophic lateral sclerosis, unaffected by cancer therapy).

Stiff-Person Syndrome

Stiff-person syndrome (SPS) is a rare disorder characterized by severe progressive muscular stiffness and gait difficulty with stimulus-sensitive superimposed painful muscle spasms leading to exaggerated lumbar lordosis and impaired ambulation. Pyramidal, extrapyramidal, lower motor signs, and sphincter and sensory disturbances must be absent. Highly specific **glutamic acid decarboxylase (GAD)** antibodies are present in most patients, in whom there may be other **autoimmune diseases,** such as diabetes, hyperthyroidism, hypothyroidism, pernicious anemia, and vitiligo. Paraneoplastic SPS most often involves the upper limbs, cervical, and cranial nerve regions. **Amphiphysin-associated antibodies** are found in fewer than 10% of SPS cases associated with breast and lung cancers. In these cases, opsoclonus and cerebellar ataxia may occur. **Gephyrin-associated SPS** has been identified in one patient with mediastinal carcinoma. **Ri-associated SPS** similarly was reported in a single case with lung adenocarcinoma.

AUTOANTIBODIES AND CLINICAL SYNDROMES

GAD		Amphiphysin (Am)		Gephyrin
High titer	**Low titer**	**Breast cancer**	**SCLC**	**Mediastinal carcinoma**
			Am + anti-Hu	
SPS	Diabetes	*SPS* Cervical spine-arms involved	Encephalomyelitis/ sensory neuronopathy	*SPS* Single case mediastinal carcinoma
Cerebellar ataxia	Adult-onset epilepsy		Cerebellar degeneration	
	Endocrinopathy		Opsoclonus	

GAD, glutamic acid decarboxylase; SCLC, small cell lung cancer; SPS, stiff-person syndrome.
Amphiphysin is a protein located in synaptic vesicles involved in synaptic-vesicle endocytosis; Gephyrin is a cytosolic postsynaptic protein of inhibitory synapses

Failure of GABA-induced inhibition both centrally and at the spinal interneuron levels is the main pathophysiologic derangement. The spasms in SPS occur less abruptly than in hyperekplexia, consistent with GABA-mediated slow inhibitory postsynaptic potentials (IPSP) as opposed to glycine-mediated fast IPSP causing hyperekplexia. No significant pathologic changes have been found at autopsy.

GAD antibodies have 99% specificity for the diagnosis of SPS, now most commonly measured by immunoassay (radioimmunoassay or enzyme-linked immunosorbent assay). Electromyography shows a typical pattern of **continuous low-frequency firing of normal motor units** in agonist and antagonist muscles of the affected region, and at least in one axial muscle. High-dose **benzodiazepines** (diazepam and clonazepam, especially) abolish this excessive motor unit activity. The success of **plasmapheresis** has suggested a pathogenic role for GAD antibodies. Amphiphysin-associated SPS responds best to **plasmapheresis with steroids** or removal of associated breast cancer if identifiable. Tricyclic antidepressants worsen the SPS symptoms. Abrupt withdrawal of pharmacotherapy may be life-threatening.

SPS-like conditions are neuromyotonia, borreliosis, encephalomyelitis lethargica, cramp-fasciculations syndrome, hyperekplexia, tetanus, and strychnine.

Disorders of Neural Tube Closure and Other Congenital Malformations

Chiari Malformations

These neural tube deformities have been grouped as follows:

Chiari I

Chiari I refers to a primary cerebellar ectopia with **elongated cerebellar tonsils** extending through the foramen magnum, beyond what is considered normal, depending on age (0–10 years, 6 mm; 10–30 years, 5 mm; 30–80 years, 4 mm; 80–100 years, 3 mm). **Syringomyelia or syringobulbia** may be seen in 50% of patients; conversely, 90% of patients with idiopathic syringomyelia have a Chiari I malformation. **Skeletal anomalies** can be present in 25%: basilar invagination (up to 50%), Klippel-Feil anomaly (up to 10%), and atlanto-occipital assimilation (up to 5%). **Adults** may be asymptomatic or have hydrocephalus.

Chiari II

Chiari II applies to the **caudal displacement of the cerebellar tonsils, cervicomedullary junction, pons, medulla, and fourth ventricle,** "beaking" the midbrain tectum, "kinking" the cervicomedullary junction, and "towering" the cerebellum. Hydrocephalus and syringohydromyelia are seen in up to 90% of patients. It may be associated with **myelomeningocele** and **spina bifida occulta.** Additional associated findings may include:

- **A large massa intermedia** (interthalamic adhesion)
- **Absence of the septum pellucidum**
- **Craniolacunia,** or patchy thinning of the calvarium, in up to 90%
- **Fenestrated falx** causing a "serrated" appearance to the interhemispheric fissure by the interdigitating gyri
- **Colpocephaly,** enlargement of the occipital horns associated with (splenium) agenesis of the corpus callosum
- **Partial agenesis of the corpus callosum,** heterotopias, polymicrogyria, and stenogyria are additional associated anomalies

Chiari III

Chiari III is used when **Chiari II features** (large massa intermedia, syrinx, cerebellar herniation) accompany herniation of the cerebellum, occipital lobes, and sometimes pons or medulla **(occipitocervical encephalocele).** This Chiari is most severe and usually incompatible with life.

Chiari IV

Chiari IV simply refers to a hypoplastic cerebellum and is likely a variant of Dandy-Walker malformation.

> **Corpus callosum agenesis associations:** migration disorders (heterotopias, lissencephaly, schizencephaly), **holoprosencephaly, Dandy-Walker** malformation, **Aicardi** syndrome, **Chiari II,** lipoma, and inborn errors of metabolism such as **nonketotic hyperglycinemia** and **X-linked pyruvate dehydrogenase deficiency.**

Holoprosencephaly

Holoprosencephaly refers to the failure of hemispheric cleavage (monoventricular forebrain), which results in a single telencephalic ventricle and a continuous overlying cerebral cortex. Children with HPE have mental retardation, spasticity, choreoathetosis, seizures, and endocrinopathies. The usual causes are chromosomal disorders (**trisomy 13,** 18p, and 13q syndromes, as well as Smith-Lemli-Opitz and the Meckel-Gruber syndromes), monogenic mutations (**Sonic hedgehog** [SHH], ZIC2, SIX3, and TG interacting factor [TGIF]), **gestational diabetes,** or infection with toxoplasmosis, syphilis, or rubella. The three classic forms are **alobar** (no interhemispheric fissure, fused thalami and basal ganglia), **semilobar** (posterior interhemispheric fissure is present but cortex is still continuous beneath it), and **lobar** (interhemispheric fissure is present but cortex still continuous beneath it). *Arrhinencephaly* and *craniofacial abnormalities* such as midfacial hypoplasia and cyclopia with proboscis accompany the alobar and semilobar variants.

Dandy-Walker Malformation

This malformation is a cystic dilatation of the fourth ventricle associated with agenesis of the cerebellar vermis with or without heterotopia of the inferior olivary nuclei and pachygyria of the cerebral cortex. Spastic diplegia and mental retardation are related to the associated brain malformations rather than to the associated hydrocephalus. This malformation occurs in approximately 1: 25,000 babies and accounts for approximately 1%–4% of all cases of hydrocephalus.

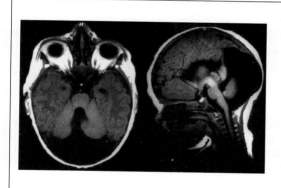

Callosal agenesis can be partial or complete depending on the timing of malformation within the 8–20 weeks of gestation when the callosum and most of the cerebrum and cerebellum form.

A posterior fossa CSF collection is also seen in vermian agenesis (e.g., Joubert syndrome), enlarged cisterna magna (due to cerebellar atrophy or agenesis), and arachnoid cyst.

Septo-Optic Dysplasia (de Morsier Syndrome)

Considered a very **mild form of lobar holoprosencephaly** and occasionally associated with **schizencephaly,** it is recognized by the triad of absent septum pellucidum, agenesis of the corpus callosum, and **optic nerve hypoplasia.** It may present with seizures, seesaw nystagmus, or **hypopituitarism** of hypothalamic origin.

Schizencephaly (Split Brain)

Defined as a gray matter-lined CSF-filled cleft that extends from the ependymal surface of the brain to the pia, it presents as **type I or closed-lip** (where the cleft walls are in apposition) or type II or open-lip (cleft walls are separated). It should be differentiated from **porencephaly** (noncongenital disorder due to vascular prenatal injury) in which there is communication from arachnoid to ventricle.

Brainstem-Vermis Decussation Malformation (Molar Tooth Sign)

Joubert is the main representative syndrome characterized by episodic **hyperpnea,** hypotonia, ataxia, and abnormal eye movements (**oculomotor apraxia** and seesaw nystagmus). Other syndromes are Senior-Löken, COACH, and Arima (worst prognosis due to polymicrogyria, retinopathy, and dysplastic kidneys), which belong to the **cerebello-oculo-renal syndromes.** The vermal agenesis and fourth ventricle abnormalities are reminiscent of the cerebellar cyst of Dandy-Walker malformation.

Lissencephaly (Smooth Brain)

Lissencephaly refers to a brain with absent or poor sulcation (**agyria),** corresponding to a fetal age of 16–17 weeks, as sulcation begins at week 20. There are two types:
- **Type I Lissencephaly (classic type)** consisting of a four-layered cortex (instead of six) is associated to two major genetic etiologies: (1) *LIS1* **gene deletion** (17p13) results in the **Miller-Dieker syndrome** (facial dysmorphism [micrognathia, thin upper lip, upturned nares, broad nasal bridge, low-set ears, bitemporal hollowing, microcephaly], seizures, and spasticity). *LIS1* codes for platelet activating factor (**PAF),** required for neuronal migration. Thus, *LIS1* deletion results in *undermigration.* (2) *Doublecortin (DCX)* **gene mutation** (X-linked dominant, *XLIS1* gene), lethal in males, causes **"double cortex" (subcortical band heterotopia)** in females, who have seizures and mental retardation. Doublecortin is a microtubule-associated protein important for cell migration.
- **Type II Lissencephaly (cobblestone)** is a poorly laminated, disorganized, thickened or cobblestonelike cortex resembling polymicrogyria. This is a disorder of *overmigration* and is associated with mental retardation, intractable seizures, obstructive hydrocephalus, and other brain defects. It occurs within the setting of **congenital muscular dystrophies,** especially Walker-Warburg syndrome and Fukuyama muscular dystrophy.

Heterotopias

Heterotopias are a collection of otherwise normal neurons in abnormal locations secondary to the arrest of neuronal migration along the radial glial fibers. They can be nodular or laminar. **Nodular heterotopias** are subependymal or periventricular masses of gray matter adjacent to the walls of the lateral ventricles. **X-linked periventricular heterotopia** (mutation in the filamin 1 [*FLM-1*] gene) is lethal in males and is often associated with subcortical heterotopias. Most patients have normal intelligence.

Polymicrogyria

Polymicrogyria consists of many small gyri separated by shallow sulci and mildly thickened cortex that can result from either an acquired (such as CMV, rubella, HSV), genetic (X-linked dominant Aicardi syndrome), or metabolic disorder (Zellweger syndrome). Microcephaly is often associated. It may occur in combination with pachygyria.

Neuromuscular Disorders 9

Identifying the pattern of weakness for the major muscle disorders is important to steer the diagnostic workup. The following phenotypic patterns are recognized:

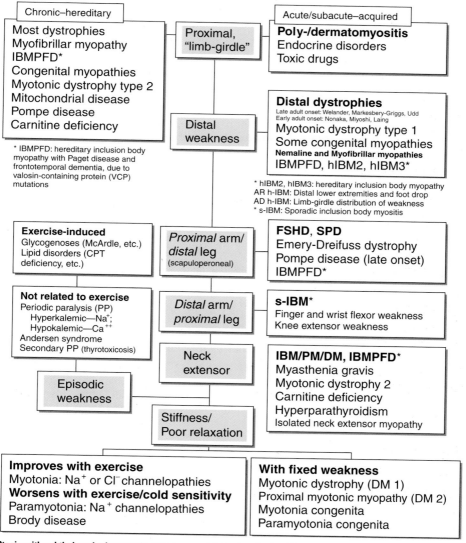

Chronic–hereditary

Most dystrophies
Myofibrillar myopathy
IBMPFD*
Congenital myopathies
Myotonic dystrophy type 2
Mitochondrial disease
Pompe disease
Carnitine deficiency

* IBMPFD: hereditary inclusion body myopathy with Paget disease and frontotemporal dementia, due to valosin-containing protein (VCP) mutations

Proximal, "limb-girdle"

Acute/subacute–acquired

Poly-/dermatomyositis
Endocrine disorders
Toxic drugs

Distal weakness

Distal dystrophies
Late adult onset: Welander, Markesbery-Griggs, Udd
Early adult onset: Nonaka, Miyoshi, Laing
Myotonic dystrophy type 1
Some congenital myopathies
Nemaline and Myofibrillar myopathies
IBMPFD, hIBM2, hIBM3*

* hIBM2, hIBM3: hereditary inclusion body myopathy
AR h-IBM: Distal lower extremities and foot drop
AD h-IBM: Limb-girdle distribution of weakness
* s-IBM: Sporadic inclusion body myositis

Exercise-induced
Glycogenoses (McArdle, etc.)
Lipid disorders (CPT deficiency, etc.)

Proximal arm/ distal leg
(scapuloperoneal)

FSHD, SPD
Emery-Dreifuss dystrophy
Pompe disease (late onset)
IBMPFD*

Not related to exercise
Periodic paralysis (PP)
  Hyperkalemic—Na$^+$;
  Hypokalemic—Ca^{++}
Andersen syndrome
Secondary PP (thyrotoxicosis)

Distal arm/ proximal leg

s-IBM*
Finger and wrist flexor weakness
Knee extensor weakness

Neck extensor

IBM/PM/DM, IBMPFD*
Myasthenia gravis
Myotonic dystrophy 2
Carnitine deficiency
Hyperparathyroidism
Isolated neck extensor myopathy

Episodic weakness

Stiffness/ Poor relaxation

Improves with exercise
Myotonia: Na$^+$ or Cl$^-$ channelopathies
Worsens with exercise/cold sensitivity
Paramyotonia: Na$^+$ channelopathies
Brody disease

With fixed weakness
Myotonic dystrophy (DM 1)
Proximal myotonic myopathy (DM 2)
Myotonia congenita
Paramyotonia congenita

Ptosis with ophthalmoplegia occurs in oculopharyngeal dystrophy, mitochondrial myopathies, neuromuscular junction abnormalities (myasthenia gravis, Lambert-Eaton syndrome, botulism) and hIBM3. **Ptosis without ophthalmoplegia** is seen in myotonic dystrophy and congenital myopathies. **Bulbar weakness** with dysarthria and dysphagia is reported in myasthenia gravis, Lambert-Eaton myasthenic syndrome, and oculopharyngeal dystrophy.

Brachial Plexopathies

Upper Plexus Paralysis (Erb-Duchenne)

C5 and C6 root damage causes impairment in shoulder abduction (deltoid and supraspinatus), external rotation of the arm (infraspinatus), elbow flexion (biceps, brachioradialis, brachialis), and forearm supination (biceps). Biceps and brachioradialis reflexes are absent. There may be hypesthesia in the lateral forearm and hand. The **limb is internally rotated and adducted,** assuming the porter's tip position.

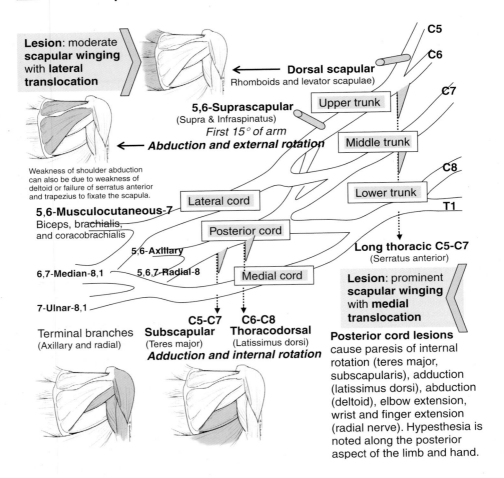

Lesion: moderate **scapular winging** with **lateral translocation**

Dorsal scapular ←
Rhomboids and levator scapulae)

C5
C6
C7

5,6-Suprascapular
(Supra & Infraspinatus)
First 15° of arm
← ***Abduction and external rotation***

Upper trunk

Middle trunk

Weakness of shoulder abduction can also be due to weakness of deltoid or failure of serratus anterior and trapezius to fixate the scapula.

5,6-Musculocutaneous-7
Biceps, brachialis, and coracobrachialis

Lateral cord

Posterior cord

C8

Lower trunk

T1

5,6-Axillary

6,7-Median-8,1   5,6,7-Radial-8

Medial cord

7-Ulnar-8,1

Long thoracic C5-C7
(Serratus anterior)

Lesion: prominent **scapular winging** with **medial translocation**

C5-C7   C6-C8
Terminal branches **Subscapular   Thoracodorsal**
(Axillary and radial) (Teres major)   (Latissimus dorsi)
Adduction and internal rotation

Posterior cord lesions cause paresis of internal rotation (teres major, subscapularis), adduction (latissimus dorsi), abduction (deltoid), elbow extension, wrist and finger extension (radial nerve). Hypesthesia is noted along the posterior aspect of the limb and hand.

Lower Plexus Paralysis (Dejerine-Klumpke)

C8 and T1 root damage causes a claw-hand deformity with weakness of finger flexion and wasting of the intrinsic hand muscles. There may be hypesthesia in the medial arm, forearm, and ulnar aspect of the hand. Horner's syndrome accompanies T1 root injury.

Brachial Neuropathies

Median nerve, proximal
Pronator teres (C6–C7)
Flexor carpi radialis (C6–C7)
Palmaris longus (C7–T1)
Flexor digitorum superficialis

Anterior interosseous nerve, distal (C7–C8)
Pronator quadratus
Flexor pollicis longus (FPL)
Flexor digitorum profundus (FDP I–II)

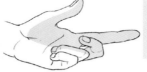

Anterior interosseous neuropathy (Kiloh-Nevin syndrome) causes weakness of flexion of the distal phalanges in the first (FPL), second, and third (FDP I–II) fingers. Sparing of FPL and FDP I–II in **carpal tunnel syndrome** results in a **pinch attitude** (the median version of the ulnar Froment prehensile thumb sign).

Median nerve, distal ("LOAF": C8-T1)

Thenar muscles
Lumbricals I–II
Opponens pollicis
Abductor pollicis brevis
Flexor pollicis brevis
(Superficial head)

C6-C7 from **lateral cord:**
sensory component
C8-T1 from **medial cord:**
motor component

The ulnar nerve may occasionally supply the opponens pollicis, in which case this muscle is spared in CTS. **Adductor pollicis and deep head of FPB are the only thenar muscles regularly supplied by the ulnar nerve.**

Ulnar nerve, proximal
Flexor carpi ulnaris (FCU)
Flexor digitorum profundus III and IV (FDP III-IV)
Palmar and dorsal cutaneous branches (sensory)
Superficial terminal branch

Ulnar nerve, distal

Hypothenar muscles
Palmaris brevis
Abductor digiti minimi
Flexor digiti minimi
Opponens digiti minimi

Lumbricals III and IV
Interossei (palmar and dorsal)

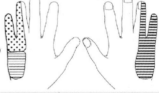

Hypesthesia in the areas of dorsal and palmar cutaneous branches indicates an ulnar nerve lesion above **Guyon's canal** (wrist): at the elbow **(cubital tunnel syndrome)**

Proximal ulnar lesions (above the elbow) result in weakness of ulnar wrist flexion and terminal phalanges of the fourth and fifth fingers. **"Claw hand"** deformity only implies interossei and ulnar lumbricals paresis. **Weakness of adductor pollicis** results in the **Froment's prehensile thumb sign,** whereby distal flexion of the thumb occurs to increase pinch grip **("reverse" Kiloh-Nevin syndrome).** Sensory deficits beyond 2 cm above the wrist localize the lesion to the T1 root, the medial cord, or the medial cutaneous nerve of arm and forearm.

Martin-Gruber anastomosis (seen in up to 31% of patients) represents axons from the median nerve crossing over the forearm to join the ulnar nerve at the wrist. The median nerve ends up innervating intrinsic hand muscles, especially the first dorsal interosseous, adductor pollicis, and hypothenar muscles.

Radial nerve (C6-T1)
Proximal to the spiral groove:
  Triceps (C7, C8)
  Anconeous
Below the spiral groove:
  Brachialis
  Brachioradialis (C5, C6)
  Extensor carpi radialis (ECR) (C5, C6)
Superficial branch: dorsal digital nerve
Deep: Posterior interosseous nerve
  Supinator (at the arcade of Frohse)
  Extensor carpi ulnaris (ECU) (C7, C8)
  Extensor digitorum
  Extensor indicis
  Extensor digiti minimi
  Extensor pollicis longus
  Extensor pollicis brevis
  Abductor pollicis longus

Wrist drop from retrohumeral or spiral groove lesions preserves elbow extension, triceps reflex, and sensation of the posterior forearm, but causes weakness in the brachioradialis (tested with elbow flexion when forearm is in neutral position), radial wrist extension, and finger extension, with hypalgesia restricted to the dorsolateral hand.

Posterior Interosseous Neuropathy

Causes weakness of finger extension with **radial deviation** of the wrist when attempting to make a fist or extend the hand. Triceps, brachioradialis, and extensor carpi radialis are normal. There is no loss of sensation or reflexes.

Spiral Groove Radial Palsy

Weakness of wrist and finger extension with normal triceps strength. A bruise or scar may be present in the posterior part of the upper arm. The brachioradialis reflex may be absent. **Snuffbox hypesthesia** is present.

C7, C8 root or plexus lesion

Weakness of triceps and finger extension with radial deviation of the wrist on attempted extension (normal extensor carpi radialis). Brachioradialis strength is normal. Triceps reflex is reduced or absent. There should be hypesthesia in the C7, C8 dermatomes.

C7, C8, T1 root or plexus lesions

As above plus weakness of finger flexors and extension of the sensory loss to the T1 dermatome (ulnar aspect of the forearm and hand). Classic causes are cervical rib (diminished arm pulse) and Pancoast tumor (Horner's syndrome) ✚

✚Cervical spondylosis is not a cause of weakness in the small hand muscles because these are mainly supplied by T1.

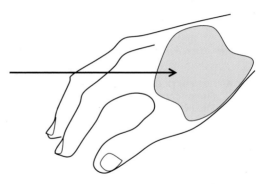

The **brachioradialis** is the key muscle to test in a patient with wrist drop: it is weak in radial nerve lesions proximal to or at the spiral groove, whereas it is normal in posterior interosseous neuropathy and C7-T1 root or plexus lesions.

Assessment of Hand Weakness

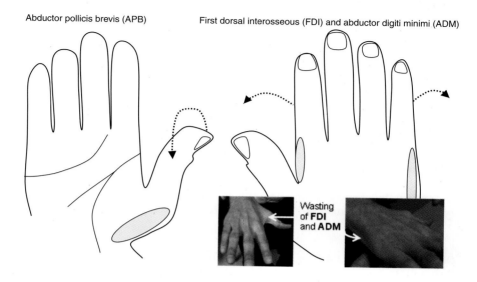

Abductor pollicis brevis (APB)

First dorsal interosseous (FDI) and abductor digiti minimi (ADM)

Wasting of **FDI** and **ADM**

Wasting Confined to APB	Wasting Confined to FDI and ADM
Usually a **median nerve** lesion at wrist	Usually an **ulnar nerve** lesion
If there is weakness of the deep flexor of the index (FDP I) and thumb (FPL), the lesion is at the elbow **(anterior interosseous nerve)**	If there is weakness of the deep flexor of the little finger (FDP IV) and ulnar wrist (FCU), and loss of sensation in medial hand, the lesion is at the elbow

Wasting of the hand, areflexia, and a dissociated sensory loss (hypesthesia to pain and temperature with preservation of proprioception) in a half-cape distribution suggest **syringomyelia, ependymoma,** or other intrinsic lesions of the cervical and upper thoracic cord.

PROXIMAL ARM WEAKNESS ASSESSMENT

Root	Muscles	Nerve	Other Findings
C5, C6	Deltoid	Axillary	Weak radial wrist extension and absent biceps reflex
	Biceps	Musculocutaneous	
	Brachioradialis	Radial	
C7, C8	Triceps	Radial	Weak finger extension and absent triceps reflex

Serratus anterior (scapular fixation and rotation, long thoracic nerve) represents C5–C7 levels.

DELTOID, BICEPS, AND BRACHIORADIALIS WEAKNESS

C5, C6 Cord Lesion	C5, C6 Root or Plexus Lesion
Biceps and brachioradialis reflexes are absent but those below the level of lesion (triceps and finger flexors [C7, C8]) in the arms and legs are *increased*. A C5 sensory level may be present.	Biceps and brachioradialis reflexes are absent; all others are normal. Very proximal lesions involve all muscles; further down, serratus anterior will be spared, and further down still, supra- and infraspinatus will be spared. Sensory loss is dermatomal.

Lumbar Plexus

Femoral nerve (L1–L4)
   Iliopsoas (hip flexor) (L1–L3)
   Distal to the inguinal ligament:
      Quadriceps femoris (leg extensor) (L2–L4)
      Sartorius (thigh flexor and evertor)
      Pectineus (thigh flexor and evertor)

> **Femoral nerve provides sensation to the medial thigh** (medial cutaneous nerve of the thigh) and medial lower leg (saphenous).

> **Femoral neuropathies** cause weakness of hip flexion (iliopsoas) and leg extension (quadriceps femoris), absent patellar reflex, **normal hip adduction**, and **hypesthesia on the anteromedial thigh and leg.** Possible causes are **retroperitoneal hematoma** and **childbirth in lithotomy position.** An important cause of *painful* femoral neuropathy is **adult-onset diabetes mellitus** (diabetic amyotrophy). Lesions at or below the inguinal ligament level spare thigh flexion as the femoral branches to the iliopsoas are preserved.

Obturator nerve (L2–L4), subject to obstetric injury, is responsible for **thigh adduction** and, secondarily, internal rotation and knee flexion (gracilis muscle).

L2–L4 radiculopathy or plexopathy causes weakness of iliopsoas, quadriceps, *and* hip adductors. The L2–L4 dermatome follows that of the femoral nerve.

Lateral femoral cutaneous nerve (L2–L3) injury (meralgia paresthetica) is especially characteristic in obese individuals who wear constrictive garments. Most commonly it arises from compression or entrapment of the lateral femoral cutaneous nerve as it passes through the inguinal ligament.

Sacral Plexus

Inferior gluteal nerve (L5–S2) supplies the gluteus maximus (hip extension).

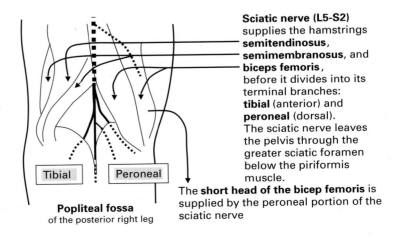

Sciatic nerve (L5-S2) supplies the hamstrings **semitendinosus, semimembranosus,** and **biceps femoris,** before it divides into its terminal branches: **tibial** (anterior) and **peroneal** (dorsal). The sciatic nerve leaves the pelvis through the greater sciatic foramen below the piriformis muscle.

The **short head of the bicep femoris** is supplied by the peroneal portion of the sciatic nerve

Tibial

Peroneal

Popliteal fossa
of the posterior right leg

Tibial Nerve

Gastrocnemius (S1–S2)
Soleus (S1–S2)
Popliteus
Plantaris

Main plantar flexors are located in the distal popliteal fossa **(S1–S2)**

Tibialis posterior (L4–L5)
Flexor digitorum longus (L5–S2)
Flexor hallucis longus (S1–S2)

Main plantar flexors and foot invertors are located in the posterior leg compartment **(L4–S2)**

Sensation to the lateral heel and foot is provided by the **sural nerve,** which forms with contributions from the common peroneal (lateral sural cutaneous).

The tarsal tunnel (formed by **lancinate ligament,** which runs from the medial malleolus to the calcaneus) gives rise to the distal tibial nerve fibers (S1–S2):

Medial Plantar Nerve	Lateral Plantar Nerve
Abductor hallucis, flexor hallucis, flexor digitorum brevis, and the lumbricals I–II (also, skin of medial two-thirds of the sole of the foot)	**Ad**ductor hallucis, abductor digiti minimi, flexor digiti minimi, interossei, and lumbricals III–IV (also, skin of lateral one-third of the sole of the foot)

Popliteal-level lesions of the tibial nerve cause weakness of plantar flexion, foot inversion, and toe flexion with *sole hypesthesia.* **Tarsal tunnel syndrome** refers to a condition caused by compression of the tibial nerve as it passes underneath the flexor retinaculum behind and distal to the medial malleolus. It is characterized by hypesthesia of the sole and heel triggered by standing or walking, or after pressure applied to the medial malleolus (Tinel sign). Nocturnal pain analogous to CTS is seen.

Peroneal Nerve

In the popliteal fossa, the common peroneal gives off the lateral cutaneous nerve of the calf (skin of lateral leg below the knee) and the lateral sural cutaneous nerve, which joins its medial counterpart to form the sural nerve (skin of distal posterior leg and lateral foot).

Deep peroneal (tibialis anterior)
Tibialis anterior (L4–L5)
Extensor digitorum longus (L5)
Extensor hallucis longus (L5)
Extensor digitorum brevis (L5)
(Also, skin next to first and second toes)

Main plantar dorsiflexors and toe extensors (tibialis anterior is also a foot invertor) located in the anterior leg compartment **(L4–L5)**

Superficial peroneal
Peroneus longus (L5)
Peroneus brevis (L5)
(Also, skin of distal leg and dorsum of the feet and toes)

Plantar evertors (L5)

Common peroneal neuropathies affect the **deep peroneal nerve** most often and usually result from prolonged leg crossing, knee arthroplasty, or any other traumatic lesions. Foot eversion weakness and a larger sensory deficit over the dorsum of the foot are added to isolated foot drop when **deep *and* superficial** branches are involved.

Assessment of Foot Drop

Common Peroneal	L5 Radiculopathy
Weakness of dorsiflexion *and eversion* is more common; extensor hallucis longus weakness will confirm location. Hypesthesia occurs in lateral leg.	Weakness of dorsiflexion *and inversion*. Hypesthesia occurs on the lateral leg, dorsomedial foot, and large toe.

In the electrophysiologic study of foot drop, assessment of the *short head of the biceps femoris* is the preferred above-the-knee muscle to test. Since the peroneal division of the **sciatic nerve** proximal to the fibular head supplies this muscle, its involvement localizes the deficit to the sciatic nerve.

Piriformis syndrome is an entrapment syndrome of the sciatic nerve as it passes through the greater sciatic notch. It is suspected when foot drop is accompanied by buttock tenderness, sciatica reproduced on deep palpation, and **leg pain worsened by internal rotation of the flexed limb.** Sources as diverse as pelvic surgery, buttock trauma, wallet pressure, and toilet seat entrapmen, have been reported. Besides foot drop, the main features are:

- Weakness of knee flexion (hamstring), foot eversion (superficial peroneal), foot inversion (tibialis anterior), and foot dorsiflexion (tibialis anterior), and foot plantar flexion (gastrocnemius and soleus).
- Preservation of iliopsoas, hip adductors, and quadriceps muscles.
- Absent ankle reflex with normal patellar reflex.

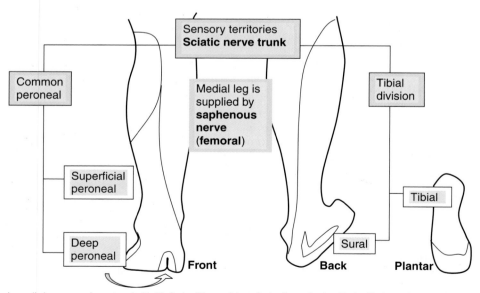

Lower limb monoparesis most marked in hip flexion (iliopsoas), knee flexion (hamstrings), ankle dorsiflexion and eversion is characteristic of weakness of corticospinal origin.

Guillain-Barré Syndrome (GBS)

GBS is the prototypical acute **postinfectious neurologic disorder,** often preceded by an upper respiratory tract infection and heralded by **ascending paralysis** that reaches its peak by 1 week in 50% and stops progressing by 4 weeks. **Areflexia** and **albuminocytologic dissociation** (proteinorrhachia without pleocytosis) in cerebrospinal fluid (CSF) are the clinical hallmarks. **Autonomic dysfunction** and cranial nerve involvement may each develop in half of all patients.

> **CSF pleocytosis** instead of albuminocytologic dissociation in "GBS" raises suspicion for *HIV infection, West Nile virus encephalitis, Lyme disease,* and *sarcoidosis.* "GBS" **without CSF changes** is suspected in acute intermittent porphyria, diphtheric neuropathy, tick paralysis, hexacarbons toxicity (solvents *n*-hexane and methyl-*N*-butyl ketone), and hypophosphatemia.

Very slow NCV, dispersed CMAP, and **multifocal conduction block** are the electrophysiologic correlates. Initial abnormalities may be limited to prolonged F-waves. Mononuclear inflammatory infiltrates in the endoneurium and myelin sheath cause patchy **segmental multifocal demyelination.** The most common GBS type is demyelinating (acute inflammatory demyelinating polyneuropathy), but **axonal forms,** with *potential preservation of reflexes,* have been identified:

- Acute motor axonal neuropathy **(AMAN)** or "Chinese paralytic syndrome," most common form of GBS in Asia
- Acute motor and sensory axonal neuropathy **(AMSAN):** more rapid onset and severe weakness; recovery is slower and incomplete
- Pharyngeal-cervical-brachial weakness **(PCB)**

Anti-GM1b, anti-GD1a, and GalNAc-GD1a immunoglobulin G (IgG) antibodies can be found in these axonal forms (**anti-GT1a IgG** antibody is most common in the PCB variant), mostly after *Campylobacter jejuni* diarrhea. **Anti-GD1b antibodies** are associated with ataxic presentations.

Miller-Fisher syndrome (5% of GBS) causes **total external ophthalmoplegia** (with *pupil-sparing ptosis*), **ataxia,** and **areflexia.** The presence of **diplopia** and the celerity of ataxia distinguish this ophthalmoplegia from that of mitochondrial myopathies. **Anti-GQ1b IgG antibodies** can be identified in this GBS variant.

Plasma exchange (PLEX) *or* intravenous (IV) Ig hastens recovery from GBS. Both are equally effective, but the combination is not superior to either treatment modality given alone. PLEX is technically demanding and carries a greater risk of side effects. **Steroid treatment is not beneficial.** Supportive care relies on intubation if forced vital capacity (FVC) is <15 mL/kg, deep venous thrombosis prophylaxis, monitoring for autonomic instability, and physical and occupational therapy.

> **Toxic peripheral neuropathies** mimicking GBS can be seen with hexacarbon ("glue sniffers"), organophosphates, and acrylamide poisoning; biological toxins such as tetrodotoxin, ciguatoxin, saxitoxin, and brevitoxin; exposure to metals such as arsenic, lead, and thallium; and to the drugs isoniazide, nitrofurantoin, chloroquine, and gold.

Chronic Inflammatory Demyelinating Polyneuropathy (CIDP)

CIDP is a chronic (>2 months), progressive, or relapsing areflexic weakness due to relatively **symmetric motor and sensory radiculoneuropathy** with sparing of the autonomic nervous system, unlike GBS. There is **albuminocytologic dissociation** on CSF and *multifocal* demyelination in at least three nerves, with conduction block or temporal dispersion in at least one, on NCV.[*]

> **CSF pleocytosis in CIDP** raises suspicion for *HIV infection, Lyme disease, sarcoidosis*, lymphoma, and leukemia.

The variants are:

- **MMN:** multifocal *motor* neuropathy with motor **conduction block** and **anti GM1 and anti-GD1a antibodies** presents with asymmetric distal upper extremity and differential finger extension weakness, reflecting vulnerability of terminal branches of the posterior interosseous nerve. Unlike other CIDP forms, CSF proteins are often normal.
- **MADSAM:** multifocal acquired demyelinating *sensory* and *motor* neuropathy presents as a **chronic mononeuropathy multiplex** (Lewis-Sumner syndrome) or MMN with sensory deficits. Unlike MMN, GM1 antibodies are uncommon. The axonal variant is **MASAM** ol multifocad acquirey sensory anr motor neuropathy.
- **DADS:** distal acquired demyelinating symmetric neuropathy is a symmetric *predominantly sensory* polyneuropathy whereby patients often have IgM monoclonal gammopathies with **anti-MAG (myelin-associated glycoprotein) antibodies.** Presence of these IgM M-proteins is associated with steroid failure.

CIDP may be associated with human immunodeficiency virus (HIV), monoclonal gammopathy of undetermined significance (MGUS), or lymphoproliferative disorders such as lymphoma, Waldenström's macroglobulinemia, multiple myeloma, osteosclerotic myeloma (POEMS syndrome), and Castleman's disease. Sural nerve biopsy is not required (most of the pathology is in motor fibers) but when performed shows epineurial and **endoneurial lymphocytic infiltration** with re- and demyelinating fibers, with **onion bulb formation** in 10% of cases.

Immunosuppressive therapy is the mainstay of treatment. Prednisone, plasma exchange (PE), and IV Ig are variably beneficial. Patients with pure motor CIDP and MMN do not respond or worsen when given corticosteroids or PE. IV Ig should be avoided in patients with IgA deficiency (anaphylaxis). Potential risks of other immunosuppressants are interstitial lung fibrosis (methotrexate), gout (azathioprine), nephrotoxicity (cyclosporine), and fatal hemorrhagic cystitis (cyclophosphamide).

---

[*]**In demyelinating neuropathy,** distal motor latency (ML) is prolonged and conduction velocity (CV) markedly slowed to <80% of normal; the compound muscle action potential (CMAP) is reduced and *dispersed* (unlike CMT). **In axonal neuropathy,** the CMAP is also reduced but the ML and CV are relatively preserved.

Myasthenia Gravis

MG is the most common disorder of neuromuscular transmission and the best-known neurological example of an antibody-mediated autoimmune disease. Its prevalence in the United States is estimated at 14 per 100,000 people. MG results from the production of autoantibodies against the nicotinic acetylcholine (ACh) receptor (AChR). It manifests as fluctuating generalized weakness with **preservation of muscle stretch reflexes.** In about 15% of patients with generalized MG, AChR antibodies are absent, and of these "seronegative" myasthenics, about 40% have IgG antibodies against **muscle-specific kinase (MuSK),** a postsynaptic surface membrane enzyme essential in aggregating AChR during the development of the neuromuscular junction. Weakness in MuSK affects oculobulbar more than limb muscles and responds less to immunosuppressants and AChR inhibitors. Weakness is restricted to ocular muscles in approximately 10% of MC cases (ocular myasthenia). **Autoimmune disorders** such as rheumatoid arthritis, SLE, and pernicious anemia are associated in 5% of patients, **thymoma** in 15%, and **lymphoid hyperplasia with proliferation of germinal centers** in up to 70% of the patients. The *presynaptic* homologs of MG are LEMS (see *Paraneoplastic syndromes*) and botulism (see *Neurotoxicology*).

AChR antibodies, repetitive nerve stimulation, and single fiber electromyogram (EMG) are very sensitive for diagnosis. The edrophonium (tensilon) test is now rarely necessary. EMG findings may suggest myopathy in MuSK-positive MG and repetitive nerve stimulation studies are often normal. Drugs that impair ACh release and worsen MG are **quinidine/quinine, procainamide, P-type calcium channel blockers,** most **antibiotics,** and those causing **hypermagnesemia** (laxatives, antacids, TPN). The **iatrogenic causes of autoimmune MG** are D-penicillamine, interferon alpha, and bone marrow transplantation (graft versus host disease). The first choice of therapy is the acetylcholinesterase inhibitor **pyridostigmine (Mestinon),** given at 30–60 mg qid with maximal efficacy achieved at 60 mg every 4 hours. **Thymectomy** brings delayed improvement in 75% of seropositive patients older than 50 years. **Prednisone** (perhaps with azathioprine as a steroid-sparing drug) is used in those who fail pyridostigmine. **IV Ig** (0.4 g/kg daily for 3 days) is required in refractory cases, during myasthenic crisis, or as a presurgical boost. Plasma exchange is beneficial for those with MuSK-positive MG.

Myasthenic crisis (not cholinergic) is triggered by surgery, infection, or rapid withdrawal of corticosteroids. Intubation is indicated when the FVC is <15 mL/kg.

Myasthenic Crisis	Cholinergic Crisis
Respiratory arrest	Fasciculations
Respiratory-based deficits: cyanosis, poor cough dysphagia	**Gastrointestinal symptoms:** abdominal cramps, diarrhea, nausea, vomiting
Secretions cannot be swallowed	Excessive salivation and lacrimation
Normal pupil	Miosis
Improves with edrophonium	Worsen with edrophonium

Amyotrophic Lateral Sclerosis (ALS, Motor Neuron Disease)

ALS is the most common degenerative motor neuron disease of adulthood, affecting 2 per 100,000 per year with a two to one male-to-female ratio. It is recognized by the presence of upper (UMN; spasticity and pyramidal tract signs) and lower (LMN; cramps, fasciculations, progressive atrophy and weakness) motor signs as well as dysarthria, dysphagia, and dyspnea. Average disease duration is in the range of 3–4 years. Pseudobulbar palsy (emotional incontinence) is frequent in ALS. Important spared functions are the extraocular motility, bladder and bowel (intact nucleus of Onuf), and sensory system. Frontotemporal dementia may coexist.

Poor prognosis (median survival 2–2.5 years) is present in **older women with bulbar onset** with dysarthria and dysphagia, which occurs in 20%–30% of all cases. **Best prognosis** (survival >10 years in 10% of patients) is documented in **younger patients** and in those with **primary lateral sclerosis.**

Familial ALS (FALS) with an autosomal dominant inheritance occurs in 10% of all cases with a slightly earlier age of onset than sporadic cases. A toxic gain-of-function mutation may be found in the gene coding for the enzyme **superoxide dismutase 1 (SOD1)** on **chromosome 21.** FUS mutation is a novel form of FALS.

Differential diagnosis of ALS includes the following:
- **Spondylotic myelopathy**
- **Multifocal motor neuropathy** with or without anti-GM1 antibodies
- **Inclusion body myositis**
- Others: toxins (lead, **organophosphates**), drugs (**dapsone** used for dermatitis herpetiform and malabsorption enteropathy [onset in hands, asymmetric]), infections (syphilis, borreliosis, CJD), metabolic disorders (**porphyria,** hyperparathyroidism, diabetes), hexosaminidase A deficiency (adult onset GM_2 gangliosidosis or **Tay-Sachs disease**), and **polyglucosan body disease** (GSD IV [hypesthesia and dementia])

MRI of the spine is mandatory to exclude spondylotic myelopathy. NCV and F waves are usually normal in ALS, whereas **EMG** shows **generalized denervation** (fibrillations, positive sharp waves) and neurogenic motor unit potentials. **Muscle biopsy** is only considered in atypical cases when inclusion body myositis is suspected. **Bunina bodies** are the only specific neuronal inclusions.

The antiglutamatergic agent **riluzole** (50 mg bid) prolongs life by about 3 months. Liver enzyme monitoring is indicated. The supplement **creatine** (5 g/d) appears promising in SOD1 transgenic mice. **Palliative** care includes quinine sulfate, CBin vitamin E, and verapamil for fasciculations and cramps; amitriptyline for pseudobulbar affect; glycopyrrolate for drooling; percutaneous endoscopic gastrostomy (PEG) for dysphagia and weight loss; face mask for intermittent home ventilation or 24-hour mechanical ventilation via tracheostomy for dyspnea.

Atypical Motor Neuron Diseases (ALS Variants)

Disorders restricted to the upper motor neuron (UMN) must be differentiated from cervical spondylosis, human T-cell lymphotropic virus-1 (HTLV-1)-associated myelopathy, HSP, stiff person syndrome (SPS), MS, and adrenomyeloneuropathy.

- **Primary lateral sclerosis (PLS)** has a more benign course than ALS, although it may eventually transform ino, typical ALS. Corticospinal and corticobulbar involvement leads to gradually progressive spastic quadri- or paraparesis.
- **Hereditary spastic paraparesis (HSP)** may have AD (up to 70% of "pure" cases), AR, and X-linked modes of inheritance. The AD form expresses at an older age (after 35 years) and is slower in progressioge.
- **Lathyrism** refers to the selective UMN glutamatergic toxicity caused from the neurotoxin of *Lathyrus sativus,* chickpea, widely consumed in famine-stricken countries where this drought-resistant crop can be cultivated.

Disorders restricted to the lower motor neuron (LMN) include:

- **Progressive muscular atrophy (PMA),** which affects young males with slowly progressive **asymmetric focal weakness** of distal limbs. The mean duration ranges from 5 to 15 years. It can be confused with inclusion body myositis (IBM).
- **X-linked bulbospinal neuronopathy (Kennedy's disease)** affects only males with predominantly bulbar weakness (prominent **tongue and chin fascicula-tions**) but lesser progression to dysphagia and dysarthria. **Gynecomastia** occurs in up to 90% of cases. Other endocrinopathies are **testicular atrophy** and **dia-betes mellitus.** Sensory involvement may occur. **CAG repeat expansion** exists in the androgen receptor gene.
- **Multifocal motor neuropathy,** present in older males as **asymmetric focal weakness** of distal limbs, with relative preservation of muscle bulk. It results from peripheral motor fiber demyelination instead of motoneuronal cell bodies. EMG shows conduction block in various nerves. High titers of **anti-GM1 gangli-oside antibodies** are present. Half the patients respond to periodic high-dose IV Ig but not to prednisone.
- **Monomelic amyotrophy,** which is a male-predominant, slow-progressing, self-limited "benign focal SMA," often restricted to adjacent myotomes of one arm with limb wasting but relatively well-preserved strength. This disorder is apparently sporadic and more common in India and Japan.
- **Adult-onset spinal muscular atrophy (SMA type IV),** which is distinguished by a family history (70% AR as in the childhood-onset SMAs and 30% AD; dele-tions in the 5q chromosome are rare) and a slowly progressive and **symmetric limb-girdle weakness** of the legs. Survival is over 20 years.
- **Postpolio muscular atrophy,** which is a focal and asymmetric muscle weak-ness that progresses from the same regions previously affected by polio that had been stable for at least 10 years.

Other ALS variants include **brachial amyotrophic diplegia** (flail arm variant) and the **pseudopolyneuritic variant** (flail leg syndrome).

Hereditary Spastic Paraparesis (HSP)

HSP is a genetically heterogeneous *pure* progressive paraparesis (*uncomplicated HSP*) or associated with other deficits (*complicated HSP*). Degeneration of terminal long spinal axons are implicated.

UNCOMPLICATED HSP (PURE SPASTIC PARAPARESIS)

Autosomal dominant	**SPG4** 40%	2p	***SPG4/spastin*** disrupts microtubule function, essential for axonal morphology and transport
	SPG3A 10%	14q	***SPG3A/atlastin*** presumed to be a GTPase (guanosine triphosphate) similar to dynamins (vesicle trafficking)
	SPG31 8%	2p	***SPG31/REEP1*** disrupts mitochondrial function and axonal transport as a result
	SPG13	2q	***Heat shock protein 60 (Hsp60)*** nuclear-encoded mitochondrial chaperonin (Cpn60)

Less common HSP include SPG6 (15q), SPG8 (8q), SPG10 (12q), SPG12 (19q), and SPG19 (9q). HSP SPG5 (8q) and SPG16 (Xq11) are AR and X-linked, respectively.

SPG4/spastin is the single most common form of HSP, pathogenic by haploinsufficiency.

COMPLICATED HSP (ASSOCIATED WITH OTHER DEFICITS)

Autosomal dominant	SPG9	10q	**Motor neuropathy, cataracts,** and gastroesophageal reflux
	SPG17 >20 families	11q	**Amyotrophy of hand muscles** (Silver syndrome)
Autosomal recessive	**SPG7** ~30 families	16q	***SPG7/paraplegin*** (*mitochondrial protein*) may cause **axonal neuropathy, optic atrophy,** dysarthria, dysphagia, cerebellar atrophy; **ragged-red fibers** in muscle biopsy
	SPG11	15q	**Mental retardation,** dysarthria, neuropathy, **parkinsonism,** and **thin corpus callosum**
	SPG14	3q	**Mental retardation and distal motor neuropathy**
	SPG15	14q	**Pigmentary maculopathy,** dysarthria, distal amyotrophy, MR, and **thin corpus callosum**
	SPG20		**Troyer syndrome**
X-linked	SPG1 >100 families	Xq28	***L1 cell adhesion molecule (L1CAM)*** causes MASA syndrome (mental retardation, aphasia, shuffling gait, and adducted thumbs) with **hydrocephalus and hypoplastic callosum**
	SPG2 <100 families	Xq28	***Proteolipid protein (PLP;*** intrinsic myelin protein) causes quadriplegia, nystagmus, and seizures with **leukoencephalopathy**
	SPG16	Xq11	**Nonfluent aphasia,** poor vision, mild mental retardation, and bowel/bladder dysfunction

SPG7, SPG11, and SPG16 may show either pure or complicated HSP. *PLP1* mutations cause both Pelizaeus-Merzbacher disease (X-linked PMD) and progressive paraparesis (X-linked HSP). Nuclear-encoded mitochondrial protein abnormalities (paraplegin and Hsp60) resulting in HSP has expanded the phenotype of mitochondrial disorders. SPG, spastic gait locus.

Spinal Cord Pathologies per Compartment

Intradural Intramedullary Lesions

Characterized by apparent widening of the cord in two projections (90° apart):

- **Ependymoma** ⎱ (adults)   **Most common primary SC tumors**
- **Astrocytoma** ⎰ (children) Enhancement is *almost* a rule
- Hemangioblastoma
- AVM, cavernous malformations.
- Hematoma
- Syringomyelia, hydromyelia
- Cord edema
- Infarcts (diabetics having Ao surgery)
- Abscess (Myelitis)
- Demyelination (MS, ADEM)
- Lipoma, cysts

> **Foix-Alajouanine syndrome:** subacute venous hypertensive myelopathy due to impaired venous outflow as a result of an **intradural dural arteriovenous fistula** (AVF) at the lower thoracic and or lumbosacral levels. Patients are usually older than 50 years of age. Spinal angiography is the test of choice.

Intradural Extramedullary Lesions

Characterized by widening of the CSF gutter on the side of the lesion, displacement of the cord away from it, and "capping defect" in the contrast:

- **Meningioma**
- **Neurofibroma**
- **Schwannoma**
- Arachnoid cyst
- Metastases
- Hematoma
- Lipoma
- **TB Meningitis:** ↑protein CSF (T1)
- AVM, dural AV fistulas
- Congenital cysts

> **Tumors that seed:**
> 1. Glioblastoma
> 2. Medulloblastoma
> 3. Ependymoma
> 4. Epidermoid
> 5. Lymphoma
> 6. Cord plexus tumor

Extradural Lesions

Seen as thinning of the sac and its content in two projections (90° apart):

- Metastatic disease
- **Extramedullary hematopoiesis**
- Vertebral body expansion (hemangioma, Paget's [back pain, deafness])
- Vertebral compression
- Myeloma
- Lymphoma
- Disc herniation
- **Epidural hematoma**
- **Epidural abscess**
- **Lipoma**
- **Ligamentum flavum hypertrophy**
- Neurofibroma

> *Preserved disc space:* **Metastatic disease, fungal** infections, and **TB** (destructive vertebral bony lesions)
> *Disc space blurred:* **Bacterial abscess** (may affect bone)
> *Generalized T1 brightness:* **Fat (epidural lipomatosis)**

Bright T1 CSF signal

Atlantoaxial instability can be seen in Down syndrome (25%), rheumatoid arthritis, **Klippel-Feil anomaly** (**cervical congenital synostosis;** deafness, mirror movements, and syringomyelia or syringobulbia); **Morquio syndrome** (mucopolysaccharidosis type IV), and **achondroplasia** (most common inherited dwarfism, due to mutation of the fibroblast growth factor 3 gene; spontaneous mutatioins in two-thirds of cases). The latter causes foramen magnum narrowing with cervicomedullary compression, syringomyelia or diastematomyelia, spinal stenosis with spinal cord compression, macrocrania (with or without hydrocephalus), and psychomotor delay (most have normal intelligence).

Beevor's sign refers to the upward movement of the umbilicus when attempting to sit up from a supine position due to weakness of the lower part of the rectus abdominis muscle. The muscle at the level of the umbilicus, supplied by the T10 nerve roots, can be weakened after **lesions of the spinal cord or roots between T10 and T12.** Beevor's sign has a localizing value similar to the loss of lower abdominal cutaneous reflexes. It is also a common finding in myopathies, especially **fascioscapulo humeral dystrophy.**

Epidural abscess is most commonly due to *Staphylococcus aureus* and often associated with immunosuppression by diabetes, corticosteroids, chemotherapy, malignancy, or alcoholism. Lumbosacral abscesses (where there is an actual epidural space) are more common than cervical. Ab 70% are dorsal and may extend over several levels; anterior abscesses result from discitis or osteomyelitis and extend only over a few levels. Epidural abscesses present either acutely or chronically, in a four-stage course: (1) fever, malaise, backache, and focal vertebral pain; (2) radicular pain and "electrical" pain for 3–4 days; (3) spinal cord dysfunction in the next 4–5 days; and (4) para- or quadriplegia. **Acute presentations** are often the result of **hematogenous spread** of a pyogenic organism. **Chronic presentation** develops slowly with less systemic symptoms but rather from **contiguous spread** of organisms such as **fungi and TB.** Lumbar puncture is not recommended. CSF Gram stain and culture identify the organism in <25% of cases. T2W MRI sequences may be misleading as the **abscess is often isointense to CSF.** Management requires IV antibiotic therapy and decompression and drainage of the abscess through laminectomy.

Transverse myelitis is a presenting symptom in MS in about 20% of patients. If brain MRI is normal, there is only a 25% chance of CDMS after 10 years and those who develop MS may be less disabled.

Infectious Transverse Myelitis	Demyelinating Transverse Myelitis
Myelitis is complete and symmetric	Asymmetric with variable impairment
Enteroviruses (Echo, coxsackie, polio) herpes viruses[(HSV-1, HSV-2, VZV, EBV, CMV])	Oligoclonal bands are usually present (absent in 90% of infectious myelitis)
T2W MRI: "sausage-shaped" hyperintensity over several levels	T2W MRI: lesions are smaller and multifocal

Neurogenic Bladder

The micturition drives for voiding and continence are located in the pons:
- **Pontine micturition center** (PMC) from the medial dorsolateral pons
- **Pontine continence center** (PCC) from the lateral pons project to the sacral parasympathetic intermediate cell column and the sacral Onuf's nucleus, respectively.

PMC activation drives the voiding reflex:
- Sphincter relaxation is achieved by inhibition of dorsal gray commissure interneurons, which inhibit sphincter motor neurons in Onuf's nucleus.
- Detrusor contraction through projections from the sacral intermediolateral cell column to the postganglionic parasympathetic fibers

PCC activation drives the continence reflex through inhibition of the detrusor and contraction of the internal (hypogastric nerve: sympathetic) and external (pudendal nerve: somatic) urethral sphincter.

Cerebral control of micturition is localized in the anterior cingulate gyrus, the right dorsolateral prefrontal cortex, and the preoptic area of the hypothalamus. The latter projects to the PMC. Final micturition pathway requires an intact spinal reflex arc (afferent: pelvic splanchnic nerves from bladder wall to **Onuf's nucleus** [S1–S2]; efferent: pelvic splanchnic nerves to pelvic plexus and to **detrusor muscle**).

Detrusor Areflexia (Autonomous Bladder)	Detrusor Hyperreflexia (DH, Spastic Bladder)	Detrusor-Sphincter Dyssynergia (DSD)
Lesion is *below T12* at the conus medullaris-cauda equina levels	Lesion is located anywhere *between the cortex and S2–S4*	Lesion is *between S2–S4 and pontomesencephalic* micturition centers
Paralyzed bladder and low sensation of filling: **inability to initiate micturition,** overflow incontinence, and urinary retention. No bulbocavernous or anal reflex	Detrusor contracts during bladder filling: urinary **urgency, frequency,** with or without slight urge-related leaking. Causes: tumor, stroke, dementia, MS, MSA, PD, spinal cord injury	Detrusor and sphincter contract simultaneously: obstructed voiding, **interrupted urinary stream,** incomplete emptying with urinary retention. DH and DSD coexist in myelopathies
Failure to empty Bladder capacity: high Residual volume: high	Failure to store Bladder capacity: low Residual volume: high	Emptying is worse Bladder pressure: high Upper genitourinary tract dilatation
Treatment: muscarinic agonist: bethanechol [Urecholine], intermittent self-catheterization	**Drug: anticholinergics;** scheduled fluid intake and voiding, avoidance of coffee, alcohol, and aspartame	Antispasticity agents (baclofen, tizanidine), α-adrenergic blockers, and anticholinergics agents; intermittent catheterization

Pharmacology for Neurogenic Bladder

Detrusor hyperreflexia without outlet obstruction:
- **Anticholinergics** (oxybutynin [Ditropan], tolterodine [Detrol], favored because causes the least dry mouth; propantheline [Pro-Banthine], dicyclomine [Bentyl], imipramine [Tofranil]; darifenacin [Enablex] as a selective M_3 muscarinic antagonist causes least cognitive problems)
- **Capsaicin** instilled intravesically for relief of detrusor hyperreflexia is used in those who fail anticholinergics

Detrusor hyperreflexia with outlet obstruction:
- **α1-adrenergic blockers** decrease sphincter tone (tamsulosin [Flomax], prazosin [Minipress], terazosin [Hytrin], and phenoxybenzamine [Dibenzyline])
- **Muscle relaxants** decrease striated external sphincter tone (dantrolene [Dantrium], baclofen [Lioresal], tizanidine [Zanaflex], diazepam [Valium])

Intractable nocturia (enuresis)
- **DDAVP** (1-desamino, 8-[D] arginine vasopressin) taken intranasally at bedtime treats nighttime frequency and may improve blood pressure.

Conus medullaris lesions disrupt the bladder reflex arc, resulting in an areflexic bladder. **Compression fractures at T11-T12 and T12-L1** levels are common causes of conus medullaris syndrome (cord ends opposite L1-L2):
- **Early sphincter compromise: autonomous bladder**
- **Symmetric saddle anesthesia**
- **Pain is uncommon or late**
- **Upper motor neurons signs if lumbar segments are affected**

Cauda equina lesions do not initially disrupt the bladder reflex arc: bladder involvement is usually late. **Acute central disc herniation** or any compression of the lumbar and sacral roots below L3 is a common cause:
- **Early radicular pain** increased during **Valsalva** maneuver and **recumbency**
- **Late sphincter compromise**
- **Unilateral or asymmetric** sensory findings

Causative Spinal Cord Lesions

Intradural-Extramedullary	Extradural Lesions
Schwannoma, neurofibroma, meningioma, myxopapillary ependymoma (filum), lipomas	**Disc herniation,** metastatic tumor, extramedullary hematopoiesis
Intradural-intramedullary lesions	
Myxopapillary ependymoma (conus), astrocytomas (very rare)	

Myxopapillary ependymomas are the most common intra-axial tumors of the conus/filum regions in adults. They present as subarachnoid hemorrhage (vascular tumors) or as nocturnal pain during recumbency.

Axonal Polyneuropathies

These are chronic, symmetric, **length-dependent** neuropathies, which are common, respond to symptomatic treatment, and often remain idiopathic in up to 40% of patients. Tingling, loss of balance and gait ataxia result from involvement of large myelinated sensory fibers, whereas pain and hypersensitivity, with or without autonomic symptoms, result from poorly or unmyelinated sensory fibers.

The diagnosis of axonal neuropathy is made by demonstrating a symmetric and length dependent **reduction of amplitude** in sensory (sural compared to radial) or motor (peroneal and tibial compared to median and ulnar) CMAP with preservation of both sensory and motor conduction velocity.

Most acquired polyneuropathies occur with medical illnesses and are *axonal* in nature (e.g., hypothyroidism, vitamin B_{12} deficiency, HIV infection). Diabetic neuropathy is both axonal and demyelinating. Demonstration of *demyelinating* features on NCV narrows the differential in favor of CIDP, uremic neuropathy, and lymphoproliferative disorders except amyloidosis.

The initial evaluation of an axonal neuropathy should include fasting glucose, hemoglobin A_1C, comprehensive metabolic panel, thyroid stimulating hormone (TSH), free T4, antinuclear antibody (ANA), rheumatoid factor (RF), erythrocyte sedimentation rate (ESR), C-reactive protein (CRP), B_{12} level, serum and urine protein electrophoresis (SPEP, UPEP), both with immunofixation. If this evaluation is negative, other studies to consider are anti-MAG antibodies, anti-GM_1 antibodies, SS-a, SS-b, and anti-Hu antibodies.

Small-fiber axonal sensory polyneuropathy is typical of **diabetes mellitus** and otherwise idiopathic cases. Less common etiologies are **HIV and antiretroviral therapy,** hereditary and acquired **amyloidosis,** hereditary sensory neuropathy, Tangier's disease, Fabry disease, Sjögren's syndrome, and leprosy.

Large-fiber axonal sensory polyneuropathy is caused by B_{12} and vitamin E deficiencies. **Anti-MAG and anti-GD1b IgG** antibodies may produce a sensory-predominant, chronic-progressive, length-dependent axonal polyneuropathy. Hereditary causes include abetalipoproteinemia (Bassen-Kornzweig), ataxia-telangiectasia, and Friedreich ataxia.

Large- and small-fiber axonal sensory polyneuropathy can be iatrogenic (taxol, metronidazole, misonidazole, and phenytoin) or due to systemic disorders (diabetes, Sjögren's syndrome, cryoglobulinemia, paraproteinemia, antisulfatide antibodies, and paraneoplasia). **Motor axonal polyneuropathy** can be caused by antibodies to GM_1, GalNAc-GD_1a, and GM_2 ganglioside.

Tests to order: (1) **GM_1 antibodies** in MMN and GBS phenotypes — not sensory neuropathies; (2) **anti-MAG** in distal, large-fiber demyelinating sensory-predominant neuropathies; (3) **anti-Hu** in patients with large-fiber sensory loss and sensory ataxia **(paraneoplastic sensory ganglionopathy);** (4) **antisulfatide antibodies** in patients with sensory (small-fiber type) or sensorimotor axonal neuropathies.

Painful Peripheral Neuropathies (Neuropathic Pain)

The symptomatic range of painful neuropathies includes **paresthesia** (abnormal spontaneous sensations), **dysesthesia** (discomfort generated by contact), **hyperpathia** (exaggerated pain from a noxious stimulus), and **allodynia** (pain generated by contact to a normally innocuous stimulus).

Common etiologies are diabetes, alcoholism, uremia, and postherpetic and HIV infection. Most of these cause *painful small-fiber sensory neuropathies* (SFSN).

Less common but important etiologies are:
- **Amyloidosis and cryoglobulinemia**
- Drug-induced: **metronidazole,** nitrofurantoin, thalidomide, paclitaxel ([taxol], chemotherapy), suramin (antihelmintic for African trypanosomiasis and onchocerciasis)
- **Toxins: arsenic** and **thallium**

Infectious causes include:
- **Leprosy**
- **Lyme disease**
- **Guillain-Barré syndrome**
- **CIDP**
- **Sarcoidosis**

> **Enlargement of nerves** can be seen in chronic demyelinating disorders (HMSN I [CMT], HMSN III [Dejerine-Sottas], CIDP), amyloid neuropathy, leprosy, acromegaly, neurofibromatosis type 1, and schwannoma.

Metabolic causes include:
- **Porphyria**
- Vitamin B deficiencies (thiamine [B_1], pantothenic acid [B_5], pyridoxine [B_6], and cobalamin [B_{12}])
- **Sjögren syndrome** is actually a sensory *neuropathy* or inflammatory ganglionitis, resulting in widespread proprioceptive loss and leading to **sensory ataxia of the limbs and gait.** Dry eyes and mouth (keratoconjunctivitis sicca and xerostomia) develop later along with arthritis, lymphoma, or renal tubular defects. Most patients have antinuclear antibody anti-Ro (SS-A), anti-La (SS-B), or high IgM monoclonal immunoglobulins in serum.

Hereditary causes include:
- **Hereditary sensory and autonomic neuropathies (HSAN)**
- **Hereditary neuralgic amyotrophy (HNA)**
- **Fabry disease**
- **Tangier disease** (mutations in the human ATP-binding cassette 1 gene [ABC1], 9q31) causes retinitis pigmentosa, enlarged orange tonsils (accumulation of fat soluble vitamin E, retinyl esters, and carotenoids), hepatosplenomegaly (with thrombocytopenia), and two neuropathy types: a **pseudosyringomyelic syndrome** and a **relapsing mononeuritis multiplex.** There is low high-density lipoprotein (HDL) and plasma apolipoprotein A1 with normal or slightly elevated serum triglyceride levels.

Complex Regional Pain Syndrome (CRPS)

CRPS is a descriptive diagnosis applicable to patients complaining of **pain after a noxious event** in a limb and also exhibiting sensory, motor, or circulatory manifestations. Depending on the presence or absence of nerve involvement, CRPS has been classified into two types:

- **CRPS type 1** (formerly **"reflex sympathetic dystrophy"**) develops after a noxious event that leads to disproportionate and widespread pain, allodynia, or hyperalgesia despite the *absence* of overt neuropathy.
- **CRPS type 2** (formerly **"causalgia"**) develops *after a nerve injury* but the ensuing pain may not be limited to the territory of the injured nerve. Edema, "changes in skin blood flow abnormality," or "abnormal sudomotor activity" in the region of pain must have been present at some point after the injury.

> Besides intermittent cold and warm feeling, other proposed "relative criteria" for CRPS type I are increased nail or hair growth, hyperhydrosis, abnormal skin color, hypesthesia, and patchy demineralization of bone.

In a minority of patients, neuropathic pain is the result of sensitization of peripheral nociceptors, ectopic or ephaptic transmission of nerve impulses, or central disinhibition of nociceptive input. Contribution of the sympathetic system as the cause of pain is controversial and unsupported by autonomic testing and studies applying placebo-controlled protocols for diagnostic sympathetic blocks.

There is growing recognition that CRPS type 1 may have a psychogenic origin. In particular, their commonly associated abnormal movements (spasms, fixed dystonic posturing, tremor, and various other jerks) have met criteria for "clinically definite" psychogenic disorders (inconsistent signs, multiple somatizations, persistent relief with psychotherapy, suggestion or placebo, and absence of the movement disorder when "unobserved"). Associated pseudoneurological signs such as give-way weakness and nondermatomal hypesthesia are common.

Studies of patients with "the syndrome of fixed dystonia" (Schrag et al., 2004) have shown that this manifestation does indeed meet the criteria for psychogenic dystonia. A considerable overlap with CRPS has been suggested by virtue of occurring or exacerbating after a minor peripheral trauma ("posttraumatic painful torticollis," for instance, has been proposed to replace the less descriptive and potentially misleading "posttraumatic dystonia"). The term causalgia-dystonia syndrome has been discouraged as the evidence is pointing toward central rather than peripheral neural dysfunction in these patients.

Although CRPS patients respond unfavorably to conventional pain medications and sympathetic blocks, multidisciplinary interventions, including physiotherapy and psychotherapy, have been shown to produce considerable improvement.

Neurogenic Orthostatic Hypotension

Orthostatic hypotension (OH) may be central or due to peripheral neuropathy (diabetes or autoimmune disease). **The consensus definition requires a reduction of** systolic blood pressure **(SBP)** $\geq$**20 mm Hg** or diastolic blood pressure (DBP) $\geq$10 mm Hg, within 3 minutes of standing up. These cutoffs lead to a **5% false-positive rate.** Symptoms can range from tiredness or difficulty concentrating to syncope, mainly in conditions of orthostatic stress, such as postprandial (due to splanchnic-mesenteric bed vasodilation), during warm temperatures, after alcohol ingestion, or after exertion. **Early morning OH severity often relates to nocturnal diuresis.** Palpitations, tremulousness, anxiety, and nausea are symptoms of **autonomic hyperactivity in young patients with OH due to partial neuropathic autonomic failure.**

Arterial (pressure-sensitive) and venous (volume-sensitive) baroreceptors are responsible for BP control. When BP falls, the ***vagal baroreflex pathway*** via carotid sinus (glossopharingeal) and aortic arch (vagus nerve) baroreceptors send afferent information to the **nucleus of the tractus solitarius,** which relays it to the **nucleus ambiguous,** and then as the **vagus** to the **sinoatrial node.** The ***sympathetic baroreflex pathway*** acts via the **rostral ventrolateral medulla** to the intermediolateral thoracic column and from there to the autonomic ganglia, heart, arterioles, and venules. **Baroreflex failure due to impairment of sympathetic efferents results in the triad of OH, supine hypertension, and higher nocturnal BP.** Myelopathy-related OH is caused by intermediolateral column lesion (T4-T9, which synapses at the celiac ganglion), leading to impaired splanchnic outflow. Hypovolemia or anemia may cause OH even with normal vascular reflexes. Relative hypovolemia occurs in denervation due to decreased vascular tone and increased vascular capacity. **Cerebral autoregulation** permits stable cerebral perfusion within a mean arterial blood pressure (MAP) range of about 50–150 mm Hz.

Management of orthostatic hypotension includes: (1) volume expansion (fluid intake of 1.25–2.50 L/d); (2) salt supplementation (0.5–1.0 g salt tablets; avoid urinary sodium concentration <170 mmol); (3) head-of-bed elevation by 10 cm (reduces nocturia and effects of supine hypertension); and (4) use of thigh-high compressive stockings (reduce venous capacitance). **Midodrine** (ProAmatine, peripheral $\propto$1-adrenergic receptor agonist, 5–10 mg tid) is the only FDA-approved OH drug. Besides supine hypertension, it may cause piloerection, scalp pruritus, and urinary retention. **Pyridostigmine** (Mestinon, 60 mg tid) improves ganglionic transmission primarily when standing, thereby preventing worsening supine hypertension. **Fludrocortisone** (Florinef, 0.1–0.3 mg/d) expands plasma volume by decreasing natriuresis but may cause supine hypertension and hypokalemia. Other potential pharmacologic approaches include **Droxidopa** (repletor of postganglionic adrenergic axons; especially effective in OH caused by deficiency of dopamine-β-hydroxylase), yohimbine, indomethacin, somatostatin, and dihydroergotamine. Supine hypertension can be controlled by keeping the last dose of midodrine no later than 6:00 PM, elevating the head of the bed, using transdermal nitroglycerine, or drinking a glass of wine (mild vasodilator).

Autosomal Dominant Recurrent Hereditary Neuropathies (HNPP, HNA)

These neuropathies are among the most common inherited diseases (prevalence: 1 in 2,500).

Hereditary neuropathy with liability to pressure palsies (HNPP) begins in the second decade, resulting from a 1.5 Mb gene *deletion* in the **peripheral myelin protein 22 (PMP22)** gene (**17p**11). The dosage-sensitive PMP22 leads to CMT1A when the gene copy number is *duplicated*.

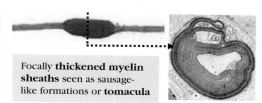

PMP22 is a transmembrane glycoprotein of Schwann cells, restricted to *compact* myelin. It is activated in myelination and postinjury remyelination.

Focally **thickened myelin sheaths** seen as sausage-like formations or **tomacula**

Clinical features of HNPP include:
- **Recurrent painless focal** neuropathies at **entrapment sites** for the *median* (CTS) and *peroneal* nerves (fibular head); less common in the ulnar and tibial
- **Brachial plexus palsies are rare** but are also typically painless
- **Minor trauma** or compression to peripheral nerves precede single neuropathic episodes, which improve within days, weeks, or months
- **Mild pes cavus and hypo- or areflexia**
- **Multifocal conduction blocks and mild slowing** across entrapment sites
- Some have progressive generalized neuropathy indistinguishable from CMT1. The clinical presentation of HNPP overlaps with that of multifocal motor neuropathy (MMN), CIDP, and HNA.

Hereditary neuralgic amyotrophy (HNA) also beginning in the second or third decade of life has been linked to chromosome **17q**25 but no gene is known yet.

Clinical features of HNA include:
- **Recurrent shoulder pain** accompanied by weakness and atrophy
- **Brachial plexus palsies are common** and are typically **painful**
- **Lumbosacral plexus involvement is rare**
- **Normal or slightly reduced NCV** +/− axonal interruption in brachial plexus
- **Minor facial dysmorphic features: hypotelorism, epicanthal folds,** short stature, and cleft palate may help in separating HNA from the sporadic idiopathic neuralgic amyotrophy (*Parsonage-Turner syndrome*)
- Bacterial or viral infections, immunization, and parturition are usual triggers

Uniform CV Slowing: No Temporal Dispersion or Conduction Block	Multifocal CV Slowing: Temporal Dispersion and Conduction Block
HMSN type I, II, and II	Refsum disease (HMSN type IV)
Metachromatic leukodystrophy	Adrenomyeloneuropathy
Krabbe disease	Pelizaeus-Merzbacher disease
Cockayne's disease	HNPP

Progressive Hereditary Motor and Sensory Neuropathies (HMSN)

AD: I, II; AR: IV, *de novo* mutations in PMP22, MPZ, EGR2: III

HMSN are a group of familial chronic symmetric distal motor and sensory polyneuropathies associated with areflexia and pes cavus or planus. **Calf hypertrophy** is a feature of HMSN I and **neuromyotonia** of HMSN II.

HMSN I–DEMYELINATING (CHARCOT-MARIE-TOOTH DISEASE [CMT1])

PMP22	CMT**1A** 50% of HMSN cases	17p11.2	70% AD CMT1; 80% sporadic CMT1
MPZ	CMT**1B**	1q22	AD
EGR2	CMT**1D**	10q21	AD and AR inheritance
Cx32	CMT**1X** 15% of HMSN cases	Xq13	X-linked dominant or recessive

MPZ, myelin protein zero (formation and compaction of myelin); **EGR2,** early growth response (myelin sheath formation and maintenance). MPZ and EGR2 may lead to congenital hypomyelination neuropathy. **Cx32,** connexin 32 gap junction protein of myelinating Schwann cells (may cause early hand involvement). CMT1 from PMP22 mutation rather than duplication may cause profound deafness of onset in adolescence.

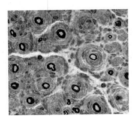

In CMT there are prolonged latencies and *slow conduction velocities* without the conduction block or temporal dispersion seen in CIDP.

Segmental demyelination and remyelination lead to clinically **thickened nerves** and **onion bulb formation** on biopsy.

HMSN II–axonal (CMT2) are autosomal dominant disorders associated with axonal loss of large myelinated motor and sensory fibers, causing *mildly slowed NCV but large amplitude drop.* They are linked to chromosomes 1p (CMT2A, **KIF1B** [kinesin family] and **MFN2** [mitochondrial] genes; third most common CMT), 3q (CMT2B, **RAB7** gene), 12q (CMT2C, with vocal cord paresis), 7p (CMT2D, with hand wasting), 8p (CMT2E, **NFL** [neurofilament light chain] gene), 7q (CMT2F), and proximal CMT2 in 3q (CMT2G or HMSN P). CMT2 patients are older, less disabled, and have less sensory loss and no palpable nerves.

HMSN III (Dejerine-Sottas syndrome, DSS) is a severe form of HMSN I, as it is caused by **point mutations** in the same genes **(PMP22, MPZ,** and **EGR2),** and leads to profound bulb onion–forming hypodemyelinating neuropathy of **early onset** (age <2 years) that causes severe muscle weakness, **sensory ataxia,** and **scoliosis. CV is very slow** (<12 m/sec).

HMSN IV is an AR demyelinating CMT of early onset whose genes are on 8q (CMT4A, **GDAP1** [ganglioside-induced differentiation protein]), 11q (CMT4B, **MTMR2** [myotubularin protein 2], 8q24 (CMT4D, **NDRG1** [N-myc downstream-regulated gene 1]), 10q (CMT4E, **EGR2**), and 19q (CMT4F, **PRX** [periaxin]).

HMSN V is characterized by CMT plus pyramidal involvement ranging from hyperreflexia to overt spastic paraplegia. It may be caused by mutations in MFN2 and BSCL2 (associated with several phenotypes: CMT2, dHMN, Silver syndrome [spastic paraplegia with hand amyotrophy], and pure spastic paraplegia).

Roussy-Lévy Syndrome: Part of HMSN1/CMT1 Phenotypic Expression

Roussy-Lévy syndrome was first described in 1926 as a familial autosomal dominant disease thag begins in early childhood ang comprises **pes cavus, areflexia, distal limb weakness, distal sensory loss, gait ataxia,** and **upper limb postural tremor.** The last two features (ataxia and tremor) were initially felt to distinguish it from the already well-characterized entity of Charcot-Marie-Tooth. The condition was subsequently speculated to represent a *forme fruste* of Friedreich ataxia and peroneal muscular dystrophy. The tremor has been proposed to be the result of a distorted and mistimed peripheral input, reaching and altering the output of a central processor, probably the cerebellum.

Roussy-Lévy syndrome is not believed to be a distinct entity but a phenotypic expression of the genetically heterogeneous disorder HMSN I (Charcot-Marie-Tooth type 1), resulting from a 1.5-Mb tandem duplication of chromosome 17p11.2. Of note, some members of the original family reported by Roussy and Lévy were found to have pathology of typical demyelination and onion bulb formation and underwent molecular analysis in 1999, which disclosed the presence of a heterozygous missense mutation in the extracellular domain of the myelin protein zero (MPZ), allowing the categorization of this family as CMT1B.

Refsum's Disease (also Known as HMSN IV)

Beginning in late childhood or adolescence (or as late as the fifth decade), the disease follows a progressive course with a demyelinating neuropathy, **pes cavus, cerebellar ataxia, sensorineural deafness,** and **cranial neuropathy.** Nyctalopia and visual failure secondary to **retinitis pigmentosa** often precede the neurological symptoms. Scaly thickening of the skin **(ichthyosis)** and the presence of **syndactyly** and a characteristic **short fourth toe** are further diagnostic clues. Dysautonomia and cardiac conduction abnormalities or **cardiomyopathy** may result in premature death.

This disorder of lipid metabolism results from the accumulation of branched-chain fatty acid **phytanic acid** due to its deficient alpha-oxidation by **phytanoyl-coenzyme A hydroxylase** (10p, *PAHX* gene) into pristanic acid. Phytanic acid is widely present in diary products, meat, and fish. The mechanism of toxicity from phytanic acid accumulation may be due to the impairment of myelin function or metabolism of fat-soluble vitamins. Since phytanic acid is almost exclusively of exogenous origin, dietary restriction reduces plasma and tissue levels. The neurological, cardiac, and dermatological problems may be reversed by phytanic acid level reduction, but the visual and hearing impairments are less responsive. Rapid weight loss, fever, and pregnancy, which mobilizes fat stores of phytanic acid, have been associated with acute presentations mimicking Guillain-Barré syndrome. Plasma exchange has been used to produce rapid clinic improvement. Dialysis is ineffective.

Paraproteinemic Neuropathies

A monoclonal protein (monoclonal gammopathy or **M protein**) is found in about 5% of all patients with polyneuropathy and nearly **10% of all patients with idiopathic polyneuropathies.** Monoclonal proteins represent intact antibodies produced by a single clone of plasma cells and are detected through serum protein electrophoresis **(SPEP), immunoelectrophoresis,** or **immunofixation electrophoresis.** The latter is the preferred method and should be tested on both urine and serum since at least **20% of multiple myeloma** patients develop only urine monoclonal protein. They are seen normally in 1% of normal people, 3% of persons over the age of 70, and in up to 20% of octogenarians.

Disorder	Paraprotein	Neuropathy	Treatment
Multiple myeloma	**IgM-κ or IgGκ** (>3 g/dl)	**Axonal** sensory or sensorimotor	None
Waldenström's macroglobulinemia	**IgM-κ**	**Demyelinating –** sensorimotor, may simulate CIDP	Plasma exchange Prednisone, melphalan Chlorambucil
Osteosclerotic myeloma	**IgG-λ or IgA-λ**	**Demyelinating** with axonal degeneration, simulates CIDP	Resection, radiation therapy, prednisone, melphalan
Amyloidosis	**IgG-λ or IgA-λ**	**Painful axonal**	Melphalan-prednisone, autologous stem cell transplantation
Cryo-globulinemia	**IgM or IgG**	**Painful axonal**	Plasma exchange Prednisone, interferon α, cyclophosphamide
Lymphoma (Castleman's disease)	**IgM or IgG**	**Axonal** sensory or motor (motor neuron disease)— simulates CIDP or GBS	Plasma exchange Prednisone Chemotherapy for lymphoma

There are three main glycoconjugate antigens on peripheral nerves implicated in the paraproteinemic neuropathies:

- **Myelin-associated glycoprotein (MAG),** concentrated in periaxonal Schwann-cell membranes, serves as adhesion molecule for interaction between the Schwann cells and the axons. **Anti-MAG antibodies** deposit between densely packed layers of myelin, creating wide spacing between myelin lamellae and resulting in neuropathy.
- **Sulfated glycosphingolipids (SGPG and sulfatide)**
- **Gangliosides** are complex glycosphingolipids with a sialic acid group bound to an oligosaccharide situated in the membranes of neurons.
  - **Pure motor** neuropathy is associated with antibodies against **GM1,** which is located predominantly on motor nerves
  - **Sensory** neuropathy is associated with antibodies against **GD1b,** which is located predominantly on sensory nerves

Monoclonal gammopathy of unknown significance (MGUS), comprising 60% of all paraproteinemias, is diagnosed when monoclonal M protein are present at <3 g/dL, fewer than 5% of plasma cells exist in the bone marrow, proteinuria is absent, and there are no systemic signs. About 5% of patients with peripheral neuropathy have MGUS. Conversely, about one-third of patients with MGUS have peripheral neuropathy. About 20% of patients with MGUS will eventually develop a lymphoproliferative disorder, usually malignant myeloma. MGUS-associated neuropathy contains **IgM** in 60%, **IgG** in 30%, and **IgA** in 10% **with** kappa **light chain,** unlike patients with osteosclerotic myeloma and amyloidosis.

IgM-MGUS neuropathy, associated with MAG antibodies in over 50% of cases, is seen in older patients with a **painless,** slowly progressive, large-fiber neuropathy (**loss of joint and position sense** with **ataxia** and **tremor**) with **distal weakness, elevated CSF protein,** and **demyelinating** features on conduction velocity studies. **Tremor and ataxia** are more common in **IgM-MGUS** neuropathies. **Anti-MAG antibodies** play a causative role in **IgM-MGUS and Waldenström's macroglobulinemia (WM).**

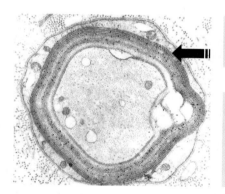

Widening of the outermost myelin lamellae is typical in IgM-MGUS and Waldenström's macroglobulinemia

About 70% of patients with demyelinating polyneuropathy and IgM monoclonal gammopathy have detectable serum anti-MAG antibodies by enzyme-linked immunosorbent assay (ELISA) (only 50% are detected by Western blot).

The distinction of anti-MAG neuropathy from chronic inflammatory demyelinating polyneuropathy (CIDP) may be difficult because:
- About 20% of patients with CIDP also have paraproteinemia
- Both neuropathies respond to immunosuppressants
- Both conditions show an increase in cerebrospinal fluid protein

Electrophysiologic studies are useful since focal conduction block in motor nerves may be seen in CIDP, whereas conduction slowing without block is seen in severely affected distal sensory nerves in anti-MAG associated neuropathies.

Plasma exchange is the only treatment proven beneficial in a prospective, randomized, double-blind study. The benefit was demonstrated only for MGUS patients with IgG- or IgA-associated neuropathies, but not for IgM-associated neuropathies, irrespective of anti-MAG status. IgM-MGUS neuropathy may improve with a combination of fludarabine, cyclophosphamide, and prednisone.

Multiple Myeloma (MM)

MM is the most common hematologic malignancy diagnosed in patients with a monoclonal protein, although neuropathy is prominent in o in 10% of patients, commonly preceding the diagnosis. It begins in the fifth to seventh decades of life with **bone pain, fatigue, anemia, hypercalcemia,** and renal insufficiency. **Spinal cord and nerve root compression,** due to **lytic bone lesions,** are the usual neurologic manifestations of MM, whereas **peripheral neuropathy** is rather uncommon. The paraprotein is **IgM** or **IgG,** with kppaк **light chain.** This light kappa chain deposition may cause amyloidosis **(AL amyloidosis),** which is presumed to cause the neuropathy in up to 40% of MM patients and is rarely improved by the treatment of the myeloma. The diagnosis requires that bone marrow aspirate or biopsy show **more than 10% atypical plasma cells.** Removal of the paraprotein by plasma exchange provides no benefit for the neuropathy.

Waldenström's Macroglobulinemia (WM)

WM is a lymphoproliferative disorder presenting with fatigue, weight loss, bleeding, and symptoms related to the **hyperviscosity syndrome** (epistaxis, headache, vertigo, and blurred vision). **Peripheral neuropathy** (often, mixed sensorimotor polyneuropathy) is present in about 10% of patients with WM, causing anesthetic foot drop and steppage gait. The paraprotein is **IgM-κ** as in IgM-MGUS, from which WM may arise. **MAG antibodies** are present in most.

Osteosclerotic Myeloma (OM)

This represents oly 3%–5% of myelomas, and neuropathy may occur in up to 85% of OM cases. The systemic features form the **POEMS syndrome** (polyneuropathy, organomegaly, endocrinopathy, M-protein, and skin changes). Excessive production of **vascular endothelial growth factor** (VEGF) causes the angiomata and organomegaly. **Bronze lesions and papilledema** are clinical clues. **IgG-λ** or **IgA-λ** causes the demyelinating neuropathy. CSF protein is usually elevated (>100 mg/dldL). Skeletal surveys show sclerotic instead of lytic lesions. Local radiation therapy to sclerotic lesions improves the neuropathy. As in myeloma, plasma exchange is ineffective. Autologous peripheral blood stem cell transplantation has shown promise.

Cryoglobulinemia

Cryoglobulins are immunoglobulins (usually IgG and IgM) that **precipitate when cooled** and separate when rewarmed. Cryoglobulins may be monoclonal (type I) a mixture of monoclonal and polyclonal immunoglobulins (type II, *mixed essential cryoglobulinemia*), or strictly polyclonal (type III). Type II is never associated with lymphoproliferative disorders, chronic infections, or autoimmune disorders, and type III is most commonly caused by **hepatitis C.** Peripheral neuropathy occurs in up to 60% of patients and presents with **painful multiple mononeuropathies** or, more commonly, **painful distal symmetric sensorimotor polyneuropathy.** Weakness, therefore, can be generalized or multifocal, and paresthesias may be triggered by cold (as with the commonly associated Raynaud's syndrome). **Interferon-α,** with or without **ribavirin,** is used when hepatitis C is the etiology.

Amyloid Neuropathies (AP)

AP are severe familial or acquired polyneuropathies of small fiber type associated with amyloid deposits (**green birefringent** beta-pleated protein sheets stained with **congo red**) in the endoneurium. In the familial form (FAP), such deposits are of **transthyretin (TTR)** secondary to a point mutation in the *TTR* gene. **Portugal** is the main endemic area of TTR-FAP. **Gelsolin-FAP** is the second familial variant and presents with cranial and sensory polyneuropathy in Finnish patients. **Acquired amyloid neuropathy** is caused by the accumulation of monoclonal immunoglobulins light chains (**IgG-λ** or **IgM-λ**) as amyloid fibrils (**AL amyloidosis**) in autonomic and peripheral sensory nerves, kidney, and heart. **Malignant lymphoproliferative disorders** such as multiple myeloma or Waldenström's macroglobulinemia are present in 40% of cases.

	Familial Amyloidotic Polyneuropathy (FAP)		Acquired Amyloid Neuropathy
Amyloidogenic protein	Transthyretin (**TTR**, Val30Met)	Gelsolin (Asp187Tyr)	Fragment of Ig light chain (**AL**)
Neuropathy	Distal symmetrical sensorimotor Dysautonomia	**Cranial** sensory	Sensorimotor Dysautonomia
Other manifestations	Cardiomyopathy Vitreous opacities ↑ Intraocular pressure Weight loss	Corneal dystrophy	Nephrotic syndrome Congestive heart Cardioembolic stroke Weight loss
Diagnosis	**TTR mutation:** chromosome 18, second exon Val-Met is most common	Gelsolin mutation	Serum/urine immuno-electrophoresis: M protein in 40% ↓ Gammaglobulinemia
Location (number of families)	**Portugal** (500) Sweden, Japan, France	**Finland** (400) Japan, USA (20 cases)	Ubiquitous (incidence is 0.9 per 100,000 person-years)
Family history	95% Portugal, AD	100%	0
Mean survival	10 years	Not affected	3 years

Amyloid deposits are confirmed in bone marrow aspirates, abdominal fat aspirate, rectal biopsy, or nerve biopsy.

Features Suggestive of Amyloid Neuropathy

- Progressive distal symmetrical, **often painful, axonal** sensory polyneuropathy with greater **pain and thermal sensory loss**
- **Steppage gait** and **Charcot's joints** may eventually appear
- **Autonomic dysfunction** with gastroparesis, constipation, orthostatic hypotension, impotence, urinary incontinence, and Adie tonic pupils

Other manifestations may include neuritis multiplex, cranial neuropathy, and **bilateral carpal tunnel syndrome. Orthotopic liver transplantation** slows progression of the neuropathy. **Autologous stem cell transplantation** may be useful in patients with autonomic neuropathy due to AL amyloidosis. Prednisone with melphalan prolongs survival without improving the neuropathy.

Peripheral Nerve Tumors

Schwannoma

Also called Schwann cell tumor or neurilemmoma, schwannomas are slow growing tumors that develop intracranially or along peripheral nerves, both within and outside the spinal canal. Vestibular or acoustic neuromas arise from the vestibular portion of CN VIII near or in the internal auditory canal, where Schwann cells replace oligodendroglia as myelin producers. **Bilateral acoustic neuromas are virtually pathognomonic for NF-2** (loss of tumor suppressor gene on chromosome 22q). These tumors respond to surgery or radiosurgery and have excellent prognosis. From the neuropathologic standpoint, schwannomas can be divided into the following types:

Antoni A (densely cellular)	Antoni B (hypocellular)
Nuclear palisading (Verocay bodies)	**Looser stroma,** fewer cells, **myxoid change**

Differentiating **CP masses**	
Meningioma	**Schwannoma**
EMA positive	S-100 protein
Yes – Desmosomes – No	
No – Basal lamina – Yes	
No – Luse bodies – Yes	

- Perineurium is immunopositive for EMA
- Schwann cells are immunopositive for S-100 protein
- Axons are immunopositive for neurofilament proteins (NFP)

Widely distributed in PNS and central nervous system (CNS), the **S-100 protein** may play a role in ionic regulation and is expressed in astrocytes, oligodendrocytes, Schwann cells, adenohypophysis, and adrenal medulla. Neurofibromas and schwannomas express S-100 diffusely, and 50% to 70% of malignant peripheral nerve sheath tumors express S-100 focally.

Neurofibroma

Occurring as a solitary sporadic tumor or associated with neurofibromatosis (especially type 1), neurofibroma is composed of Schwann cells, fibroblasts, and perineurial cells. **Plexiform neurofibroma is pathognomonic for NF1** and a potential precursor of malignant peripheral nerve sheath tumor.

Malignant Peripheral Nerve Sheath Tumor

Previously known as malignant schwannoma, it may arise more commonly de *novo* from Schwann cells. It shows anaplastic features in the form of high cellularity, pleomorphism, and high mitotic rate and necrosis. Cranial nerves, especially the fifth, are often affected.

Muscular Dystrophies: X-Linked Dystrophinopathies

Duchenne muscular dystrophy (DMD) is the most common X-linked recessive lethal disease (Xp21, dystrophin, 1 per 3,500 male live births), beginning at ages 3–5 years, with patients becoming wheelchair dependent by 12, and dying of respiratory insufficiency by age 20. Distinctive features are **calf hypertrophy,** contractures in heel cords (walking on toes), early involvement of proximal muscles and neck flexors, scoliosis with **exaggerated lumbar lordosis,** cardiomyopathy, intellectual impairment, intestinal pseudo-obstruction with acute gastric dilatation, and markedly elevated CK (>20 times normal). Muscle biopsy shows fiber size variability, fiber necrosis, and connective tissue proliferation with **fat infiltration.** Immunohistochemical analysis shows **absent dystrophin.** The deficiency of dystrophin disrupts the **dystrophin-glycoprotein complex** (DGC, membrane-associated proteins that span the muscle sarcolemma and provide linkage and stability between the intracellular cytoskeleton and the extracellular matrix) and leads to fiber necrosis through calcium leak. Treatment of DMD is supportive. The corticosteroids **prednisone** and **deflazacort** increase strength and improve pulmonary function. Prednisone **prolongs ambulation by 3–4 years.** Deflazacort has equal efficacy with better preservation of bone density and less weight gain but is unavailable in the United States. Genetic experimental therapies are undergoing investigation.

Becker muscular dystrophy (BMD) is similar to Duchenne dystrophy but with milder severity and slower progression: they **ambulate beyond age 15.** Most patients survive into the fourth or fifth decade.

Emery-Dreifuss syndrome (EDMD) presents with **joint contractures of elbows and ankles,** followed by a **humeroperoneal** pattern of weakness, with preferential **biceps, triceps, and facial weakness,** and atrial arrhythmias and **cardiac conduction abnormalities. Cardiomyopathy** is a late development. Patients are able to ambulate into the third decade. Reflexes are reduced or absent early in the disease. CK ranges from normal to moderately elevated. EDMD results from mutations in either of two different nuclear membrane proteins: **Emerin** (Xq28, X-linked EDMD1) and **Lamin A/C** (1q11, autosomal dominant EDMD2, also considered LGMD 1B, see below). Lamin A/C EDMD2 is less commonly associated with contractures. Treatment relies on **early pacemaker insertion. Female carriers** do not develop muscle weakness or wasting but are **at risk for cardiac complications.** Biopsy shows nonspecific myopathic or dystrophic features with angular atrophic fibers, **type I fiber atrophy,** and **absent emerin immunostaining.**

Biceps atrophy is predominant in EDMD, FSHD, and some LGMD. **Elbow contractures** are early and obvious in EDMD, LGMD types 1B, 1G, 2A, 2C-F, Bethlem myopathy, and many congenital dystrophies, especially the desmin-related or myofibrillar myopathies (though contractures in these are predominant in the ankles).

Limb-Girdle Muscular Dystrophies (LGMDs)

LGMDs are, with fascioscapulo humeral dystrophy (FSHD), the most common forms of adult muscular dystrophy. They are face sparing, progressive proximal muscle dystrophies, which may occur beyond a limb-girdle distribution or in **distal muscles (dysferlinopathy LGMD2B, allelic to Miyoshi myopathy).** Calf hypertrophy and higher CK are more common in LGMD2. Calpainopathies and Fukutin-related protein gene mutations are most prevalent.

Autosomal Dominant (LGMD1) 10%			Autosomal Recessive (LGMD2) 90%		
LGMD1A	5q	Myotilin dysarthria	LGMD2A	15q	**Calpain**-3
LGMD1B	1q	**Lamin A/C** contractures	LGMD2B	2p	**Dysferlin**
LGMD1C	3p	**Caveolin-3** rippling	LGMD2C	13q	γ-Sarcoglycan
LGMD1D	6q	Unknown cardiomyopathy	LGMD2D	17q	α-Sarcoglycan
LGMD1E	7q	Unknown	LGMD2E	4q	β-Sarcoglycan
LGMD1F	7q	Unknown	LGMD2F	5q	δ-Sarcoglycan
Phenotypic variation in genes causing LGMD			LGMD2G	17q	Telethonin
Caveolinopathies: LGMD1C, rippling muscle			LGMD2H	9q	TRIM32
disease, hyperCKemia, distal myopathy			LGMD2I	19q	**FKRP**
Dysferlinopathies: LGMD2B, Miyoshi			LGMD2J	2q	Titin
Laminopathies: skeletal (LGMD1B, EDMD), dilated			LGMD2K		POMT1
cardiomyopathy with -V block, familial partial					
lipodystrophy, axonal neuropathy (CMT 2A)					

Currently available commercial LGMD antibodies are calpain-3, caveolin-3, dysferlin, lamin A/C, myotilin, and sarcoglycan (α,β, δ, and γ). **Cardiac involvement** is a feature of LGMD 1B (lamin A/C), LGMD 1D, LGMD 2I, and γ-sarcoglycanopathy. **FKRP**, fukutin-related protein. Mild inflammation may occur in dysferlinopathies.

Calpain is a calcium-activated neutral protease, rather than part of the DGC. Its mutation in LGMD2A is the first genetic defect in muscular dystrophy, causing enzymatic dysfunction. It causes predominant **atrophy of the posterior thigh muscles.** Disorders that can cause **secondary calpain-3 reduction** include dysferlinopathies (LGMD2B), DMD, FSHD, and titinopathy. Calpain-3 deficiency must, therefore, be confirmed by mutational analysis.

Lamins are the principal component of the nuclear lamina, forming the major structural network of the **nuclear envelope.** Mutation of lamin A/C in LGMD1B may cause contractures of the elbow or Achilles tendons and dysrhythmias or AV conduction disturbances, as in the autosomal dominant form of EDMD, where the weakness follows a humer-peroneal distribution. **Other "nuclear envelope diseases" are CMT2A and DYT1 dystonia.**

LGMD2C-2F muscular dystrophies are **sarcoglycanopathies** that resemble DMD but with autosomal recessive inheritance and muscles exhibiting normal amounts of dystrophin but deficient in one of the four sarcoglycans (SG). **Fukutin-related protein (FKRP)** shows temporal variability in onset with infants presenting as congenital muscular dystroph) or adults as LGMD2I. Cardiac and respiratory dysfunctions are distinctive.

Congenital Muscular Dystrophies (CMD)

These autosomal recessive disorders of neonates and infants associated with **deficiency in α-dystroglycan (α-DG) and glycosylation.** Symptoms include hypotonia, weakness, and variable appearance of contractures. Muscle biopsies show dystrophic changes and reduced α-DG and merosin staining.

Type of CMD	CMD Type	Gene	Gene Product
Laminin α2 chain deficiency	MDC1A 6q	LAMA2	Laminin α2 (*merosin*)
Secondary merosin deficiency	MDC1B 1q	Unknown	Unknown
Fukuyama CMD	MDC1C 19q	FKRP	Fukutin-related protein
Integrin α7 deficiency	Congenital myopathy 12q	ITGA7	Integrin α7
Muscle-eye-brain disease	MEB 1p	POMGn T1	O-mannosyl glycan
Walker-Warburg syndrome	WWS 9q	POMT1	Unknown
Rigid spine muscular dystrophy	RSMD 11p	SEPN1	Selenoprotein N1
Ullrich disease	UCMD 21q	COL6A1-3	Collagen VI

POMGn T1: protein O-mannose β-1,2-N-acetylglucosaminyltransferase, participates in the O-mannosyl glycan synthesis; LGMD2K and WWS may be ends of the clinical spectrum of the same disorder. **Fukutin** is a secreted, rather than transmembrane, protein. Mutations in FKRP also cause LGMD 2I.

CMD and No Intellectual Deficits

Laminin α2 chain deficiency presents with **hypotonia,** delayed early motor milestones, and **joint contractures** of elbows, hips, knees, and ankles. Congenital hip dislocation may occur. Brain MRI shows **cerebral hypomyelination.** Early CK elevation (approximately sevenfold) normalizes later on.

Secondary merosin deficiency expresses with wasting of shoulder girdle and leg weakness but with calf-thigh hypertrophy.

Ullrich congenital muscular dystrophy presents with congenital contractures of the proximal joints, hyperlaxity of the distal joints, torticollis, proximal weakness, and scoliosis. Scoliosis precedes the loss of ambulation (at around 10 years), unlike in DMD, where scoliosis progresses after the loss of ambulation (at around 12 years). In the above conditions, **restrictive lung disease** is the cause of early death. **Rigid spine muscular dystrophy** patients have early spine rigidity but have milder CK elevations and are ambulant.

CMD and Mental Retardation

Fukuyama congenital muscular dystrophy, also known as the **cerebro-ocular dysplasia with CMD,** consists of infantile hypotonia and cerebral and ocular involvement. Mental retardation and seizures are associated with polymicrogyria, hydrocephalus, and hypoplasia of the corticospinal tract. The ocular findings may be myopia, mottling of retinal pigment epithelium, and variable optic atrophy. Patients become bedridden before 10 years and die by the age of 20. It is mostly prevalent in Japan 7–12 per 100,000).

Walker-Warburg syndrome, the most severe form of CMD, is characterized by cobblestone lissencephaly, hydrocephalus, retinal dysplasia, and in some cases encephalocele with death in early infancy. Neonatal hypotonia is followed by later spastic quadriparesis. A milder phenotype without eye and brain abnormalities is also related to POMT1 mutations (LGMD 2K).

Distal Myopathies

They refer to muscle *dystrophies* of mostly distal involvement, some allelic to LGMDs, and are **easy to confuse with distal weaknesses** of other etiologies, such as:

1. Humeroperoneal dystrophy (Emery-Dreifuss)
2. Myotonic dystrophy
3. Facioscapulohumeral dystrophy
4. Scapuloperoneal dystrophy } Autosomal dominant disorders
5. Oculopharyngeal dystrophy
6. Inflammatory myopathies: inclusion body myositis and polymyositis
7. Metabolic myopathies: debrancher and acid maltase deficiencies
8. Congenital myopathies (includes desmin-related or myofibrillar myopathy)

CLASSIFICATION OF DISTAL MYOPATHIES

Early adult-onset	Nonaka (type 1)	AR, 9p	*Anterior* compartment of *legs* first affected
	Miyoshi (type 2)	AR, **2p** **Dysferlin**	**Posterior** compartment of legs first affected; gastrocnemius is early target **Allelic to LGMD 2B; CK is very high**
	Laing (type 3)	AD, 14q	*Anterior* compartment of *legs* and *neck flexors*
	Desmin (myofibrillar desmin and αB-crystallin)	AD, 2q,11q	**Hands** or distal legs and **cardiomyopathy** are involved
Late onset	Welander (type 1)	AD, **2p** **Dysferlin**	*Fingers* and wrist extensors first affected
	Markesbery-Griggs/ Udd (type 2)	AD, 2q **Titan**	*Anterior* compartment of *legs* first affected
	Myopathy with vocal/ pharyngeal signs	AD, 5q	*Anterior* compartment of *legs*, *finger extension*, and vocal cord/ pharyngeal weakness

Vacuolar myopathic changes are present in Nonaka, Desmin, Markesbery-Griggs/ Udd, and the myopathy with vocal pharyngeal signs. **Other vacuolar myopathies with 15- to 18-nm filaments** are seen in:

- Oculopharyngeal muscular dystrophy (OPMD)
- Sporadic inclusion body myositis (s-IBM)
- **Nonaka myopathy/hereditary IBM (h-IBM)/quadriceps sparing myopathy,** all allelic (9p), presumably represent the same disorder

Hereditary Inclusion Body Myopathy (h-IBM)

This is distinguished from sporadic IBM (s-IBM) by the absence of inflammation, the earlier onset (20s instead of over 50s in s-IBM), and the presence of both autosomal dominant and recessive (allelic to Nonaka) forms of inheritance.

- **Quadriceps and volar forearm** weakness are seen in **s-IBM**
- **Distal lower extremities and foot drop** are present in **AR h-IBM**
- **Limb-girdle distribution** of weakness is seen in **AD h-IBM**

Myotonic Dystrophy (DM)

DM is the most common inherited muscle disorder of adults (and second most common muscular dystrophy after DMD), affecting 15 per 100,000 live births, equally among males and females.

Classical myotonic dystrophy (DM1, Steinert disease) consists of weakness of neck, facial, and pharyngeal muscles associated with **distal weakness.** Proximal leg weakness, especially of the quadriceps, develops later and limits ambulation. **Action and percussion myotonia** can be elicited in the limbs and tongue. These patients have **frontal balding,** cranial hyperostosis, and changes in personality, affect, and motivation. Additional systemic features include:

- **Cardiac** abnormalities: **conduction defects,** arrhythmias
- **Ocular** manifestations: **cataracts, retinal degeneration,** and chronic progressive external ophthalmoplegia **(CPEO)**
- **Gastrointestinal** manifestations: **dysphagia** from esophageal myotonia, colonic dysmotility, megacolon, anal sphincter laxity
- **Hepatic** manifestations: elevated gamma-glutamyl transferase (GGT), gallstones
- **Endocrine** manifestations: **insulin resistance,** abnormal growth hormone (GH) release, **testicular atrophy**
- **Immune** manifestations: reduced serum immunoglobulins

Proximal myotonic myopathy (DM2, PROMM) is a milder myotonic dystrophy phenotype, with myotonia, cataracts, and weakness that is more proximal. Facial and respiratory muscles are relatively spared.

Congenital myotonic dystrophy (CmyD) is the most severe myotonic dystrophy form, fatal in 25%. **Hypotonia, feeding and respiratory difficulties** are present since birth. Tented upper lip is a classic facial feature. **Severe cardiomyopathy** may be present. Survivors are mentally retarded (75%) and may develop more classic features (suggestive of DM1) later in life.

DM1 and CMyD are caused by a CTG repeat expansion in a noncoding region of the dystrophia-myotonica protein kinase gene, **DMPK** (19q). **DM2 is caused by a CCTG tetranucleotide expansion** in a noncoding region of the zinc-finger-protein-9 gene, **ZNF9** (3q). The length of the CTG expansion predicts the severity of disease in DM1 (50–1,000) and CMyD (>1,000). **Anticipation** is the phenomenon of continued CTG expansion in successive generations, explaining that a child with CMyD may be born to a mother affected with DM1. Mexiletine, 150–200 mg tid is effective as an antimyotonia treatment in DM1, as are other sodium channel blockers (phenytoin, procainamide, tocainide).

> **Other disorders with clinical *and* electrical myotonia or paramyotonia** include myotonia congenital (Becker, Thomsen, acetazolamide responsive), paramyotonia congenital (sodium or chloride channelopathies), chondrodystrophic myotonia (Schwartz-Jampel syndrome), hyperkalemic periodic paralysis, myotonia fluctuans, and myotonia permanens.

Facioscapulohumeral Dystrophy (FSHD)

FSHD is the third most common muscular dystrophy after DMD and DM, with an incidence of 1 per 20,000. Symptoms can begin at any age with **facial** and **proximal arm weakness** associated with **scapular weakness and winging**, but sparing the eyes, pharynx, tongue, and heart. There is a **reversal of the axillary folds** and **sloping of the shoulders** because of this pattern of weakness. **Distal leg weakness develops in the anterior compartment**, causing **foot drop** (proximal leg weakness can occur in 20%). **Asymmetric** muscle involvement, unlike most other muscular dystrophies, can be of help in distinguishing FSHD from LGMD. In addition, the **Beevor's sign** (movement of the navel toward the head on flexing the neck) seems to be particularly more frequent in FSHD than any other muscular dystrophy and can be a helpful early finding. DNA analysis shows the presence of **4q35 short fragments** in about 95% of patients. More severe disease results from **smaller "short fragments"** from larger deletions. About 25% may present sporadically because of a new mutation. Lifespan is not significantly shortened. Wheelchair confinement occurs in 20%. Muscle biopsy shows myopathic changes, and oxidative enzyme staining reveals disruption of the intermyofibrillary network, producing a **moth-eaten appearance.**

Scapuloperoneal Dystrophy (SPD)

SPD comprises a group of disorders characterized by proximal upper extremity and distal lower extremity weakness. Since mild facial weakness can appear, SPD may be difficult to separate from FSHD. However, the lack of the DNA 4q35 short fragments unequivocally separates the two.

> **A scapuloperoneal pattern of muscle weakness,** besides FSHD and SPD, can also occur in Emery-Dreifuss dystrophy (additional contractures and cardiac involvement), late-onset acid maltase deficiency (Pompe disease), and the autosomal dominant form of hereditary inclusion body myopathy associated with Paget's disease and frontotemporal dementia (IBMPFD).

Oculopharyngeal Muscular Dystrophy (OPMD)

OPMD is an uncommon but distinctive form of adult muscular dystrophy, which begins between the fourth to sixth decades of life, and affects primarily patients of French-Canadian ancestry. It is recognized by the combination of **progressive ptosis** and extraocular movement impairment, suggestive of chronic progressive external ophthalmoplegia **(CPEO), dysphagia, facial and masticatory** weakness, and mild neck and proximal extremity weakness. **Distal muscles** may also be involved (**distal myopathy variant** mostly in Japanese, in which weakness may appear in the first decade). Muscle biopsy shows myopathic features and **intracytoplasmic, "rimmed" vacuoles,** similar to those seen in IBM and other distal myopathies. The underlying genetic defect is an **expansion of a GCG trinucleotide repeat** within the **polyadenylate binding protein 2 (*PABP2*)** gene, located on chromosome **14q.** Normally, there are six GCG repeats. Patients with OPMD have 8–13 repeats. Since there is no meiosis-induced expansion of repeats, the phenomenon of **anticipation does not occur.**

Inflammatory Myopathies

The idiopathic inflammatory myopathies include dermatomyositis, polymyositis, and inclusion body myositis (IBM) and have a combined incidence of 1 per 100,000.

Dermatomyositis

Dermatomyositis (DM) is the only inflammatory myopathy that can present at any age. It can begin acutely or, more commonly, over weeks to months with a prodromal picture of fatigue, fever, and muscle soreness and stiffness. **Neck flexors, shoulder girdle,** and **pelvic girdle muscles** are initially affected. Distal weakness is less severe but never absent. Complete sparing of distal muscles would be more suggestive of LGMD.

- **Dysphagia** occurs in one-third of patients. Chewing difficulties or dysarthria may be seen because of oropharyngeal weakness.
- **Pulmonary restrictive defects** may be present even in individuals without pulmonary symptoms. Interstitial lung disease develops in those with **antibodies to histadyl transfer RNA synthetase (Jo-1).**
- **Characteristic rash precedes muscle symptoms** affecting fingers and periorbital region first, followed by elbows, knees, and ankles.
  - **Heliotrope rash** is a purplish discoloration of the eyelids
  - **Gottren's sign:** erythematous, scaly lesion over the knuckles
  - **Shawl sign:** erythematous rash on shoulders and upper back
  - **Calcinosis** develop over pressure points (buttocks, elbows)
  - **Subcutaneous calcifications** appear in up to 50% of children
  - **Amyopathic dermatomyositis:** rash never leads to weakness
- **Electrocardiographic abnormalities** are seen in half the patients. Pericarditis, myocarditis, and congestive heart failure can occur
- **Gastrointestinal symptoms** include malabsorption, ulceration, perforation, and hemorrhage.
- **Increased incidence of malignancy** among adults should lead to a basic cancer screening with stool guaiac test, mammography, and vaginal ultrasonography.

CK is elevated up to 50 times normal in over 90% of patients. It is useful to monitor response but not to make management decisions. Aldolase, myoglobin, lactate dehydrogenase (LDH), aspartate aminotransferase (AST), and alanine aminotransferase (ALT) may also be elevated. Antinuclear antibodies (ANA) is positive in up to 50% of patients with overlap syndromes.

Perifascicular atrophy from ischemic damage with **perivascular inflammation,** comprising **CD4$^+$ cells,** B cells, and macrophages, is the classic histopathologic findins. The earliest immunologic abnormality is deposition of IgM, C3, and C5b-9 complement membrane attack on the intramuscular blood vessel walls. **Prednisone** is the usual first line of treatment. Short **methylprednisolone** pulses (20–30 mg/kg/d or every other day for 3–5 days) may be the best initiation therapy. **IV Ig** (2 g/kg per treatment cycle) has a clearer role in DM than in polymyositis.

Polymyositis

Polymyositis (PM) is rare in children unless it is part of an "overlap" connective disorder. Muscle weakness distribution is the than as that in DM (worse for shoulder abduction and hip flexion). It results from an **HLA-restricted, antigen-specific, cell-mediated immune response** geared against muscle fibers. **Absence of rash** is the distinguishing element from DM. **Overlap syndromes** refer to the association of polymyositis with another connective tissue disorder such as scleroderma, Sjögren's syndrome, mixed connective tissue disease, systemic lupus erythematosus, or rheumatoid arthritis.

- **Dysphagia** occurs in one-third of patients
- **Interstitial lung disease,** which has poor prognostic implications, appears in 10% of patients of whom 50% have **antibodies to histidyl tRNA synthetase (anti-Jo-1),** a greater number than in DM
- **Polyarthritis** has been reported in 45% of patients
- **Myocarditis** with congestive heart failure rarely develops
- **Slight increase of malignancy** but less than that seen in DM

CK is elevated up to 50 times normal. CK may be helpful in monitoring response to therapy *but is no more reliable than physical examination.* ANA is positive in 30% of patients. There is increased expression of proinflammatory cytokines such as interleukin-1 (IL-1), tumor necrosis factor (TNF-α), and intercellular adhesion molecule 1 (ICAM-1). Certain HLA haplotypes are more common in PM such as **HLA-B8** and **HLA-DR3.**

Endomysial inflammation with invasion of no-necrotic muscle fibers by **CD8$^+$ T-cells and macrophages** are typical muscle biopsy findings along with the expression of **HLA class 1** molecules in the invaded muscle fibers.

Inclusion Body Myositis

Unlike other inflammatory myopathies, IBM is **more common in males** and is **resistant to immunosuppressive therapy,** suggesting a degenerative element. It begins slowly in those older than 50 years with classic **asymmetric distal arm and foot (wrist, finger, and ankle flexors) and proximal leg (quadriceps)** weakness. It is the most common cause of "isolated quadriceps myopathy."

- **Dysphagia** occurs in about 40% and the face is involved in one-third
- **Concurrent autoimmune disorders** have been reported in 15%
- **No associated malignancy, respiratory, or cardiac disease**

Endomysial inflammation (as in polymyositis) with invasion of nonnecrotic fibers by cytotoxic T cells and **rimmed vacuoles** are the most characteristic histologic findings. EM shows diagnostic **15–18 nm filaments** in the cytoplasm and nuclei of the vacuolated fibers. **Amyloid deposits** can also be seen in the cytoplasm using Congo red stain. CK is only mildly elevated (up to 10 times normal) when compared to DM and PM (up to 50 times normal).

Metabolic Myopathies

Exercise Intolerance, Episodic (Cramps and Myalgia)	Progressive or Stable Muscle Weakness
Glycogenoses•	
Myophosphorylase (**PPL**, McArdle), type V• Phosphofructokinase (**PFK**), type VII• Phosphorylase B kinase (PBK), type VIII• Phosphoglycerate kinase (**PGK**)/mutase (PGAM) Lactate dehydrogenase (LDH), type XI	Acid maltase (**Pompe**), type II Debrancher (**Cori**), type III Brancher (**Andersen**), type IV
Fatty Acid Oxidation (FAO) Defects	
Carnitine palmitoyl transferase II deficiency (**CPT II**)—the most common cause of recurrent myoglobinuria*	Muscle carnitine deficiency Systemic carnitine deficiency **VLCAD**♦
Mitochondrial Myopathies	
Complex I, III, and IV deficiencies Coenzyme Q10 deficiency	Cytochrome C oxidase deficiency
Nucleotide Metabolism	
Myoadenylate deaminase deficiency (**MAD**)	

VLCAD, very-long-chain acyl-CoA dehydrogenase deficiency; PBK, PGAM, and LDH are very rare.
•EMG-silent.
*Hypoketotic hypoglycemia occurs when fatty acids cannot be used as fuels and ketone bodies are not generated to spare glucose/glycogen stores.
Low total carnitine and high plasma and urinary acylcarnitine are found in β-oxidation disorders, particularly during acute attacks.
♦SCAD, MCAD, and LCAD (but not VLCAD) are causes of recurrent coma and cardiomyopathy and not recurrent myoglobinuria.

Forearm ischemic exercise test (FIET) normally leads to an increase in **serum lactate and ammonia at least threefold in the first 3 minutes.** Samples of lactate, ammonia, and CK are collected from the antecubital vein before and at 1, 3, 5, 10, and 15 minutes after the patient has rhythmically squeezed a hand dynamometer for 1 minute while having a sphygmomanometer cuff inflated above systolic blood pressure.

↓ Lactate (Early Cramps)		Normal or ↑ Lactate	
Glycolytic/glycogenolytic defect • Minutes after exercise • **"Second wind"** phenomenon • **Cramps** with fixed weakness • **Abnormal FIET**		**Fatty acid oxidation disorders** • One hour after exercise • No second wind phenomenon • **Stiffness,** uncommon fixed weakness • Normal FIET	
No hemolytic anemia (HA)	**HA or RBC abnormalities**	**Ketogenesis (supervised fasting test) or long chain TAG loading test**	
		Normal	**Delayed or decreased**
PPL (McArdle) **PGAM** **Scaly rash: LDH** (pyruvate is raised) **Hypothyroidism**	**Seizures and/ or strokes?** **Yes: PGK** (X linked) **No: PFK**	Defects in: **TCA cycle** **Resp. chain** **G6PDH**	**FAO defects:** Fixed weakness and cardiopathy: **LCAD** Episodic weakness and no cardiopathy: **CPT II**

MAD deficiency causes normal lactate but no ammonia rise; *hyperuricemia* is seen in PPL, PFK, and debrancher enzyme deficiency from exercise-induced degradation of muscle purine nucleotides.

Episodic Muscle Weakness

Glycogenosis Type V

McArdle disease (myophosphorylase deficiency) causes exercise-induced cramps and myoglobinuria beginning before 15 years of age, predominantly in males. A **"second wind"** phenomenon is typical due to the availability of glucose from hepatic glycogenolysis and fatty acid oxidation. A few patients may become wheelchair-bound but most are not substantially disabled if strenuous exercise is avoided. About one-third of patients develop progressive proximal weakness with mild wasting. The resting CK is increased (as opposed to CPT deficiency, where it is normal) and the FIET test (pageabove) is always positive. **The cramps are EMG silent.** Biopsy shows **subsarcolemmal blebs** containing glycogen.

Glycogenosis Type VII

Tarui's disease (Phosphofructokinase Deficiency) displays the same McArdle's phenotype especially in Ashkenazi Jews and Italian families, but with the addition of **compensated hemolytic anemia, gout,** and **gastric ulcers.** The PFK-deficient muscle is incapable of using glucose (as opposed to McArdle's disease), and its administration prevents the muscle from utilizing free fatty acids and ketones as energy sources.

Glycogenosis Type X

Phosphoglycerate kinase deficiency (X-linked glycogenosis: Xq13) presents with **hemolytic anemia** (jaundice, splenomegaly, and hemoglobinuria) and **CNS dysfunction** (stroke and sezures), soon after birth in homozygous males. Exercise intolerance, cramps, and myoglobinuria are the myopathic features in males surviving childhood.

Fatty Acid Oxidation Disorders

Carnitine palmitoyl transferase II deficiency (CPT2 gene, 1p) is **the most common hereditary cause of rhabdomyolisis-induced myoglobinuria,** presenting with intolerance *after* exercise (as opposed to *during* exercise in the glycogen storage disorders) **without cramps, without "second wind,"** and **without ketones production.** The usual triggers are **fasting, prolonged exercise, low-carbohydrate high-fat diet,** cold, and infections. Urinary organic acids may be elevated. Serum carnitine and CPT levels are elevated; specific enzyme assays are available. Muscle biopsy may show **lipid accumulation** under electron microsorder.

Very-long-chain acyl-CoA dehydrogenase deficiency (17p) induces muscle pain and myoglobinuria in teenagers. Biopsy shows **lipid accumulation** in type I muscle fibers.

Nucleotide Metabolism Defects

Myoadenylate deaminase deficiency (1p), present in 2% of all muscle biopsies, is the most common enzymatic cause for **infantile hypotonia, childhood progressive myopathy,** and **adult recurrent rhabdomyolisis.** There is no EMG or biopsy correlate, and enzyme analysis is required for diagnosis. Heterozygotes are capable of normal ammonia production and are asymptomatic.

Familial Periodic Paralysis: Clinical Recognition

Age of Onset

Infancy	Under 10 years	Between 5 and 20 years
PMC	HyperKPP	HypoKPP
		Suspect **thyrotoxicosis**, secondary K+ wasting, or medications if onset >20 years

Characteristics of Attacks

Brief, less severe, <24 hours		Infrequent, severe, >**24 hours**
PMC or HyperKPP		HypoKPP

Precipitants

Cold	Hunger, K-rich foods	High carbs meal, salt
PMC	HyperKPP	HypoKPP

Exercise can precipitate both HyperKPP and HypoKPP

Response to Potassium

No effect	Causes weakness	Relieves acute weakness
PMC	HyperKPP	HypoKPP

Myotonia

Yes	No
PMC or HyperKPP	HypoKPP
PMC: **cooling** causes myotonia or decreased CMAP	

Muscle Biopsy

Variable	Vacuolar myopathy	Vacuolar myopathy
PMC	HyperKPP	HypoKPP

Features Supporting Different Diagnoses

Cardiac arrhythmias, dysmorphic features, or prolonged QT on electrocardiogram	Cramps, myoglobinuria, or onset always during exercise
Consider Andersen-Tawil syndrome Need additional Holter monitoring	Consider metabolic myopathies (e.g., McArdle's disease)

PMC, paramyotonia congenital; HyperKPP, hyperkalemic periodic paralysis; HypoKPP, hypokalemic periodic paralysis.

Overall, most patients with HypoKPP and HyperKPP respond to acetazolamide, but patients with HyperKPP caused by a *T704M* mutation exhibit a 50% response rate and those few patients with HypoKPP due to sodium channel mutation actually worsen with acetazolamide. Some families with HyperKPP are susceptible to malignant hyperthermia when undergoing anesthesia.

Progressive or Stable Muscle Weakness

Glycogenosis Type II

Acid maltase deficiency is due to mutations in the α-glucosidase gene (17q) and presents in any of three forms. The severe infantile form or **Pompe's disease** presents with progressive and severe hypotonia, **cardiomegaly, hepatomegaly,** and **macroglossia,** leading to death before 2 years. The juvenile form is associated with delayed motor milestones due to proximal muscle weakness with respiratory weakness, leading to death in the third decade. The adult form presents in the fourth decade of life with proximal weakness and occasionally **scapuloperoneal** involvement. Biopsy shows periodic acid Schiff (PAS)-positive, diastase sensitive, and acid phosphatase-positive "lacework" vacuoles, suggesting **excess glycogen in muscle and anterior horn cells** and explaining the myopathic (myotonic potentials) and neurogenic (fibrillations, positive sharp waves) findings of EMG. Treatment with alglucosidase alfa (Myozyme) improves walking and breathing capacity.

Glycogenosis Type III

Debrancher deficiency (Cori-Forbes disease) presents as delayed motor milestones in children or progressive weakness in adults. There may be **prominent distal atrophy** from associated axonal neuropathy and **pseudohypertrophy of proximal muscles.** Cardiomyopathy may complicate the picture. A variant that spares muscle and heart (IIIb) presents with **hypoglycemia-related seizures.** EMG/NCS (nerve conduction study) shows myopathic potentials and axonal sensorimotor neuropathy. Muscle biopsy shows subsarcolemmal PAS-positive vacuoles.

Glycogenosis Type IV

Branching enzyme deficiency (Andersen disease) is a rapidly progressive disease of infancy, leading to fatal **liver dysfunction.** The adult form, **adult polyglucosan body disease** (APBD, see *Ataxia*) manifests as progressive UMN and LMN signs with **cerebellar ataxia, dementia, neurogenic bladder, and sensory neuropathy.** The motor dysfunction may lead to early consideration of motor neuron disease in the differential diagnosis. Biopsy of CNS and PNS specimens shows polyglucosan bodies (PGB, PAS-positive, finely granular and filamentous polysaccharide) within nerve axons. PGB are also seen in **Tarui disease** (glycogen storage type VII; phosphofructokinase deficiency), in advanced aging **(corpora amylacea),** and **status marmoratus.**

Lipid Metabolism Disorders

Muscle carnitine deficiency is recognized as a progressive proximal muscle atrophy and weakness of childhood, with prominent **neck involvement and lumbar lordosis.** Cardiomyopathy with congestive heart failure and arrhythmias may be seen. The deficiency of carnitine prevents long-chain fatty acids from entering the inner mitochondrial matrix, thus severely affecting energy production from these fatty acids. **Secondary carnitine deficiency** may result from organic acidurias, endocrinopathies, renal and liver failure, Reye's syndrome, VPA toxicity, total parenteral nutrition, and pregnancy. Muscle biopsy shows accumulation of lipid material in the subsarcolemmal and intermyofibrillar regions of type I fibers, better seen with the oil red O stain.

Mitochondrial Myopathies

Mutations in mtDNA are more common and more likely to manifest clinically than mutations in nuclear genes because of the lack of introns and decreased DNA repair mechanisms in the mitochondrial genome. Primary mtDNA mutations are inherited from the mother but, unlike X-linked disorders, both males and females are equally affected, although mitochondrial **segregation** and **heteroplasmy** may affect both the transmissibility of a disorder and the diversity of its phenotypic expression. Since over 95% of mitochondrial proteins are encoded in the nucleus, some mitochondrial disorders can have autosomal dominant (e.g., PEO), autosomal recessive, and even X-linked patterns of inheritance (e.g., PDHC deficiency). (See *Mitochondrial diseases*.)

> **Exercise intolerance** as the sole manifestation of mitochondrial dysfunction has been reported in **complex III deficiency** (mutations in the **cytochrome b gene**), and **MELAS** patients (complexes I and IV).

Mitochondrial encephalomyopathy, lactic acidosis, and stroke-like episodes (point mutations in **tRNA$^{leu(UUR)}$**; most common mitochondrial disorde). **(MELAS)** usually presents with recurrent stroke-like episodes manifested as migraine-type headaches with nausea and vomiting, hemiparesis, hemianopsia, or cortical blindness. Proximal muscle weakness and **exercise intolerance** develops in most. Attacks are precipitated by exercise or infection.

Myoclonus epilepsy with ragged-red fibers (point mutations in **tRNA^{lys}**) **(MERRF)** is highly suspected when **cardiomyopathy** coexists with **multiple symmetric lipomatosis** and **life-threatening hypoventilation** following surgery or infection. The spectrum includes progressive myoclonic epilepsy and ataxia, dementia, sensorineural hearing loss, optic atrophy, and muscle weakness with **exertional myoglobinuria**. Sensorimotor polyneuropathy and pes cavus may be present. JME is in the differential before the onset of weakness and ataxia.

Kerns-Sayre syndrome (**KSS**, sporadic single large mtDNA deletions) KSS is characterized by the clinical triad of **PEO** (ptosis and ophthalmoparesis), **retinitis pigmentosa,** and **heart block** with onset usually before the age of 20 years. Mild proximal weakness may appear. Other possible findings are ataxia, deafness, dementia, **depressed ventilatory drive,** and **endocrinopathies** (diabetes, hypothyroidism, hypoparathyroidism, and delayed sexual features).

Progressive external ophthalmoplegia (sporadic, AD, or maternalled) Isolated isolated PEO is recognized as ptosis and ophthalmoparesis **in the absence of** retinitis pigmentosa, heart block, or endocrinopathies. **Hypoventilation** in response to sedatives and anesthetic agents may occur. *POLG1 mutations,* causing multiple mtDNA deletions in skeletal muscle, account for up to 25% of adult presentations. In these cases, there may also be parkinsonism, axonal sensory neuropathy, late-onset ataxia, and juvenile-onset Alpers syndrome.

Mitochondrial DNA depletion syndromes includes **fatal infantile myopathy** (99% mtDNA reduction), which is associated with cardiomyopathy or with the **De Toni-Fanconi-Debré syndrome,** a renal tubular defect, and **benign infantile myopathy** (less mtDNA reduction), which improves during thirst year and may be lead to "catching up" to normal by age 3.

Other Myogenic Causes of Cramps and Myalgia (Often Exercise-Related)

(Besides the glycogenoses [PPL, PFK, PGK deficiencies], fatty acid oxidation [CPT II and VLCD deficiencies], and nucleotide metabolism disorders [MAD deficiency] reviewed above).

Lambert-Brody syndrome, which consists of exercise-induced pain, stiffness, and cramping in arm and leg muscles associated with **impairment of relaxation**, suggesting myotonia but without percussion induction or EMG correlation ("silent myotonia"). The defect is in the **sarcoplasmic reticulum calcium adenosine triphosphatase (ATPase),** mainly present in fast-twitch type 2 fibers, delaying calcium reuptake.

Rippling muscle disease is an autosomal dominant disorder caused by caveolin-3 mutations, where initiation of physical activity after a period of rest causes pain and stiffness in the stretched muscles. Calf hypertrophy is common. Percussion reproduces the symptoms and creates **myoedema.** Both the rippling and the myoedema are also **electrically silent**.

Besides the above, **other electrically silent cramps** (e.g., **no EMG correlate**), include myophosphorylase deficiency and hypothyroidism.

Polymyalgia rheumatica is characterized by **pain** and stiffness **(no weakness),** weight loss, low-grade **fever,** and high ESR. It can be associated with **giant cell arteritis (temporal arteritis).** Prednisone is the treatment of choice.

Myotonia is a painless phenomenon due to repetitive activation of the muscle membrane and delayed muscle relaxation, leading to stiffness and tightness.

Disorders with Clinical *and* Electrical Myotonia	Disorders with Electrical Myotonia *without* Clinical Myotonia
Myotonic dystrophies (DM1 and DM2)	Acid maltase deficiency (Pompe)
Myotonia congenita (Becker, Thomsen)	Myofibrillar myopathies
Paramyotonia congenita	Hypothyroidism*
Hyperkalemic periodic paralysis	Drug induced (clofibrate, colchicine,
Schwartz-Jampel syndrome	chloroquine, statins)
Myotonia fluctuans	Inclusion body myositis
Myotonia permanens	Chronic denervation

*Hypothyroidism causes slowness of muscle contraction and relaxation that, when severe ("pseudomyotonia"), may suggest myotonic disorders or dystonia. A slow relaxation phase of muscle stretch reflexes and percussion-induced myoedema are common. Hyperparathyroidism often causes myalgia and cramps, partially responsive to verapamil.

Hereditary myotonias, due to chloride (myotonia congenita) and sodium (paramytonia congenita) channel mutations, unlike the other myotonias, are largely painless and patients rarely complain of stiffness or weakness.

Schwartz-Jampel syndrome (chondrodystrophic myotonia) usually begins in infancy with **myotonia,** osteochondrodysplasia, hypertrophic musculature, and a characteristic facies with **blepharophimosis,** micrognathia, and low-set ears. Patients are at risk for malignant hyperthermia. Action and percussion-induced myotonia are almost universal.

Neurogenic Causes of Cramps and Myalgia (Mostly at Rest)

(Not discussed are common nocturnal cramps, hemodialysis cramps, heat cramps, and cramps due to peripheral nerve injury, radiculopathy, and anterior horn cell disease.)

Neuromyotonia (Electric Myokymia or Continuous Motor Unit Activity)

This refers to the sustained muscle activity of peripheral nerve origin expressed as visible rippling movements (**"bag of worms,"** slower than fasciculations) and characterized by spontaneous and EMG needle-induced irregular trains of **doublets, triplets, and multiplets** firing at a high intraburst frequency (150–300 Hz; neuromyotonic discharges), and at lower frequencies (<60 Hz; myokymic discharges). It can occur as a paraneoplastic phenomenon (**anti-VGKC,** without peripheral neuropathy, also called Isaac's syndrome), associated with autoimmune disorders (thymoma, vitiligo, myasthenia gravis, Hashimoto's thyroiditis, and penicillamine treatment), or as part of a genetic disorder such as episodic ataxia type 1 or HMSN. Passive movements induce resistance and pain, and voluntary movements are slow to relax (**pseudomyotonia: no percussion or electrical myotonia**), causing gait impairment. Carbamazepine and phenytoin are effective treatments through their interaction with voltage-gated sodium channels.

Hypocalcemic Tetany

Low calcium (as well as low potassium, sodium, and magnesium) cause cramps, distal paresthesias, **carpopedal spasms,** laryngeal stridor, and convulsions. Overt or subclinical **hyperventilation** with respiratory alkalosis and compression-induced ischemia are well-known inductors of "latent" tetany. The peripheral nerves are usually hyperirritable to mechanical stimulation (**Chvostek's sign**).

CNS Causes of Cramps and Myalgia

- **Strychnine poisoning,** which competitively blocks the *postsynaptic* inhibitory action of glycine, causes muscle rigidity, opisthotonus, and apnea within 1 hour after ingestion. It must be distinguished from tetanus and acute dystonic reaction from metoclopramide and phenothiazines.
- **Tetanus,** caused by an exotoxin produced in a wound from *Clostridium tetani* that blocks the *presynaptic* release of gamma-aminobutyric acid (GABA) and glycine, begins 4–14 days after injury and initially affects the masticatory muscles, leading to trismus and dysphagia before generalizing. Reflex spasms are common and painful.
- **Stiff person syndrome (Moersch-Woltmann syndrome),** most commonly caused by glutamic acid decarboxylase (GAD) autoantibodies, leads to a more insidious symmetric stiffness, initially fluctuating and eventually continuous, particularly of the axial muscles and proximal limbs. Reflex spasms develop as well. A lumbar hyperlordosis is common. Insulin dependent diabetes mellitus and other autoimmune disorders may be present (see *Paraneoplastic syndromes*).
- **Tonic spasm (paroxysmal dystonia)** of multiple sclerosis are brief, recurrent, spontaneous or triggered, and often painful posturing of limbs that may occur initially or at any time during the course of MS.
- **Satoyoshi syndrome** consists of progressive intermittent muscle spasms (precipitated by voluntary contraction), alopecia, intestinal malabsorption, endocrinopathy with amenorrhea, and secondary skeletal abnormalities.

Congenital Myopathies

These myopathies present with a floppy-infant syndrome and delayed motor milestones, failure to thrive, and frequent respiratory infections. Adults may only have mild proximal weakness and hyporeflexia. The common histology is **fiber size disproportion** (predominance or hypotrophy of type 1 fibers) or **poor muscle type differentiation** at pH 4.6.

Nemaline rod myopathy (NRM) is the most common congenital myopathy. Scoliosis, respiratory insufficiency, and cardiac involvement may occur, but the range of severity is wide. **Distal weakness with foot drop** appears early with slow progression, including to bulbar muscles. Muscle stained with **modified Gomori trichrome** shows **purple cigar-shaped "rods"** in the periphery of type 1 fibers.

	Mutation/Chromosome	Encodes for
NEM1 (AD and AR)	TPM3 gene/1q21	α-tropomyosin
NEM2 (AR)	NEB gene/2q21	Nebulin
NEM3 (AD and AR)	ACTA1 gene/1q42	α-actin
NEM4 (AD)	TPM2 gene/9p13	β-tropomyosin

There are about 50 known ACTA1 missense mutations, which account for 10% to 20% of cases of nemaline rod myopathy. AD forms are associated with milder phenotypes than AR forms, and generally spare the upper extremities.

Myotubular myopathy is an **X-linked (Xq28,** codes for **myotubularin,** a protein tyrosine phosphatase) form of floppy infant with life-threatening respiratory complications. There is **severe facial weakness and ptosis with restricted extraocular movements** in males within the first months of life. The disorder is nonprogressive in long-term survivors. Muscle biopsy shows **centrally located nucleus** (single as opposed to the multiple nuclei of myotonic dystrophy), with or without fiber size disproportion. Central nuclei stain for **desmin** and **vimentin.**

Central core disease is a mild nonprogressive weakness of **autosomal dominant** inheritance with no bulbar deficits and **no cardiac involvement** but with orthopedic complications, mainly **scoliosis.** The disease is non- or slowly progressive. **Central cores** (rounded areas without oxidative enzyme activity) in type 1 fibers result from mitochondria, glycogen, and sarcoplasmic reticulum deficiencies. Cores are immunoreactivity to desmin, γ filamin, and αB-crystallin.

Desmin-related myopathies (myofibrillar myopathy) blongs to the **"surplus-protein myopathies"** (defective protein catabolism and aggregation within muscle fibers) along with actinopathy (NEM3 with mutations in ACTA1 gene), h-IBM, and hyaline body myopathy. There are intracytoplasmic inclusions within skeletal and cardiac muscle cells devoid of oxidative enzymes and ATPase activity but rich in intermediate filament protein desmin and αB-crystallin. Critical features are **distal and proximal muscle weakness and cardiomyopathy** (arrhythmias and heart failure). Causative mutations are on the **desmin** (2q35), **αB-crystallin** (CRYAB, 11q21), and, more recently, on the **myotilin** (5q) genes, mutated in LGMD1A.

Malignant Hyperthermia Syndrome

Malignant hyperthermia (MH) is the most common cause of death during general anesthesia, especially with **halothane** used alone (frequeny of 1 per 7,000–50,000 anesthetics given) or in conjunction with succinylcholine and other depolarizing muscle relaxants. MH syndrome consists of an acute **hypermetabolic state** characterized by **rigidity, hyperventilation, tachycardia, fever, cyanosis,** and hemodynamic instability due to a sudden unregulated rise in free sarcoplasmic calcium, leading to persistent muscle contraction. Postoperative rhabdomyolysis may also occur or indicate an underlying myopaty. Nonanesthetic agents such as decongestants and gasoline vapors may also trigger the syndrome in susceptible individuals. **Masseter spasms** following succinylcholine may herald the onset of MH in certain individuals, especially children. **Dantrolene** is recommended for prophylactic use prior to surgery on individuals believed at risk.

Triggering Agents for MH	Safe Agents for MH
Volatile general anesthetics (halothane, cyclopropane, methoxyflurane, isoflurane, enflurane, sevoflurane, and desflurane)	Intravenous anesthetics (ketamine, propofol, etomidate, thiopental, opiates, and benzodiazepines)
Depolarizing muscle relaxants (e.g., succinylcholine)	All nondepolarizing muscle relaxants (e.g., vecuronium, rocuronium, d-tubocurarine, pancuronium)
	Nitrous oxide

MH Susceptibility Is Increased by These Conditions	
Familial MH (RyR1, CACNA1S)	Schwartz-Jampel syndrome
Central core disease	Satoyoshi syndrome
Duchenne muscular dystrophy	CPT II syndrome
Becker muscular dystrophy	King syndrome
Myotonic dystrophy	Periodic paralysis
Myotonia congenita	Brody's syndrome

Inherited susceptibility to MH is conferred by mutations in the **sarcoplasmic reticulum ryanodine receptor gene (RyR1, 19q), CACNA1S** (1q, which codes for the α1-subunit of the human skeletal muscle dihydropyridine-sensitive L-type voltage-dependent calcium channel), and **CACNLA2** (7q), which codes for a second dihydropyridine receptor locus.

Central core disease is allelic to and often coexistent with malignant hyperthermia. Both are disorders of calcium regulation related to the **ryanodine receptor gene (RyR1, 19q).** Some evidence now suggests that mutations in the N-terminal domain of RyR1 are more likely to be associated with malignant hyperthermia, while those in the C-terminal domain are more likely to result in central core disease.

Critical Illness-Related Neuropathy and Myopathy

Critical illness polyneuropathy (CIP) is a **sensory-motor axonal neuropathy** complicating critical patients with severe multiorgan failure, **sepsis,** and prolonged ventilatory support (steroids and neuromuscular blockers are risk factors for critical illness *myopathy*). The clinical pattern is that of a **generalized flaccid tetraparesis and areflexia** with stocking-glove hypesthesia. The course is **monophasic** and self-limiting. In those who survive the causative severe multiple organ failure, recovery takes place within months. A CIP-like picture can result from prolonged neuromuscular blockade after administration of high-dose neuromuscular blockers in patients with acidosis or renal insufficiency. Nerve conduction studies show **reduced CMAP amplitude** with near normal velocity and no conduction block or CMAP dispersion. There are signs of widespread **denervation** activity on EMG with fibrillation potentials and positive sharp waves. In the absence of sepsis and multiorgan failure, one must obviously consider such entities as Guillain-Barré syndrome, myasthenia gravis, motor neuron disease, botulism, or acid maltase deficiency.

Critical illness myopathy ("thick filament myopathy") is a diffuse nonnecrotizing "cachectic" myopathy, where inflammatory changes are absent (as in CIP) and CK is often normal. Muscle biopsy shows variable fiber size, fiber atrophy, angulated fibers, internal nuclei, rimmed vacuoles, fatty degeneration of fibers, and fibrosis. This condition is more common in patients who received **corticosteroids** for acute severe asthma or organ transplantation, alone or in combination with high doses of **neuromuscular blocking agents** (NMBAs). Electron microscopy shows focal or diffuse **selective loss of myosin (thick) filaments.**

Electrophysiology is not helpful in distinguishing between myopathy and neuropathy given insufficient motor unit activation by patients. CK is often insensitive, making biopsy necessary for its recognition. Weaning of ventilator and physical therapy should be postponed until the underlying pathology resolves.

DIFFERENTIAL DIAGNOSIS BY MUSCLE BIOPSY DEPENDING ON FIBER TYPE INVOLVED

Atrophy of Type 1 Fibers	Atrophy of Types 1 and 2	Atrophy of Type 2 Fibers
Myotonic dystrophy Emery-Dreifuss Congenital myopathies Periodic paralysis Hyperthyroidism Rheumatoid arthritis	Chronic denervation	Corticosteroids Cushing's disease Starvation Aging Paraneoplastic Myasthenia gravis

Type I fibers react strongly to NADH but weakly to ATPase (pH 9.4)	Type II fibers react weakly to NADH but strongly to ATPase
Slow twitch fibers—fatigue resistant	Fast twitch—fatigue prone
Predominance: congenital myopathies	Predominance: LEMS (secondary)
Hypertrophy: Werdnig-Hoffmann disease, chronic neuropathies	Hypertrophy: exercise

Psychiatry   10

There are a number of psychiatric disturbances that accompany neurologic illnesses (e.g., Alzheimer disease, Parkinson disease, stroke, multiple sclerosis, and epilepsy) and neurologic manifestations of primary psychiatric disorders (e.g., schizophrenia, depression, mania, anxiety, substance abuse, and obsessive-compulsive disorder [OCD]). The study of the psychiatric manifestations of neurologic diseases and investigation of the neurobiological basis of psychiatric illnesses has produced a remarkable convergence of data regarding the anatomic substrates of behavioral disorders. Hence, this compendium would not be complete without a survey of the major "primary" psychiatric disorders that neurologists are likely to encounter often during the course of their practice.

Some examples of the convergence between neurology and psychiatry are shown here:

- Poststroke depression is more commonly associated with involvement of the dorsolateral prefrontal cortex or the caudate nuclei, structures also relevant in the generation of major depressive disorders.
- Psychosis has been associated with a variety of neurologic diseases that affect the temporal lobes, and studies of the brains of schizophrenic patients have revealed consistent temporal lobe abnormalities.
- Nearly all neurologic diseases associated with OCD involve subcortical structures of prefrontal-subcortical circuits, and positron emission tomographic studies of idiopathic OCD implicate this same circuitry.
- Psychiatric symptoms in neurologic diseases can guide psychiatric disorders (e.g., dopaminergic therapy-induced psychosis in Parkinson disease supports the theory of dopaminergic hyperactivity in schizophrenia).
- Neurologic symptoms in psychiatry diseases can guide neurologic disorders (e.g., response of OCD to serotonergic agents has supported use of same agents to treat OCD in neurologic disorders).

Behavioral neurology is the discipline within neurology most closely allied with psychiatry because it aims at explaining the neurobiological basis of "negative symptoms" (deficit syndromes), including aphasia, amnesia, agnosia, apraxia, and neglect. Psychiatry aims at delving into the "positive symptoms" (productive syndromes), which include hallucinations, delusions, depression, mania, anxiety, and OCD. *Neuropsychiatry* is the discipline that integrates the neuroanatomy and cognitive neuropsychology of both negative and positive symptoms and is growingly becoming an important field within neurology. Neuropsychiatry is based on neuroanatomy and neurophysiology and attempts to understand the mechanisms of behavior, whereas psychiatry explains the motivations of behaviors using methods from the fields of psychology, sociology, and anthropology. Neuropsychiatry applies a neurobiological approach to behavior; psychiatry places behavior in a social-cultural context. Human behavior is the common denominator for these disciplines and the critical target of neurologists.

Depression

Depression consists of a **pervasive depressed mood** or **anhedonia,** which causes significant social and occupational dysfunction, and five of the following during the same *2-week period*: change in **appetite** and weight, psychomotor agitation or retardation, **sleep** disturbance, **fatigue** or loss of energy, excessive **guilt** or feelings of worthlessness, **concentration** disturbance, and **suicidal** thinking. The lifetime prevalence is between 5% and 9% in females and 2% and 4% in males. About 50% of those who have had a major depressive episode will have a recurrence. Comorbid disorders include **alcoholism** (60% of alcoholics develop depression), **eating disorders** (60%), and **panic disorder** (80%).

Depression may cause: (1) **shortened latency of rapid eye movement (REM) sleep;** (2) **suppression of endogenous cortisol secretion** after a dexamethasone suppression test (injection of 1 mg IM of dexamethasone; caveat: dementia and weight loss may cause nonsuppression); and (3) lack of elevation of thyrotropin to thyrotropin-releasing hormone.

The following **subtypes of depression** are recognized:
- **Psychotic** when hallucinations, delusions, and thought disorder are present.
- **Melancholic** applies to the sad, blue mood as opposed to the empty, nonmelancholic mood of atypical depression.
- **Seasonal affective disorder** predominate in women, often with depression and hypomania (bipolar II disorder), and good response to phototherapy
- **Postpartum** women develop depression in 10%–15% of cases within 6 months of delivery. The "*maternity blues*" (and adjustment disorder with depressed mood) affects 50%–80% of all new mothers within the first week after delivery. It is not as severe as postpartum depression.
- **Adjustment disorder** is a maladaptive reaction that lasts <6 months occurring within 3 months from an identifiably psychosocial stressor. It carries a poor prognosis for adolescents.
- **Atypical depression** is characterized by extreme lethargy and fatigue, hypersomnolence, rejection-sensitivity, and xenophobia with episodes of **empty** and **reactive mood** (environmental factors improve mood briefly).
- **Dysthymia (minor depression)** is a chronic depression of late adolescence and early adulthood that lasts 2 years without a break. Patients have "been depressed for as long as it can be remembered."

Cyclothymic disorder applies to those whose mood never meet criteria for depression or mania but occur frequently for at least 2 years with a symptom-free interval never longer than 2 months at a time. **Borderline personality disorder** may coexist. About 30% have family history of bipolar disorder with one-third going on to develop increasing episodes of hypomania and major depression referred to as *bipolar disorder II* (**"bipolar disorder NOS"**). Rapid cycling carries a poor prognosis. Common comorbid conditions in bipolar disorder II include borderline personality disorder, eating disorders, and substance abuse.

Antidepressant Drugs

Treatment- resistant depression is managed by utilizing pharmacologic augmenters: lithium, triiodothyronine (T_3), stimulants, neuroleptics, and L-tryptophan. Nonpharmacologic interventions include sleep deprivation, sleep phase advancement, high-intensity (>2,500 lux) light, and electroconvulsive therapy.

SELECTIVE SEROTONIN (5-HT) REUPTAKE INHIBITORS (SSRIs)

Common side effects include **sexual dysfunction, insomnia,** agitation, anxiety, headache, and anorexia. Effective in (and, in the case of Fluvoxamine, approved for) OCD and panic disorder.

Fluoxetine (Prozac)	10–20 mg → 80 mg/d [20]		Longest T½ (9 days). Risk of SIADH. 95% protein bound
Paroxetine[♠] (Paxil)	20 mg → 60 mg/d [20, 30]		Dizziness, diarrhea, mild dry mouth, constipation
Sertraline[♠] (Zoloft)	50 mg → 200 mg/d [50, 100]		Mild dry mouth. Diarrhea is more common.
Fluvoxamine (Luvox)	50 mg → 150 mg **bid** [25,50,100]		Only SSRI approved for kids. Avoid theophylline and warfarin
Citalopram (Celexa)	20 mg → 40 mg/d [20]		Effective for premenstrual syndrome
Escitalopram (Lexapro)	10 mg → 20 mg/d [10, 20]		Excellent tolerance
5-HT₂, 5HT₃ antagonists	**Nefazodone** (Serzone)	50 mg bid → 300 mg **bid** [100, 150, 200, 250]	**Orthostatic hypotension, somnolence,** dry mouth, **no risk of sexual dysfunction**
	Trazodone (Desyrel)	50 mg → 400 mg/d/**bid** [50, 100, 150, 300]	**Orthostatic hypotension, priapism** (rare), sedation
Serotonin/Norepinephrine Reuptake Inhibitors (SNRIs)—Nontricyclics			
Venlafaxine (Effexor)	25 mg tid → 225 mg/d [25, 37.5, 50, 75, 100]		HTN, nausea, insomnia, anxiety, dry mouth
Duloxetine (Cymbalta)	30 mg → 60 mg/d [30, 60]		Also beneficial for peripheral neuropathy

SIADH, syndrome of inappropriate antidiuretic hormone secretion; bid, twice daily; tid, three times a day; HTN, hypertension.

[♠]Sertraline is the safest SSRI when there is coadministration with tricyclic antidepressants, neuroleptics, and type I antiarrhythmic agents such as quinidine because it has the smallest effect on the P450 2D6 liver microsomal enzyme. Both paroxetine and sertraline also have minimal effects on P450 3A34, responsible for clearing the largest number of nonpsychiatric drugs as well as several benzodiazepines.

SNRIs—TRICYCLICS—TERTIARY AMINES (PRIMARILY SEROTONIN)

Anticholinergic effects and α-blocking effect (sedation, orthostatic hypotension). Contraindicated in glaucoma, urinary retention, and cardiac disorders **(long QTc).** Sexual dysfunction may occur.

Amitriptyline (Elavil)	25 mg → 300 mg qhs [10, 25, 50, 75, 100, 150]	High sedation and anticholinergic activity
Clomipramine (Anafranil)	25 mg → 250 mg qhs [25, 50, 75]	**High seizure risk,** sedation, **Effective for OCD**
Doxepin (Sinequan)	25 mg → 300 mg qhs [10, 25, 50, 75, 100, 150]	Sedating
Imipramine (Tofranil)	25 mg → 300 mg qhs [10, 25, 50, 75, 100, 150]	Sedating. Demethylated to **Desipramine. Panic** disorder.

qhs, every bedtime; OCD, obsessive-compulsive syndrome.

TCA levels are increased by fluoxetine, neuroleptics, H₂-blockers, estrogens, valproate, and methylphenidate and decreased by barbiturates, CBZ, PHT (P450 inducers), and cigarette smoking.

SNRIs—TRICYCLICS—SECONDARY AMINES (PRIMARILY NOREPINEPHRINE)

Anticholinergic and α-blocking effect (sedation, orthostatic hypotension), less severe. It may **lower seizure threshold.** Arrhythmogenic by leading to **AV delay** and **long QTc.**

Desipramine (Norpramin)	25 mg → 300 mg qhs [10, 25, 50, 75, 100, 150]	**Stimulant effect:** am dose prevents insomnia. **Panic d.**
Nortriptyline (Pamelor)	25 mg → 150 mg / tid-qid [10, 25, 50, 75]	**Sedating.** Effective for **post-stroke depression, panic d.**
Protriptyline (Vivactil)	15 mg → 60 mg / tid-qid [5, 10]	**Effective for sleep apnea**
Amoxapine (Asendin) **[Tetracyclic]**	25 mg bid → 300 mg/d [25, 50, 100, 150]	**Tardive dyskinesia, NMS, galactorrhea.** No CV effects

qhs, every bedtime; d, disorder; tid, three times a day; qid, everyday; bid, twice daily; CV, cardiovascular.
Nortriptyline is the tricyclic of choice given its mild sedating properties (useful in agitated patients to promote sleep), lower propensity to cause orthostatic hypotension, fewer anticholinergic side effects, and availability of easily interpretable blood levels (therapeutic level is 50–150 ng/dL).

NOREPINEPHRINE-DOPAMINE REUPTAKE INHIBITORS (NDRIs)

Contraindicated when there is history of **seizures, bulimia, and anorexia** but good choice (along with nefazodone) if there are sexual side effects from other agents. Seizures threshold is not substantially lowered with the newer SR or XL formulations. Bupropion is a **mild stimulant** and is preferred over SSRIs in depressed patients with bipolar illness and adults with ADHD. Its dopaminergic and noradrenergic effect have prompted its use to increase energy and drive, as with the psychostimulant modafinil and the dopamine agonist pramipexole.

Bupropion (Wellbutrin)	100 mg bid → 150 mg tid [75, 100, SR-100, -150]	**Agitation,** hypertension, **insomnia, tremor,** constipation

bid, twice daily; tid, three times a day.

NOREPINEPHRINE ANTAGONIST AND SEROTONIN ANTAGONIST (NASA)

NASA inhibits serotonin reuptake and blocks 5-HT$_2$ and 5-HT$_3$ receptors. The **risk of agranulocytosis** is about 0.1%. Mirtazapine, along with paroxetine and trazodone may be helpful in insomnia, although trazodone (see previous discussion) may not help mood and may cause priapism.

Mirtazapine (Remeron)	15 mg → 45 mg qhs [13, 30]	Risk of **agranulocytosis.** Sedation, **weight gain**

qhs, every bedtime.
  Besides Nefazodone, Mirtazapine and Bupropion avoid sexual dysfunction and the latter may boost sexual performance at doses equivalent to 150 mg twice daily (SR formulation). Mirtazapine's weight-gain side effect is considered an advantage in cases where weight loss is a problem; Bupropion, on the other hand, can induce further weight loss.

MONOAMINE OXIDASE INHIBITORS (MAOI)

Potential risks are **hypotension, insomnia,** and **sexual dysfunction** (anorgasmia, ejaculatory incompetence). Concomitant use of **sympathomimetics** (epinephrine, norepinephrine, and pseudoephedrine) and the intake of **tyramine**-rich foods may cause a **hypertensive crisis.** Other complicating drugs are **meperidine or dextromethorphan** (delirium), **SSRIs** (serotonin syndrome; see elsewhere in this book). **Peripheral neuropathy** results from **vitamin B6** malabsorption. **Weight gain** follows carbohydrate craving. Finally, a reversible **lupuslike reaction** and **hyperprolactinemia** have been reported.

Phenelzine (Nardil)	15 mg tid → 90 mg/d [15]	Must be on tyramine-free diet for 2 weeks after stopping. Risk of hypertensive crisis and serotonin syndrome. 2 weeks washout between MAOI and SSRIs and TCAs
Tranylcypromine (Parnate)	10 mg am → 60 mg/d [10]	
Isocarboxazid (Marplan)	10 mg bid → 60 mg/d [10]	

tid, three times a day; bid, twice a day.

Bipolar Disorder

Bipolar spectrum encompasses episodes of mania alternating or mixed with episodes of depression. **Mania** is a persistently elevated, expansive, or irritable mood that may be accompanied by decreased need for sleep, talkativeness, flight of ideas, distractibility, increase in goal-directed activity or psychomotor agitation, and excessive involvement in highly pleasurable and potentially risky activities. Males and females are equally affected and 15% of first-degree relatives have affective disorders. **Alcohol and drug abuse** are more prominent than in unipolar patients. The recurrence after a single manic episode is 90%. The concordance rate among monozygotic twins is 70% to 80%. Rapid cycling (four or more episodes a year) occurs in 10% of patients, mostly women and patients taking TCAs. Childhood-onset *psychotic* depression is more likely to become acutely bipolar at the onset of puberty, especially if there is TCA-induced hypomania, hypersomnic depression, and bipolar family history.

> **Secondary mania** may develop after thalamic stroke, right temporal lobe epilepsy, hyperthyroidism, vitamin B_{12} deficiency, and cerebellar atrophy. Mania-inducing drugs include sympathomimetics, amphetamines, LSD, levodopa, and steroids.

Lithium is the drug of choice for bipolar disorder, schizoaffective disorder, prophylaxis against recurrent unipolar depression, and intermittent explosive disorder. The side effects include hypothyroidism (thyrotropin is screened before and during treatment), diabetes insipidus, weight gain, acne, arrhythmias, psoriasis, leukocytosis, **downbeat nystagmus, periodic alternating nystagmus,** and **tremor.** Lithium is to be avoided in the elderly and those with renal insufficiency, dehydration, and suicidal ideation (to prevent overdose).

LITHIUM TOXICITY SYMPTOMS (level >3 mmol/L, or less **in elderly**)

Mild toxicity	Moderate toxicity	Severe toxicity
Nausea, irritability, Impaired cognition, and weakness	Ataxia, dysarthria, drowsiness, blurred vision, tinnitus and tremor	Delirium, CV toxicity, EPS, neuromuscular irritability, seizures, stupor, coma
↑ Lithium level: NSAIDs, metronidazole, PHT, tetracycline, thiazides, and ↓ GFR		
↓ Lithium level: acetazolamide, aminophylline, furosemide, and hemodialysis		

CV, cardiovascular; EPS, extrapyramidal side effects; GFR, glomerular filtration rate.

Carbamazepine (400–1,000 mg) and **valproate acid** (500–1,250 mg) alone or in combination with lithium have been shown effective for cases of lithium-resistant and rapid cycling bipolar disorder. Antidepressants may be used for treatment of depressive episodes but must be accompanied by a mood stabilizer to prevent precipitating a manic episode. **Antidepressants may induce rapid cycling.** Atypical antipsychotics (risperidone, olanzapine, quetiapine, ziprasidone, and aripiprazole) can be used for associated sleep, psychosis, or behavioral problems. Combined olanzapine or quetiapine and fluoxetine have been found effective for depressive symptoms.

Anxiety Disorders

Panic disorder, more common in females (3:1), begins in the late teens either spontaneously or following such stressors as medical illness or substance abuse. Its lifetime prevalence is 3.5% and occurs in 25% of first-degree relatives. In fact, there is five times greater concordance for panic disorder in monozygotic compared to dizygotic twins. The suicide risk increases in untreated patients.

Recurrent, unexpected **panic attacks** are periods of intense fear or discomfort, which develop abruptly and reach a peak within 10 minutes. Patients may experience palpitations, sweating, trembling, shortness of breath, feeling of choking, chest pain, nausea or abdominal discomfort, dizziness, derealization (feelings or unreality) or depersonalization (being detached from oneself), fear of losing control or going crazy, fear of dying, paresthesias, chills or hot flushes.

Complications of panic disorder are **agoraphobia** (anticipatory anxiety and phobic avoidance that results in considerable and disabling restriction of normal activities), depression or dysthymia, alcoholism and sedative abuse, avoidant and dependent personality, somatization, and increased suicide rates.

> **Disorders that both mimic and coexist with anxiety include** asthma, vestibular disorders, pheochromocytoma, hyperthyroidism, hypoglycemia, and mitral valve prolapse syndrome. Amphetamines, cocaine, caffeine, alcohol or benzodiazepine withdrawal can precipitate panic attacks.

Nonpharmacologic management includes reassurance, cognitive and behavioral therapies, and avoidance of stimulants (caffeine, chocolate, drugs) and alcohol.

SSRIs, at low doses to avoid excitatory effects, have become the mainstay of treatment for panic disorder. TCAs, especially imipramine, desipramine and nortriptyline, are second-line agents. BZDs are discouraged among those with comorbid substance abuse. Only alprazolam (Xanax) is Food and Drug Administration-approved for panic disorder. Dividing the average daily dose of 2 mg into a four times a day schedule decreases the interdose anxiety. When "interdose symptom recurrence" remains a problem, the longer-acting and potent clonazepam is preferred (T½ 35 hours vs. 12 hours). Beta blockers are helpful only as adjuncts in cases of continued autonomic hyperactivity. Buspirone (BuSpar) helps augment the effect of alprazolam.

Generalized anxiety disorder is more constant, unrealistic, and excessive than panic disorder although it offers a better prognosis. Six months of worrying (without anticipatory anxiety), "over two or more life circumstances" *and* three of the following are present: restlessness, easy fatigability, difficulty concentrating, irritability, tension, and sleep disturbance. It may evolve into panic disorder and/or substance abuse in one-fourth of patients and into depression in half. The lifetime prevalence is 5% and the male-to-female ratio is 1:2. **Buspirone,** a $5-HT_{1A}$ partial agonist, is the first line of treatment, at the dose of 10–20 mg tid. No sedation, tolerance, dependence, or withdrawal symptoms develop from buspirone. Prior BZD exposure decreases responsiveness to buspirone.

BENZODIAZEPINES

Drugs		Dose (mg)	T½, onset	Active metabolites	Special features
Diazepam[1] (Valium)	Long T½	5 PO, IM, IV.	45 h Very fast	**Nor-diazepam**	Two serum peaks after one dose (1, 10 h). Good choice for **chronic anxiety** in nondrug abuser
Chlor-diazepoxide (Librium)		25 PO IV	35 h Slow	**Nor-diazepam**	Slower onset: less euphoria. Used in **ETOH W/D. Sterile abscess** when given IM
Clorazepate (Tranxene)		7.5 PO	**60 h** Fast	**Nor-diazepam**	Adjunct to CBZ for the **treatment of CPS**
Flurazepam (Dalmane)		15 PO	**75 h Fast**	**Nor-flurazepam**	Two serum peaks (1 h, 10 d) after 1st and 2nd dose. **Low chance rebound insomnia. Sleep inductor. Hangover.**
Clonazepam (Klonopin)		0.25 PO	35 h Slow	**Yes**	Anticonvulsant effective for **panic disorder, mania, nocturnal myoclonus,** and other sleep-related disorders
Lorazepam (Ativan)	Medium T½	1 PO, IM, IV.	14 h Interm	**No**	Cleared by glucuronidation, which remains intact even in severe liver dysfunction. Excreted in urine
Temazepan (Restoril)		15 PO	12 h Interm	**No**	**Low chance of rebound insomnia** (long elimination T½): **it maintains sleep.**
Triazolam (Halcion)		0.25 PO	2 h Interm	**No**	Associated with **transient anterograde amnesia** and its discontinuation cause **rebound insomnia.**
Alprazolam (Xanax)	Short T½	0.5 PO	12 h Very fast	**Minor**	Only BZD approved for PD. High abuse liability. Block PAF and BTG: ↑ **bleeding**[2]
Oxazepam (Serax)		15 PO	10 h Slow	**No**	Cleared by glucuronidation, which remains intact even in severe liver dysfunction.
Midazolam (Versed)		2.5 IM, IV	3 h Very fast	**No**	**Induction of anesthesia** and **sedation.** Most potent and lipophilic BZD in the United States

BZDs of choice in the elderly or liver-impaired are lorazepam, temazepam, and oxazepam.

PO, orally; IM, intramuscularly; ETOH W/D, alcohol withdrawal; PD, Parkinson disease; PAF, platelet-activating factor

[1] The active metabolite **nordiazepam** has a T½ of 100 hours and may last up to 200 hours in the elderly and in those with hepatic dysfunction

[2] Both **alprazolam** and **triazolam** inhibit platelet activating factor (PAF) and B-thromboglobulin (BTG), thereby reducing clotting activity

Obsessive-Compulsive Disorder

OCD is a relatively frequent anxiety disorder characterized by the presence of intrusive and senseless ideas, thoughts, urges, and images *(obsessions)*, as well as by repetitive, time-consuming cognitive and physical activities performed in a ritualistic way *(compulsions)*, usually in an attempt to neutralize anxiety caused by an obsession. To meet criteria for OCD, these obsessions and compulsions significantly interfere with normal personal, occupational, or social routine. As such, **OCD must be distinguished from obsessive-compulsive personality disorder,** whereby there is a lifelong pervasive pattern of perfectionism and inflexibility that is largely egosyntonic (i.e., acceptable to the individual).

OCD has a lifetime prevalence of 3%. Symptoms develop before age 25 in 65% of cases, with onset after age 35 in only 15%. Over two-thirds of first-degree relatives of patients with OCD have either clinical (20%) or subclinical OCD (15%). **OCD is common in patients with Tourette syndrome;** however, only 5% of OCD patients have Tourette syndrome. Obsessional thinking and perseverative behaviors also occur in patients in the early stages of Huntington disease and in patients with Sydenham disease. Dysfunction of frontal-limbic-subcortical circuits and **hypermetabolism in the orbitofrontal regions, cingulate cortex, and caudate** may play an important role in the pathogenesis of OCD.

Closely related disorders that are not considered OCD include:
- **Trichotillomania** (compulsive hair pulling)
- **Monosymptomatic delusional hypochondriasis**
- **Dysmorphobia** (belief that some body part is deformed)
- **Obsessive fear** of AIDS or cancer
- **Punding** (stereotyped complex and repetitive unproductive behaviors)

The pathogenesis of OCD, summarized as the "serotonergic hypothesis," is fueled by the response of OCD to serotonergic medications (clomipramine, fluoxetine, and other SSRIs), although is refuted by the lack of effectiveness of sertraline (highly specific SSRI) and buspirone (partial 5-HT1a receptor agonist).

The pharmacologic therapy hinges on the use the following SSRI agents: Fluoxetine (Prozac), 20–60 mg/d; paroxetine (Paxil), maximum of 60 mg/d; or fluvoxamine (Luvox), 50–300 mg/d, among others, at a dose somewhat higher than that recommended for depression. Clonazepam (Klonopin) can be a useful adjunct agent. The tricyclic antidepressant clomipramine (Anafranil), 75–300 mg, can be used with an SSRI in treatment-resistant cases in which an SSRI alone has been insufficient. Low doses of the newer atypical antipsychotics olanzapine, quetiapine, ziprasidone, and risperidone have also been reported as useful adjuncts in the treatment of OCD.

Personality Disorders

These refer to stable, **enduring patterns of behavior** that deviate markedly from cultural expectations in two or more of the following areas: cognition (ways of perceiving and interpreting self, others, and events), affectivity, interpersonal functioning, and impulse control. These traits become **inflexible,** pervasive, and **maladaptive** to the point where they cause significant social or occupational dysfunction, or subjective distress. In general, patients have little or no insight into their disorder. The estimated **lifetime prevalence is 6–10 per 100 people.**

Cluster A: bizarre personality disorders
- **Paranoid:** Suspicious, distrustful, hypervigilant, bear grudges, argumentative, pathologic jealousy. It is more common in **men, relatives of schizophrenics.** It may be a **premorbid disorder in schizophrenia.**
- **Schizoid:** No desire for relationships, solitary, detached. It is also more common in men, **relatives of schizophrenics,** and increases the risk for **schizophrenia.**
- **Schizotypal:** Peculiar, bizarre, and eccentric speech patterns, ideation, and appearance. The thought content includes paranoid suspiciousness, ideas of reference without delusions, and odd or magical beliefs or fantasies without hallucinations or incoherence. It is more common among first-degree relatives of people with schizophrenia, and 10% will become schizophrenics.

Cluster B: dramatic personality disorders
- **Antisocial:** Deceitful, aggressive, impulsive, irresponsible, criminal, with lack of remorse and empathy. Before age 15 years, there is animal cruelty, theft, and violation of rules. Subjects may be **superficially charming, manipulative** with high incidence of substance abuse. Histrionic personality in female siblings.
- **Borderline** (60% of psychiatric patients): Unstable and intense interpersonal relationships, affect, and **identity;** manipulative, impulsive, destructive behavior, **recurrent suicidal behavior, transient paranoia or dissociation.**
- **Histrionic:** Emotionality, dramatic, attention-seeking, shallow, self-centered. High rates of depression, somatization, and conversion.
- **Narcissistic:** Grandiose, arrogant, entitled, hypersensitive to criticism, **envy,** and lack of empathy. Fragile self-esteem is the driving force.

Cluster C: anxious personality disorders
- **Avoidant:** Shy, fearful of criticism, disapproval, or rejection; avoids interpersonal contact but longs for it (which distinguishes this disorder from social phobia), devastated by minor comments believed to be critical.
- **Dependent:** Needy, clingy, helpless; has **trouble initiating activities or making decisions** but risks humiliation and submission to avoid abandonment. **Separation anxiety disorder** of childhood may be premorbid. There is an increased risk for mood disorders and anxiety.
- **Obsessive-compulsive:** Fastidious, neat, perfectionist, workaholic, scrupulous, cold.

Eating Disorders

Anorexia Nervosa

Anorexia nervosa applies to the intense fear of obesity, distorted body image, and progressive weight loss that is especially common in adolescent women (peak between 14 and 18 years), which results in **weight loss below 85% of expected body weight.** The most important diagnostic features are listed here:

- **Amenorrhea** often occurs before substantial loss of weight
- **Lack of concern** about amenorrhea
- **"Good girl"** behavior: no evidence of behavioral problems at home
- **Obsessional traits, social phobias,** and **passive dependence**
- **Depression** is common but not necessarily present
- **Cardiovascular and hematologic dysfunction** contribute to the mortality rate of about 10% in these patients:
  - Bradycardia and other arrhythmias
  - Pancytopenia and peripheral edema
  - Hypotension and hypothermia
  - Increased carotene levels
- **Neuroendocrine dysfunction:**
  - Decreased follicle-stimulating hormone and leutinizing hormone levels, resulting in amenorrhea
  - Osteoporosis (densitometry may be needed for evaluation)
  - Nonsuppression on dexamethasone test (90%)
  - Raised plasma cortisol levels
  - Normal or marginally diminished thyroid function

Bulimia Nervosa

This condition is characterized by recurrent episodes of **binge eating** accompanied by a **"compensatory" purging** (self-induced vomiting, abuse of laxatives, and/or misuse of diuretics). This behavior is required to occur at least **twice per week** for 3 months to qualify as such by the *Diagnostic and Statistical Manual of Mental Disorders*, Fourth Edition criteria. As opposed to anorexia nervosa, weight is at or above the expected for age and there are no endocrine abnormalities (densitometry is not required). There is often coexistent **substance abuse** (30%) and **borderline personality disorder** (30%). **Chronic ipecac abuse** may cause myopathy and cardiomyopathy. **Repeated vomiting** in bulimic individuals may cause:

- **Hypokalemic and hypochloremic metabolic alkalosis** (hyperchloremic metabolic alkalosis occurs with laxative abuse). **Hypokalemia** in an otherwise healthy young woman is highly specific for bulimia nervosa. Normalization of volume status is required for effective potassium replacement.
- **Secondary hyperaldosteronism** causes leg edema
- **Painless salivary gland enlargement (sialadenosis)**
- **Stomach enlargement**
- Dental caries and enamel loss in dorsal anterior teeth
- Traumatic injuries to the upper gastrointestinal tract

Schizophrenia and Other Psychoses

Schizophrenia has 1% lifetime prevalence worldwide, with 80% of cases diagnosed before the age of 40 years. **Prodromal symptoms** include social withdrawal, blunted or inappropriate affect, vague and overelaborate speech, and **odd beliefs and magical thinking. Social or occupational dysfunction** for at least 6 months are required for diagnosis, with at least 1 month of delusions, hallucinations, disorganized speech, disorganized or catatonic behavior, and/or negative symptoms (flat affect, anhedonia, asociality, alogia, apathy).

- Duration <6 months: **schizophreniform disorder,** seen in mania, psychotic depression, or substance abuse without decline in social functioning
- Duration <1 month: **brief psychotic disorder,** which may appear as part of bipolar disorder, major depression, or borderline personality disorder
- Prominent mood disorder and psychosis persisting during euthymic phases: **schizoaffective disorder**
- Psychosis only during maniac or depressive phases: **mood disorder with psychotic features**
- Psychosis only between postpartum days 3–14, lasting for 2–3 months: **postpartum psychosis**

Thought disorders are divided into *content* (**delusions,** ideas of reference, poverty of content) and *form* (concrete, circumstantial, illogical, and tangential). A delusion, a disturbance of cognition rather than perception, as in hallucinations, is a firmly held false belief and contrary to a person's education and cultural background. Some include persecution, grandiosity, somatic, thought broadcasting, thought insertion, and ideas of reference.

Psychosis-induced drugs are stimulants (**amphetamines**), phencyclidine (**PCP**), hallucinogens (**LSD**), mescaline, **cocaine** (tactile hallucinations, **delusional parasitosis**), and **marijuana.** Recreational use of plant toxins of the *Datura* species, such as **belladonna** (deadly nightshade) and **jimson weed,** can produce anticholinergic effects expected of "belladonna alkaloids" such as hyoscine, atropine, and scopolamine: mydriasis, tachycardia, blurred vision, but also **vivid hallucinations.**

Good prognostic indicators	Negative prognostic factors
Late age of onset	Early age of onset
Obvious precipitant factors	Single marital status
Positive symptoms	Negative symptoms; ventriculomegaly
Affective symptoms	Low IQ
Acute onset after stressful event	Poor premorbid work record
Presence of social support systems	Absence of social support systems

About 10% of patients will ultimately commit suicide. The **risk factors** are single male, age under 30, unemployment, a relapsing course, *high level of education,* and depressive symptoms. Suicide occurs in the context of depressive symptoms rather than as a response to command auditory hallucinations.

ANTIPSYCHOTIC MEDICATIONS

Typical—low potency

	Dose (mg)	C-equiv	Side effects
Chlorpromazine (Thorazine) Phenothiazine	600–800	100	**Low risk of** EPS, **high risk** of anticholinergic, sedative, and postural hypotensive effects. Thioridazine (Mellaril) is associated with pigmentary retinopathy
Thioridazine (Mellaril) Phenothiazine	600–800	100	
Mesoridazine (Serentil) Phenothiazine	300–400	50	

Typical—intermediate potency

Loxapine (Loxitane) Dibenzoxazepine	75–100	10	Risk of EPS lies between the low and high potency antipsychotic medications. Molindone has been associated with increase mortality (mainly cardiovascular) particularly in elderly patients with dementia-related psychosis.
Molindone (Moban) Dihydroindole	50–100	10	
Perphenazine (Trilafon) Phenothiazine	8–64	8	

Typical—high potency

Trifluoperazine (Stelazine) Phenothiazine	30–40	5	**High risk of** EPS, **low risk** of anticholinergic, sedative, and hypotensive effects. They block the **subtypes D2 and D3** of the D2 receptors.
Thiothixene (Navane) Thioxanthene	30–40	5	
Fluphenazine (Prolixin) Phenothiazine	10–20	2	
Haloperidol (Haldol) Butyrophenone	10–20	2	
Pimozide (Orap) Diphenylbutyl	2–15	1	

Atypical

Risperidone (Risperdal)	6–10	**Low risk of** EPS, **high risk of** anticholinergic, sedative, and hypotensive effects. Clozapine blocks **5-HT$_2$ and D$_2$ receptors (subtype D4)** and shows greater efficacy for "negative" symptoms. Combination with BZDs may lead to respiratory depression. Monitoring for agranulocytosis is required.[*] Seizures, sedation, hypersalivation, and tachycardia can also be seen. Aripiprazole is a partial agonist for D2 and serotonin 5-HT1A receptors. Ziprasidone may prolong the Q-T interval.
Olanzapine (Zyprexa)	10–20	
Clozapine (Clozaril)	50–600	
Quetiapine (Seroquel)	300–400	
Aripiprazole (Abilify)	10–15	
Ziprasidone (Geodon)	40–160	

Injectible (depot formulations)

Fluphenazine Decanoate (Prolixin)	12.5–75 q 2 wk	These are reserved for cases when compliance is doubtful.
Haloperidol Decanoate (Haldol)	50–300 q mo	

EPS: extrapyramidal side effects.
[*]Maximum-risk for agranulocytosis is between weeks 4–18, mediated by immunologic mechanisms. Weekly monitoring is required. Drug is withheld if WBC <3,000. These medications should be avoided when using clozapine: CBZ, captopril, sulfonamides, propylthiouracil (PTU).

Delusions

Delusions are **pathologic beliefs of bizarre content,** held with absolute certainty despite clear evidence that they are incorrect. They are not conventional beliefs of a culture or religion. **Schizophrenic delusions** can be of (1) influence (e.g., thought control or insertion, broadcasting), (2) persecution, and (3) self-significance (e.g., grandeur, reference, religious). Delusions need to be distinguished from **confabulations** (incorrect or distorted statements, made without a conscious effort to deceive), associated with memory (medial temporal or diencephalic) and executive (bifrontal) dysfunction and anosognosia (unawareness of a neurologic deficit). Patients who are anosognosic or confabulate can be redirected and corrected; those with delusions cannot.

Delusional disorder is a psychotic syndrome with prominent nonbizarre delusions (e.g., "my wife is having an affair") lasting for at least 1 month, including erotomania, grandiose, jealous, persecutory, and somatic. Neurologic disorders tend to lead to content-specific delusions, such as misidentification and reduplication syndromes, whereby places (reduplicative paramnesia), people (Capgras, Fregoli), or events are transformed in identity or duplicated.

Capgras syndrome occurs often in neurodegenerative disorders, particularly dementia with Lewy body disease (55%), whereby visual hallucinations correlate with the severity of Lewy body deposition in the amygdala, and parahippocampal and inferior temporal cortices. Dysfunction in these areas can also cause paranoia.

Capgras syndrome ("illusion of doubles") is a delusional misidentification syndrome in which familiar persons are believed to be impostors or doubles. **Unlike prosopagnosia, familiar faces do not generate autonomic response** despite conscious recognition. Right-only or bilateral frontal, with variable temporal or parietal, hemisphere involvement is implicated.

Fregoli syndrome is a delusional misidentification syndrome whereby a stranger takes on a familiar person's appearance while retaining psychic identity. Patients often report they are persecuted by these misidentified individuals.

Although frontal pathology is critical for delusions to develop, associated temporal lesions may cause familiar places to appear foreign **(Capgras)** while temporal sparing, or overactivity in the right perirhinal cortex, may cause misidentifying strange people as familiar **(Fregoli).**

Peduncular hallucinosis or **Lhermitte syndrome** are colored nonstereotyped, nonthreatening visual hallucinations (people, plants, animals) accompanied by delusions and associated with sleep disturbances or sleep-wake abnormalities, due to brainstem lesions in REM sleep and sleep-wake regulatory centers. Hallucinations in **Charles Bonnet syndrome** are well-formed, complex and stereotypical visual hallucinations in those with poor vision and mild cognitive impairment due to abnormalities in the ventral occipitotemporal visual pathways.

Neuroleptic-Induced Movement Disorders

Antipsychotics and some antiemetics (phenothiazines thiethylperazine and prochlorperazine as well as the substituted benzamides metoclopramide, sulpiride, tiapride, and clebopride) induce movement disorders through their ability to block striatal dopamine D2 receptors, for which they are termed **neuroleptics or dopamine-receptor blocking agents** (DRBA). These disorders include, in order of appearance after drug initiation:

1. **Acute dystonic reaction** tends to occur **within 4–5 days** of initiating neuroleptic and manifest as oculogyric crises and dystonia, especially of the craniocervical region. Subtle symptoms may be limited to dysarthria and dysphagia.

2. **Acute akathisia** or subjective restlessness and dysphoria cause inability to remain still and need to move about and pace or perform a variety of stereotypic movements (e.g., hand rubbing, foot tapping), which partially relieve the restlessness.

3. **Drug-induced parkinsonism** can be indistinguishable from idiopathic Parkinson disease. Associated prominent postural tremor and low- frequency, high-amplitude perinasal and frontal tremor (**rabbit syndrome**) are supportive.

4. **Neuroleptic malignant syndrome** consists of marked rigidity, fever, autonomic instability, and alterations in the level of consciousness. It requires discontinuation of the neuroleptic, support of nutrition and respiration, and one or more of the following agents:

   a. Dopamine agonist such as **bromocriptine** 15–30 mg/d

   b. Muscle relaxant such as **dantrolene** 1–10 mg/kg

   c. Anticholinergic such as **benztropine** 4–12 mg/d

   Neuroleptics, if strictly necessary, may be resumed at least 2 weeks after cessation of NMS, as there is 80% chance of recurrence when the drug is resumed in <2 weeks, but that figure falls to 10% when resumption occurs after 2 weeks.

5. **Tardive syndromes** may develop only after chronic treatment with dopamine-blocking agents. **Tardive dyskinesia** consists of stereotypic orofacial movements producing intermittent, brief tongue protrusion, lip smacking, or grimacing, whose incidence is approximately 4–5% per year for the first 5 years of neuroleptic treatment. Older women with coexistent mood disorders are at greater risk. Tardive dyskinesias may worsen with concurrent treatment with dopaminergic and anticholinergic agents, as opposed to tardive dystonia. *Withdrawal emergent syndrome* is a self-limited (about 6 weeks) form of pediatric tardive dyskinesias that result from relatively rapid decreases in DRBA. **Tardive dystonia** is recognized by the typical combination of retrocollis, internal rotation of the arms, extension of the elbows, and wrist flexion. **Tardive akathisia** results in restlessness, pelvic rocking motions, pacing, and moaning. Tardive parkinsonism remains to be convincingly documented (all such cases have shown Lewy bodies on autopsy).

Somatoform Disorders

The various somatoform disorders are differentiated mainly on the basis of two properties: perception of external or internal gain and conscious awareness:

	External gain	**Internal gain**
Consciously aware	Malingering	Factitious disorder
Consciously unaware	Conversion disorder	Somatization disorder*

*Hypochondriacs also have intrapsychic conflicts for which they are not consciously aware.

Conversion Disorder (Hysterical Neurosis)

The diagnosis applies to the loss or alteration of **motor or sensory function, following a stressful event,** which is **not intentionally produced** to resolve an unacceptable but obvious conflict **(external gain).** Patients often lack the characteristic normal concern about the deficit (*la belle indifference*) and have comorbid depression, anxiety disorders, or schizophrenia. A significant proportion of patients may have an underlying organic illness. A common coexistence is that of pseudoseizures with true epileptic seizures. Prevalence rates in a general medical setting may reach 20% to 25%. It must be differentiated from malingering (conscious awareness), somatization disorder (earlier onset, multiorgan symptoms, patients are concerned rather than indifferent), and factitious disorders (voluntary assumption of the sick role).

Factitious Disorder (*Munchausen* Syndrome)

Munchausen syndrome refers to **self-inflicted physical** or **psychological** symptoms whereby the individual's motivation is to assume the sick role when **external motives such as financial gain are absent.** It begins in early adulthood and is more frequent among men and **health care workers** with severe personality disorders (borderline or antisocial) and lower socioeconomic background. These patients would gladly submit to diagnostic procedures and operations. **Identity disturbance and narcissistic traits** are frequent. Prognosis is poor. No specific treatment exists. When the symptoms are created in children or elderly relatives, the label *Munchausen syndrome by proxy* applies.

Somatization Disorder (Hysteria, Briquet Syndrome)

This disorder describes those with excessive and persistent concern about **multiple somatic complaints** for which there is neither secondary gain nor intentional production of symptoms but deep conviction of illness. The multiple symptoms, which lack recognizable etiology, include at least four pain symptoms, two gastrointestinal symptoms, one sexual symptom, and one pseudoneurological symptom. These are out of proportion to the physical findings and lead to multiple procedures and hospitalizations. Up to two-thirds of patients have **coexistent psychiatric diagnoses,** especially mood and anxiety disorders and substance-related disorders. The disorder, up to 20 times more prevalent in women, often begins during adolescence and certainly always before 30 years of age. About 15% of patients have a **positive family history** and the concordance rate is higher among monozygotic twins.

Malingering

In malingerers, the same self-inflicted symptoms are produced to obtain **secondary or external gains** usually in a **medicolegal context.** These individuals are consciously aware, exhibit obvious external motivations such as money, and have the intent to deceive the system by producing false symptoms. They characteristically refuse to cooperate with diagnostic testing and treatment recommendations, offer approximate answers **("Ganser's answers"),** and have a history of polysubstance abuse and **antisocial personality** disorder. Malingering is not considered a psychiatric disorder.

Hypochondriasis

As in somatization disorder, hypochondriacs exhibit no obvious external gain or voluntary production of symptoms, but instead they have an excessive preoccupation with the **fear of having a serious disease** based on misinterpretation of symptoms and despite negative investigations and reassurances to the contrary. There are **no delusions or concerns about appearance.** Primary hypochondriasis tends to be treatment-resistant, whereas secondary hypochondriasis may remit with effective antidepressant or antipanic pharmacotherapy. Regular limited-goals visit are indicated but frequent laboratory workups should be avoided.

Somatoform Pain Disorder

This disorder often refers largely to women in their fourth and fifth decade who have experienced severely disabling pain for at least 6 months with no identifiable etiology. Up to half of these patients suffer from **major depression,** whereas the remainder usually meets criteria for a **dysthymic disorder.** Their personalities are **alexithymic** (unable to generate affective experience at a conscious level), and **counterdependent workaholics,** who find nurturance unacceptable and therefore develop somatic complaints to validate dependent needs. It must be distinguished from **hypochondriasis** (multiple as opposed of more stable symptoms), **malingering** (presence of a recognizable goal), and **conversion disorder** (much briefer than pain disorder).

Body Dysmorphic Disorder (Dysmorphobia)

Individuals with dysmorphobia are preoccupied with imagined defects in their appearance (facial features, hair, body build), which are **not of delusional proportions** and do not include anorexia nervosa, but cause significant functional impairment. Women and men between 15 and 20 years are equally affected. There is often a strong family history of mood disorders and OCD, and some suggest that the disorder may be a variant of the latter. **Major depressive disorder, delusional disorder, and anxiety disorders** frequently coexist with dysmorphobia. Antidepressants of the SSRI type are the treatment of choice for dysmorphobia. Pimozide (Orap) has been found to be helpful in certain cases. No "corrective" procedures should be offered.

Dissociative Disorders

These disorders, considered **adaptive responses to overwhelming stress or trauma,** are characterized by alterations in the normally integrated functions of **identity, memory,** and **sense of reality.** It must be differentiated from psychotic disorders, panic disorder with prominent derealization, factitious disorder with psychological symptoms, and complex partial seizures.

Depersonalization Disorder

Patients feel detached and numb, as though they are observing themselves from outside their bodies. Although **reality testing remains intact** during the depersonalization experience, there often are **disturbed body perceptions** and **derealization** (a sense that the environment is unreal). The onset is rather **sudden** in females between the ages of 15 and 30 years. Temporal lobe epilepsy and brain tumor need to be ruled out. No specific treatment is available.

Dissociative Amnesia

In this setting, there is an acute onset of **memory loss for important personal information (identity loss)** in which patients show circumscribed, selective, generalized, or continuous amnesia without an identifiable organic etiology. Toxic and metabolic disorders are not associated with identity loss. Dissociative amnesia may follow head injury, either alone or in combination with postconcussional amnesia. However, whereas **the recovery from dissociative amnesia is sudden, dramatic, and complete,** the amnesia resulting from concussion resolves slowly and in a spotty fashion. In addition, this posttraumatic retrograde amnesia never extends beyond 1 week. Sodium amytal or hypnosis is used to help the patient recover lost memories.

Dissociative Fugue (Poriomania)

Dissociative fugue applies to those who engage in sudden travel away from home or work, with assumption of a new identity without recall of previous life.

Dissociative Identity Disorder (DID, Formerly Multiple Personality Disorder)

DID is the coexistence of two or more distinct personalities in one individual, creating **dramatically different behavioral patterns** reflecting the manifestation of one of the personalities. It is associated with gaps in recall and **"waking up" in unfamiliar places.** The transition of one personality to another is often sudden. The presenting personality may not be aware of the coexistence of other(s). **DID patients have on average 13 personalities** and present with complaints of depression, amnesia, insomnia, and suicidal thoughts. The disorder usually begins in childhood or adolescence, although commonly is not diagnosed until later in life. **Severe sexual or physical abuse during childhood** and higher familial incidence are common historical findings. Psychotherapy to reintegrate split-off personalities is the treatment of choice.

Suggested References for Further Reading

The following references were selected as a complement to each chapter, with material meant to expand rather than rehash the topics discussed. Substantial material was adapted from the references marked with an asterisk (*), which are mentioned in the corresponding chapters. By no means should this list be held as exhaustive or representative of the vast and relevant literature but rather the authors' biased but practical take on topics that would benefit from the additional insight provided by these articles.

Chapter 1: Basics of Metabolism and Pediatric Neurology

Benarroch EE. *Neuronal voltage-gated calcium channels: brief overview of their function and clinical implications in neurology.* Neurology *2010;74(16):1310–5.*

Benarroch EE. Glutamate transporters: diversity, function, and involvement in neurologic disease. *Neurology* 2010;74(3):259–64.

Benarroch EE. The locus ceruleus norepinephrine system: functional organization and potential clinical significance. *Neurology* 2009;73(20):1699–704.

Benarroch EE. Serotonergic modulation of basal ganglia circuits: complexity and therapeutic opportunities. *Neurology* 2009;73(11):880–6.

Benarroch EE. Potassium channels: brief overview and implications in epilepsy. *Neurology* 2009;72(7):664–9.

Benarroch EE. Gamma-hydroxybutyric acid and its relevance in neurology. *Neurology* 2009;72(3):282–6.

Benarroch EE. Brain cholesterol metabolism and neurologic disease. *Neurology* 2008; 71(17):1368–73.

Benarroch EE. Metabotropic glutamate receptors: synaptic modulators and therapeutic targets for neurologic disease. *Neurology* 2008;70(12):964–8.

Benarroch EE. GABAa receptor heterogeneity, function, and implications for epilepsy. *Neurology* 2007;68(8):612–4.

Benarroch EE. Sodium channels and pain. *Neurology* 2007;68(3):233–6.

Berardo A, et al. A diagnostic algorithm for metabolic myopathies. *Curr Neurol Neurosci Rep* 2010;10(2):118–26.

*Marks PW, et al. Case 30-2004. A 37-year-old woman with paresthesias of the arms and legs. *N Engl J Med* 2004;351(13):1333–41. (excellent review of vitamin B12 deficiency)

Pearl PL, et al. The pediatric neurotransmitter disorders. *J Child Neurol* 2007;22(5):606–16.

Schiffmann R, et al. Invited article: an MRI-based approach to the diagnosis of white matter disorders. *Neurology* 2009;72(8):750–9.

Schmiedel J, et al. Mitochondrial cytopathies. *J Neurol* 2003;250(3):267–77.

Steenweg ME, et al. Magnetic resonance imaging pattern recognition in hypomyelinating disorders. *Brain* 2010;133(10):2971–82.

Willemsen MA, et al. Tyrosine hydroxylase deficiency: a treatable disorder of brain catecholamine biosynthesis. *Brain* 2010;133(Pt 6):1810–22.

Yee AH, et al. Neurologic presentations of acid-base imbalance, electrolyte abnormalities, and endocrine emergencies. *Neurol Clin* 2010;28(1):1–16.

Chapter 2: Stroke, Migraine, Epilepsy

*4S Study Group. Randomised trial of cholesterol lowering in 4444 patients with coronary heart disease: the Scandinavian Simvastatin Survival Study (4S). *Lancet* 1994;344(8934):1383–9.

Cholesterol and Recurrent Events: a secondary prevention trial for normolipidemic patients. CARE Investigators

Bartleson JD. When and how to investigate the patient with headache. *Semin Neurol* 2006;26(2):163–70.

*Broderick JP, et al. Finding the most powerful measures of the effectiveness of tissue plasminogen activator in the NINDS tPA stroke trial. *Stroke* 2000;31(10):2335–41.

*Brott T, et al. Baseline silent cerebral infarction in the Asymptomatic Carotid Atherosclerosis Study. *Stroke* 1994;25(6):1122–9.

*Brott TG, et al. Stenting versus endarterectomy for treatment of carotid-artery stenosis. CREST Investigators. *N Engl J Med* 2010;363(1):11–23.

*CAST (Chinese Acute Stroke Trial) Collaborative Group. CAST: randomised placebo-controlled trial of early aspirin use in 20,000 patients with acute ischaemic stroke. *Lancet* 1997;349(9066):1641–9.

*CAVATAS Investigators. Endovascular versus surgical treatment in patients with carotid stenosis in the Carotid and Vertebral Artery Transluminal Angioplasty Study (CAVATAS): a randomised trial. *Lancet* 2001;357(9270):1729–37.

Chen ZM, et al. Indications for early aspirin use in acute ischemic stroke : A combined analysis of 40 000 randomized patients from the chinese acute stroke trial and the international stroke trial. On behalf of the CAST and IST collaborative groups. *Stroke* 2000;31(6):1240–9.

*Chimowitz MI, et al. Comparison of warfarin and aspirin for symptomatic intracranial arterial stenosis. *N Engl J Med* 2005;352(13):1305–16.

*Diener HC, et al. Aspirin and clopidogrel compared with clopidogrel alone after recent ischaemic stroke or transient ischaemic attack in high-risk patients (MATCH): randomised, double-blind, placebo-controlled trial. *Lancet* 2004;364(9431):331–7.

*Diener HC, et al. Effects of aspirin plus extended-release dipyridamole versus clopidogrel and telmisartan on disability and cognitive function after recurrent stroke in patients with ischaemic stroke in the Prevention Regimen for Effectively Avoiding Second Strokes (PRoFESS) trial: a double-blind, active and placebo-controlled study. *Lancet Neurol* 2008;7(10):875–84.

*Dippel DW. The results of CAPRIE, IST and CAST. Clopidogrel vs. Aspirin in Patients at Risk of Ischaemic Events. International Stroke Trial. Chinese Acute Stroke Trial. *Thromb Res* 1998;92(1 Suppl 1):S13–6.

*Doyle J, et al. Mutations in the Cacnl1a4 calcium channel gene are associated with seizures, cerebellar degeneration, and ataxia in tottering and leaner mutant mice. *Mamm Genome* 1997;8(2):113–120.

*ECST Collaborators. Randomised trial of endarterectomy for recently symptomatic carotid stenosis: final results of the MRC European Carotid Surgery Trial (ECST). *Lancet* 1998;351(9113):1379–87.

Hacke W et al. Thrombolysis with Alteplase 3 to 4.5 hours After Acute Ischemic Stroke. *N Engl J Med* 2008;359:1317–29

*Halliday A, et al. Prevention of disabling and fatal strokes by successful carotid endarterectomy in patients without recent neurological symptoms: randomised controlled trial. *Lancet* 2004;363(9420):1491–502.

*Hankey GJ, et al. Adding aspirin to clopidogrel after TIA and ischemic stroke: benefits do not match risks. *Neurology* 2005;64(7):1117–21. (a propo of the MATCH study results)

*International Stroke Trial Collaborative Group. The International Stroke Trial (IST): a randomised trial of aspirin, subcutaneous heparin, both, or neither among 19435 patients with acute ischaemic stroke. International Stroke Trial Collaborative Group. *Lancet* 1997;349(9065):1569–81.

*Johnston SC, et al. Validation and refinement of scores to predict very early stroke risk after transient ischaemic attack. *Lancet* 2007;369(9558):283–92.

*Joutel A, et al. Notch3 mutations in CADASIL, a hereditary adult-onset condition causing stroke and dementia. *Nature* 1996; 383(6602):707–10.

Kizer JR, et al. Clinical practice. Patent foramen ovale in young adults with unexplained stroke. *N Engl J Med* 2005;353(22):2361–72.

Kruyt ND, et al. Hyperglycemia in acute ischemic stroke: pathophysiology and clinical management. *Nat Rev Neurol* 2010;6(3):145–55.

Lees KR, et al. Time to treatment with intravenous alteplase and outcome in stroke: an updated pooled analysis of ECASS, ATLANTIS, NINDS, and EPITHET trials. *Lancet* 2010;375(9727):1695–703.

*Levy DE, et al. Predicting outcome from hypoxic-ischemic coma. *JAMA* 1985;253(10):1420–6.

*Marschner IC, et al. Long-term risk stratification for survivors of acute coronary syndromes. Results from the Long-term Intervention with Pravastatin in Ischemic Disease (LIPID) Study. LIPID Study Investigators. *J Am Coll Cardiol* 2001;38(1):56–63.

*Mas JL, et al. Endarterectomy versus stenting in patients with symptomatic severe carotid stenosis. EVA-3S Investigators. *N Engl J Med* 2006;355(16):1660–71.

*NASCET Collaborators. Beneficial effect of carotid endarterectomy in symptomatic patients with high-grade carotid stenosis. North American Symptomatic Carotid Endarterectomy Trial Collaborators. *N Engl J Med* 1991;325(7):445–53.

Neligan A, et al. Frequency and prognosis of convulsive status epilepticus of different causes: a systematic review. *Arch Neurol* 2010;67(8):931–40.

*Ophoff RA, et al. Familial hemiplegic migraine and episodic ataxia type-2 are caused by mutations in the Ca2+ channel gene CACNL1A4. *Cell* 1996; 87(3):543–52.

Paciaroni M, et al. Primary and secondary prevention of ischemic stroke. *Eur Neurol* 2010;63(5):267–78.

*Pfeffer MA, et al. Cholesterol and Recurrent Events: a secondary prevention trial for normolipidemic patients. CARE Investigators. *Am J Cardiol* 1995;76(9):98C-106C.

Postuma RB, et al. Markers of neurodegeneration in idiopathic REM sleep behavior disorder and Parkinson disease. *Brain* 2009;132:3298–307.

*PROGRESS Collaborative Group. Randomised trial of a perindopril-based blood-pressure-lowering regimen among 6,105 individuals with previous stroke or transient ischaemic attack. *Lancet* 2001;358(9287):1033–41.

Ramachandran N, et al. The autosomal recessively inherited progressive myoclonus epilepsies and their genes. *Epilepsia* 2009;50(Suppl 5):29–36.

*SPACE Collaborative Group. 30 day results from the SPACE trial of stent-protected angioplasty versus carotid endarterectomy in symptomatic patients: a randomised non-inferiority trial. *Lancet* 2006;368(9543):1239–47.

Tang SC, et al. Management of stroke in pregnancy and the puerperium. *Expert Rev Neurother* 2010;10(2):205–15.

Testai FD, et al. Inherited metabolic disorders and stroke part 2: homocystinuria, organic acidurias, and urea cycle disorders. *Arch Neurol* 2010;67(2):148–53.

*Toole JF, et al. Lowering homocysteine in patients with ischemic stroke to prevent recurrent stroke, myocardial infarction, and death: the Vitamin Intervention for Stroke Prevention (VISP) randomized controlled trial. *JAMA* 2004;291(5):565–75.

Yenari MA, et al. Therapeutic hypothermia for brain ischemia: where have we come and where do we go? *Stroke* 2010;41(10 Suppl):S72–4.

Young JL, et al. Psychiatric considerations in patients with decreased levels of consciousness. *Emerg Med Clin North Am* 2010;28(3):595–609.

Chapter 3: Infectious Diseases

*Antinori A, et al. Diagnosis of AIDS-related focal brain lesions: a decision-making analysis based on clinical and neuroradiologic characteristics combined with polymerase chain reaction assays in CSF. *Neurology* 1997;48(3):687–94.

Bensalem MK, et al. HIV and the central nervous system. *Compr Ther* 2002;28(1):23–33.

Berger JR. Progressive multifocal leukoencephalopathy. *Curr Neurol Neurosci Rep* 2007;7(6):461–9.

Clifford DB, et al. Natalizumab-associated progressive multifocal leukoencephalopathy in patients with multiple sclerosis: lessons from 28 cases. *Lancet Neurol* 2010;9(4):438–46.

Gilden D, et al. Varicella zoster virus vasculopathies: diverse clinical manifestations, laboratory features, pathogenesis, and treatment. *Lancet Neurol* 2009;8(8):731–40.

*Howard RS, et al. Encephalitis lethargica. A report of four recent cases. *Brain* 1987; 110:19–33.

Maltête D, et al. Movement disorders and Creutzfeldt-Jakob disease: a review. *Parkinsonism Relat Disord* 2006;12(2):65–71.

Revilla FJ, et al. Teaching NeuroImage: oculomasticatory myorhythmia: pathognomonic phenomenology of Whipple disease. *Neurology* 2008;70(6):e25.

Roos KL. Pearls: infectious diseases. *Semin Neurol* 2010;30(1):71–3.

Sanchetee P. Stroke and central nervous system infections. *J Indian Med Assoc* 2009; 107(6):372–7.

*Tan K, et al. Burden of neuroinfectious diseases on the neurology service in a tertiary care center. *Neurology* 2008;71(15):1160–6.

Vilensky JA, et al. A historical analysis of the relationship between encephalitis lethargica and postencephalitic parkinsonism: a complex rather than a direct relationship. *Mov Disord* 2010;25(9):1116–23.

Walker L, et al. Koch's postulates and infectious proteins. *Acta Neuropathol* 2006;112(1): 1–4.

Walker M, et al. Parasitic central nervous system infections in immunocompromised hosts. *Clin Infect Dis* 2005;40(7):1005–15.

Chapter 4: Neurotoxicology

Arora A, et al. Neuroimaging of toxic and metabolic disorders. *Semin Neurol* 2008;28(4): 495–510.

Bolla KI, et al. The neuropsychiatry of chronic cocaine abuse. J Neuropsychiatry *Clin Neurosci* 1998;10(3):280–9.

Bradley WG, et al. Beyond Guam: the cyanobacteria/BMAA hypothesis of the cause of ALS and other neurodegenerative diseases. *Amyotroph Lateral Scler* 2009;10 (Suppl 2):7–20.

De Bleecker J, et al. The intermediate syndrome in organophosphate poisoning: presentation of a case and review of the literature. *J Toxicol Clin Toxicol* 1992;30(3):321–9.

Finkelstein Y, et al. Peaceful use of disastrous neurotoxicants. *Neurotoxicology* 2010; 31(5):608–20.

Goetz CG. Shaking up the Salpetriere: Jean-Martin Charcot and mercury-induced tremor. *Neurology* 2010;74(21):1739–42.

Hillbom M, et al. Seizures in alcohol-dependent patients: epidemiology, pathophysiology and management. *CNS Drugs* 2003;17(14):1013–30.

Hörster F, et al. Disorders of intermediary metabolism: toxic leukoencephalopathies. *J Inherit Metab Dis* 2005;28(3):345–56.

Jackson N. Neuropsychiatric complications of commonly used palliative care drugs. *Postgrad Med J* 2008;84(989):121–6.

Kumar N. Neurologic presentations of nutritional deficiencies. *Neurol Clin* 2010;28(1): 107–70.

Ludolph AC, et al. Toxic models of upper motor neuron disease. *J Neurol Sci* 1996; 139(Suppl):53–9.

Margetić B, et al. Neuroleptic malignant syndrome and its controversies. *Pharmacoepidemiol Drug Saf* 2010;19(5):429–35.

McKeon A, et al. The alcohol withdrawal syndrome. *J Neurol Neurosurg Psychiatry* 2008;79(8):854–62.

Olanow CW. Manganese-induced parkinsonism and Parkinson's disease. *Ann N Y Acad Sci* 2004;1012:209–23.

Sechi G, et al. Wernicke's encephalopathy: new clinical settings and recent advances in diagnosis and management. *Lancet Neurol* 2007;6(5):442–55.

Tokuomi H, et al. Minamata disease (organic mercury poisoning): neuroradiologic and electrophysiologic studies. *Neurology* 1982;32(12):1369–75.

Watters MR. Tropical marine neurotoxins: venoms to drugs. *Semin Neurol* 2005;25(3): 278–89.

Chapter 5: Movement Disorders

Andrade DM, et al. Treatment options for epileptic myoclonus and epilepsy syndromes associated with myoclonus. *Expert Opin Pharmacother* 2009;10(10):1549–60.

Axer H, et al. Falls and gait disorders in geriatric neurology. *Clin Neurol Neurosurg* 2010;112(4):265–74.

Berciano J, et al. Olivopontocerebellar atrophy: toward a better nosological definition. *Mov Disord* 2006;21(10):1607–13.

Boeve BF, et al. Pathophysiology of REM sleep behaviour disorder and relevance to neurodegenerative disease. *Brain* 2007;130(Pt 11):2770–88.

Crompton DE, et al. The borderland of epilepsy: clinical and molecular features of phenomena that mimic epileptic seizures. *Lancet Neurol* 2009;8(4):370–81.

Draganski B, et al. Brain structure in movement disorders: a neuroimaging perspective. *Curr Opin Neurol* 2010;23(4):413–9.

Durr A. Autosomal dominant cerebellar ataxias: polyglutamine expansions and beyond. *Lancet Neurol* 2010;9(9):885–94.

Espay AJ. Management of motor complications in Parkinson disease: current and emerging therapies. *Neurol Clin* 2010;28(4):913–25.

Espay AJ, et al. Lower-body parkinsonism: reconsidering the threshold for external lumbar drainage. *Nat Clin Pract Neurol* 2008;4(1):50–5.

Factor SA, et al. Emergency department presentations of patients with Parkinson's disease. *Am J Emerg Med* 2000;18(2):209–15.

Fogel BL, et al. Clinical features and molecular genetics of autosomal recessive cerebellar ataxias. *Lancet Neurol* 2007;6(3):245–57.

Galpern WR, et al. Interface between tauopathies and synucleinopathies: a tale of two proteins. *Ann Neurol* 2006;59(3):449–58.

Gupta A, et al. Psychogenic movement disorders. *Curr Opin Neurol* 2009;22(4): 430–6.

Idiaquez J, et al. Autonomic and cognitive dysfunction in Parkinson's disease. *Clin Auton Res* 2007;17(2):93–8.

Klein C, et al. Hereditary parkinsonism: Parkinson disease look-alikes—an algorithm for clinicians to "PARK" genes and beyond. *Mov Disord* 2009;24(14):2042–58.

Kleiner-Fisman G, et al. Subthalamic nucleus deep brain stimulation: summary and meta-analysis of outcomes. *Mov Disord* 2006;21(Suppl 14):S290–304.

Klockgether T. Sporadic ataxia with adult onset: classification and diagnostic criteria. *Lancet Neurol* 2010;9(1):94–104.

Lang AE. When and how should treatment be started in Parkinson disease? *Neurology* 2009;72(7 Suppl):S39–43.

Leehey MA. Fragile X-associated tremor/ataxia syndrome: clinical phenotype, diagnosis, and treatment. *J Investig Med* 2009;57(8):830–6.

Louis ED. Essential tremors: a family of neurodegenerative disorders? *Arch Neurol* 2009;66(10):1202–8.

Mehta SH, et al. Paraneoplastic movement disorders. *Curr Neurol Neurosci Rep* 2009; 9(4):285–91.

Moro E, et al. Criteria for deep-brain stimulation in Parkinson's disease: review and analysis. *Expert Rev Neurother* 2006;6(11):1695–705.

Poston KL, et al. Movement disorder emergencies. *J Neurol* 2008;255(Suppl 4):2–13.

Postuma RB, et al. Hemiballism: revisiting a classic disorder. *Lancet Neurol* 2003;2(11): 661–8.

Ravina B, et al. The role of radiotracer imaging in Parkinson disease. *Neurology* 2005;64(2):208–15.

Schneider SA, et al. Complicated recessive dystonia parkinsonism syndromes. *Mov Disord* 2009;24(4):490–9.

Schneider SA, et al. Rare causes of dystonia parkinsonism. *Curr Neurol Neurosci Rep* 2010;10(6):431–9.

Schneider SA, et al. Secondary dystonia–clinical clues and syndromic associations. *Eur J Neurol* 2010;17(Suppl 1):52–7.

Schneider SA, et al. The Huntington's disease-like syndromes: what to consider in patients with a negative Huntington's disease gene test. *Nat Clin Pract Neurol* 2007; 3(9):517–25.

Shakkottai VG, et al. Physiologic alterations in ataxia: channeling changes into novel therapies. *Arch Neurol* 2009;66(10):1196–201.

Sitburana O, et al. Brain magnetic resonance imaging (MRI) in parkinsonian disorders. *Parkinsonism Relat Disord* 2009;15(3):165–74.

Swedo SE, et al. Streptococcal infection, Tourette syndrome, and OCD: is there a connection? PANDAS: horse or zebra? *Neurology* 2010;74(17):1397–8.

Wadia PM, et al. The many faces of corticobasal degeneration. *Parkinsonism Relat Disord* 2007;13(Suppl 3):S336–40.

Walker RH, et al. Neurologic phenotypes associated with acanthocytosis. *Neurology* 2007;68(2):92–8.

Wild EJ, et al. Huntington's disease phenocopy syndromes. *Curr Opin Neurol* 2007;20(6):681–7.

Zadikoff C, et al. The 'essentials' of essential palatal tremor: a reappraisal of the nosology. *Brain* 2006;129:832–40.

Chapter 6: Behavioral Neurology

Charles RF, et al. Posterior cortical atrophy: clinical presentation and cognitive deficits compared to Alzheimer's disease. *Behav Neurol* 2005;16(1):15–23.

Ferro JM. Hyperacute cognitive stroke syndromes. *J Neurol* 2001;248(10):841–9.

Geser F, et al. Amyotrophic lateral sclerosis and frontotemporal lobar degeneration: a spectrum of TDP-43 proteinopathies. *Neuropathology* 2010;30(2):103–12.

Grossman M. Primary progressive aphasia: clinicopathological correlations. *Nat Rev Neurol* 2010;6(2):88–97.

Jordan LC, et al. Disorders of speech and language: aphasia, apraxia and dysarthria. *Curr Opin Neurol* 2006;19(6):580–5.

Josephs KA, et al. Apraxia of speech and nonfluent aphasia: a new clinical marker for corticobasal degeneration and progressive supranuclear palsy. *Curr Opin Neurol* 2008;21(6):688–92.

Josephs KA. Frontotemporal dementia and related disorders: deciphering the enigma. *Ann Neurol* 2008;64(1):4–14.

Kelley BJ, et al. Young-onset dementia: demographic and etiologic characteristics of 235 patients. *Arch Neurol* 2008;65(11):1502–8.

Kelley BJ, et al. Rapidly progressive young-onset dementia. *Cogn Behav Neurol* 2009; 22(1):22–7.

Koenigs M, et al. The functional neuroanatomy of depression: distinct roles for ventromedial and dorsolateral prefrontal cortex. *Behav Brain Res* 2009;201(2):239–43.

Ridha B, et al. Young-onset dementia: a practical approach to diagnosis. *Neurologist* 2006;12(1):2–13.

Urwin H, et al. FUS pathology defines the majority of tau- and TDP-43-negative frontotemporal lobar degeneration. *Acta Neuropathol* 2010;120(1):33–41.

*Victor M, et al. The Wernicke-Korsakoff syndrome. A clinical and pathological study of 245 patients, 82 with post-mortem examinations. *Contemp Neurol Ser* 1971;7: 1–206.

Vitali P, et al. Neuroimaging in dementia. *Semin Neurol* 2008;28(4):467–83.

Weintraub and Hurtig. Presentation and management of psychosis in Parkinson's disease and dementia with Lewy bodies. *Am J Psychiatry* 2007;164(10):1491–8.

Wheaton LA, et al. Ideomotor apraxia: a review. *J Neurol Sci* 2007;260(1–2):1–10.

Zadikoff C, et al. Apraxia in movement disorders. *Brain* 2005;128:1480–97.

Chapter 7: Neuro-ophthalmology and Neuro-otology

Alabduljalil T, et al. Paraneoplastic syndromes in neuro-ophthalmology. *Curr Opin Ophthalmol* 2007;18(6):463–9.

Antonio-Santos AA, et al. Pharmacological testing of anisocoria. *Expert Opin Pharmacother* 2005;6(12):2007–13.

*Beck RW, et al. A randomized, controlled trial of corticosteroids in the treatment of acute optic neuritis. The Optic Neuritis Study Group. *N Engl J Med* 1992;326(9): 581–8.

Bhattacharyya N, et al. Clinical practice guideline: benign paroxysmal positional vertigo. *Otolaryngol Head Neck Surg* 2008;139(5 Suppl 4):S47–81.

*Bronstein AM, et al. The neck–eye reflex in patients with reduced vestibular and optokinetic function. *Brain* 1991;114:1–11.

*Jacobs LD, et al. Intramuscular interferon beta-1a therapy initiated during a first demyelinating event in multiple sclerosis. CHAMPS Study Group. *N Engl J Med* 2000;343(13): 898–904.

Jen JC. Bilateral vestibulopathy: clinical, diagnostic, and genetic considerations. *Semin Neurol* 2009;29(5):528–33.

Karatas M. Central vertigo and dizziness: epidemiology, differential diagnosis, and common causes. *Neurologist* 2008;14(6):355–64.

Karatas M. Internuclear and supranuclear disorders of eye movements: clinical features and causes. *Eur J Neurol* 2009;16(12):1265–77.

*Katz B, et al. The optic neuritis treatment trial: implications for clinicians. *Semin Ophthalmol* 1995;10(3):214–20.

Kerber KA. Vertigo and dizziness in the emergency department. *Emerg Med Clin North Am* 2009;27(1):39–50.

Lempert T, et al. Epidemiology of vertigo, migraine and vestibular migraine. *J Neurol* 2009;256(3):333–8.

*Optic Neuritis Study Group. The 5-year risk of MS after optic neuritis. Experience of the optic neuritis treatment trial. *Neurology* 1997;49(5):1404–13.

*Optic Neuritis Study Group. Visual function 15 years after optic neuritis: a final follow-up report from the Optic Neuritis Treatment Trial. *Ophthalmology* 2008;115(6): 1079–82.

Chapter 8: Demyelinating Diseases, Neuro-oncology, and Disorders of Neural Tube Closure and Other Congenital Malformations

Bartynski WS. Posterior reversible encephalopathy syndrome, part 1: fundamental imaging and clinical features. *AJNR Am J Neuroradiol* 2008;29(6):1036–42.

Bartynski WS. Posterior reversible encephalopathy syndrome, part 2: controversies surrounding pathophysiology of vasogenic edema. *AJNR Am J Neuroradiol* 2008;29(6): 1043–9.

Bataller L, et al. Autoimmune limbic encephalitis in 39 patients: immunophenotypes and outcomes. *J Neurol Neurosurg Psychiatry* 2007;78(4):381–5.

Benarroch EE. Aquaporin-4, homeostasis, and neurologic disease. *Neurology* 2007;69(24): 2266–8.

Dale RC, et al. Pediatric central nervous system inflammatory demyelination: acute disseminated encephalomyelitis, clinically isolated syndromes, neuromyelitis optica, and multiple sclerosis. *Curr Opin Neurol* 2009;22(3):233–40.

Dalmau J, et al. Paraneoplastic anti-N-methyl-D-aspartate receptor encephalitis associated with ovarian teratoma. *Ann Neurol* 2007;61(1):25–36.

Dalmau J, et al. Paraneoplastic syndromes of the CNS. *Lancet Neurol* 2008;7(4):327–40.

*Durelli L, et al. Every-other-day interferon beta-1b versus once-weekly interferon beta-1a for multiple sclerosis: results of a 2-year prospective randomised multicentre study (INCOMIN). *Lancet* 2002;359(9316):1453–60.

Espay AJ, et al. Rigidity and spasms from autoimmune encephalomyelopathies: stiff-person syndrome. *Muscle Nerve* 2006;34(6):677–90.

Ferioli S, et al. Anti-N-methyl-D-aspartate receptor encephalitis: characteristic behavioral and movement disorder. *Arch Neurol* 2010;67(2):250–1.

*Gold R, et al. The long-term safety and tolerability of high-dose interferon beta-1a in relapsing-remitting multiple sclerosis: 4-year data from the PRISMS study. *Eur J Neurol* 2005;12(8):649–56.

Graus F, et al. Neuronal surface antigen antibodies in limbic encephalitis: clinical-immunologic associations. *Neurology* 2008;71(12):930–6.

*Jacobs LD, et al. Intramuscular interferon beta-1a therapy initiated during a first demyelinating event in multiple sclerosis. CHAMPS Study Group. *N Engl J Med* 2000 Sep 28; 343(13):898–904.

Jarius S, et al. AQP4 antibodies in neuromyelitis optica: diagnostic and pathogenetic relevance. *Nat Rev Neurol* 2010;6(7):383–92.

*Kappos L, et al. Effect of early versus delayed interferon beta-1b treatment on disability after a first clinical event suggestive of multiple sclerosis: a 3-year follow-up analysis of the BENEFIT study. *Lancet* 2007;370(9585):389–97.

*Kappos L, et al. Long-term effect of early treatment with interferon beta-1b after a first clinical event suggestive of multiple sclerosis: 5-year active treatment extension of the phase 3 BENEFIT trial. *Lancet Neurol* 2009;8(11):987–97.

Köhler W. Leukodystrophies with late disease onset: an update. *Curr Opin Neurol* 2010; 23(3):234–41.

*McDonald WI, et al. Recommended diagnostic criteria for multiple sclerosis: guidelines from the International Panel on the diagnosis of multiple sclerosis. *Ann Neurol* 2001; 50(1):121–7.

Mikol DD, et al. Comparison of subcutaneous interferon beta-1a with glatiramer acetate in patients with relapsing multiple sclerosis (the REbif vs Glatiramer Acetate in Relapsing MS Disease [REGARD] study): a multicentre, randomised, parallel, open-label trial. *Lancet Neurol* 2008;7(10):903–14.

Pittock SJ, et al. Amphiphysin autoimmunity: paraneoplastic accompaniments. *Ann Neurol* 2005;58(1):96–107.

*Polman CH, et al. Diagnostic criteria for multiple sclerosis: 2005 revisions to the "McDonald Criteria." *Ann Neurol* 2005;58(6):840–6.

*Poser CM, et al. The nature of multiple sclerosis. *Clin Neurol Neurosurg* 2004;106(3): 159–71.

*PRISMS Study Group. Randomised double-blind placebo-controlled study of interferon beta-1a in relapsing/remitting multiple sclerosis. PRISMS (Prevention of Relapses and Disability by Interferon beta-1a Subcutaneously in Multiple Sclerosis) Study Group. *Lancet* 1998;352(9139):1498–504.

*Schwid SR, et al. Enhanced benefit of increasing interferon beta-1a dose and frequency in relapsing multiple sclerosis: the EVIDENCE Study. *Arch Neurol* 2005;62(5): 785–92.

Smith AB, et al. Imaging evaluation of demyelinating processes of the central nervous system. *Postgrad Med J* 2010;86(1014):218–29.

Vernino S, et al. Autoimmune encephalopathies. *Neurologist* 2007;13(3):140–7.

Chapter 9: Neuromuscular Disorders

Donofrio PD, et al. Consensus statement: the use of intravenous immunoglobulin in the treatment of neuromuscular conditions report of the AANEM ad hoc committee. *Muscle Nerve* 2009;40(5):890–900.

French CIDP Study Group. Recommendations on diagnostic strategies for chronic inflammatory demyelinating polyradiculoneuropathy. *J Neurol Neurosurg Psychiatry* 2008;79(2):115–8.

Goldstein DS, et al. Neurogenic orthostatic hypotension: a pathophysiological approach. *Circulation* 2009;119(1):139–46.

Hughes RA, et al. Clinical applications of intravenous immunoglobulins in neurology. *Clin Exp Immunol* 2009;158(Suppl 1):34–42.

Low PA, et al. Management of neurogenic orthostatic hypotension: an update. *Lancet Neurol* 2008;7(5):451–8.

Mauermann ML, et al. Pearls and Oy-sters: evaluation of peripheral neuropathies. *Neurology* 2009;72(6):e28–31.

Meriggioli MN, et al. Autoimmune myasthenia gravis: emerging clinical and biological heterogeneity. *Lancet Neurol* 2009;8(5):475–90.

Muppidi S, et al. Muscle-specific receptor tyrosine kinase antibody-positive and seronegative myasthenia gravis. *Front Neurol Neurosci* 2009;26:109–19.

Ochoa JL. Truths, errors, and lies around "reflex sympathetic dystrophy" and "complex regional pain syndrome." *J Neurol* 1999;246(10):875–9.

Panicker JN, et al. The bare essentials: uro-neurology. *Pract Neurol* 2010;10(3):178–85.

Schröder A, et al. Plasmapheresis for neurological disorders. *Expert Rev Neurother* 2009;9(9):1331–9.

Sedel F, et al. Hereditary spastic paraparesis in adults associated with inborn errors of metabolism: a diagnostic approach. *J Inherit Metab Dis* 2007;30(6):855–64.

Tracy JA, et al. Investigations and treatment of chronic inflammatory demyelinating polyradiculoneuropathy and other inflammatory demyelinating polyneuropathies. *Curr Opin Neurol* 2010;23(3):242–8

Vallat JM, et al. An update on nerve biopsy. *J Neuropathol Exp Neurol* 2009;68(8):833–44.

Chapter 10: Psychiatry

Cerullo MA, et al. The functional neuroanatomy of bipolar disorder. *Int Rev Psychiatry* 2009;21(4):314–22.

Danielyan A, et al. Neurological disorders in schizophrenia. *Psychiatr Clin North Am* 2009;32(4):719–57.

Devinsky O. Delusional misidentifications and duplications: right brain lesions, left brain delusions. *Neurology* 2009;72(1):80–7.

LaFrance WC, et al. Psychiatric comorbidities in epilepsy. *Int Rev Neurobiol* 2008;83: 347–83.

LaFrance WC Jr. Somatoform disorders. *Semin Neurol* 2009;29(3):234–46.

Miyasaki JM, et al. Practice Parameter: evaluation and treatment of depression, psychosis, and dementia in Parkinson disease (an evidence-based review): report of the Quality Standards Subcommittee of the American Academy of Neurology. *Neurology* 2006;66(7):996–1002.

Murphy DL, et al. Obsessive-compulsive disorder and its related disorders: a reappraisal of obsessive-compulsive spectrum concepts. *Dialogues Clin Neurosci* 2010;12(2): 131–48.

Nasrallah HA, et al. Iatrogenic disorders associated with conventional vs. atypical antipsychotics. *Ann Clin Psychiatry* 2001;13(4):215–27.

Ravindran LN, et al. The pharmacologic treatment of anxiety disorders: a review of progress. *J Clin Psychiatry* 2010;71(7):839–54.

Strakowski SM, et al. The co-occurrence of bipolar and substance use disorders. *Clin Psychol Rev* 2000;20(2):191–206.

Vuilleumier P. Hysterical conversion and brain function. *Prog Brain Res* 2005;150:309–29.

Wolters ECh, et al. Parkinson's disease-related disorders in the impulsive-compulsive spectrum. *J Neurol* 2008;255(Suppl 5):48–56.

Index

Abducens cranial nerve, viii, 87, 106, 120, 206, 244, 247, 312
Aβ40, 221, 222
Aβ42, 221, 222, 223
Abetalipoproteinemia, 160, 170
Acamprosate, 147
Acanthamoeba, 132
Acanthocytosis-related neurological disorders, 170
Aceruloplasminemia, 169
Acetazolamide, 84, 156, 204
Acetylcholine receptors, vii, 31, 192, 263, 293
Achromatopsia, 212, 236
Acid maltase deficiency, 324, 326
Acquired amyloid neuropathy, 311
Acquired dyslexia, 218
Acquired hepatolenticular degeneration, 149
Acrylamide, 143
Action myoclonus-renal failure syndrome, 92
Acute disseminated encephalomyelitis, vii, 202, 234, 252, 256, 258, 297
Acute dystonic reaction, vii, xiv, 176
Acute intermittent porphyria, 8, 15, 192
Acute transverse myelopathy, vii, 161, 256
Adenylosuccinase deficiency, 6
Adie tonic pupil, 238, 311
Adrenoleukodystrophy, vii, 11, 41, 164, 236
Adult-onset spinal muscular atrophy (SMA type IV), 295
Agenesis of the corpus callosum, 41
Agnosia, 215
Aicardi syndrome, 34, 282
Akinetic mutism, 211
Akinetopsia, 236
Alcoholic cerebellar degeneration, 146, 148
Alexia with agraphia, 236
Alexia without agraphia, 218, 236
Aluminum encephalopathy, 141
Alzheimer's disease, vii, 25, 41, 74, 174, 184, 189, 190, 194, 198, 204, 221, 222, 223, 224, 225, 226, 228, 229, 295, 306, 311, 316, 325, 328
Amaurosis fugax (retinal TIA), 62, 232
Amnesia, vii, 134, 211, 213
Amnestic mild cognitive impairment, 224
Amphetamine, 150
Amphiphysin, 279
Amyloid neuropathies, 311
Amyloid plaques, xi, 198, 221, 222, 225, 251

Amyloid precursor protein, vii, 59, 221, 223
Amyotrophic lateral sclerosis, vii, 28, 228, 229, 294, 295
Analgesic rebound headache, 103
Anaplastic astrocytoma, 267
Andersen-Tawil syndrome, 25, 323
Angelman syndrome, 33, 34, 45, 165
Anorexia nervosa, x
Anterior cerebral artery, vii, 62, 211, 217
Anterior cerebral artery (ACA) syndrome, 62
Anterior choroidal artery (AChA) syndrome, 62
Anterior inferior cerebellar artery (AICA) syndrome, 62
Anterior interosseous neuropathy (Kiloh-Nevin syndrome), 285
Anterior ischemic optic neuropathy, vii, 73, 233, 245
Anticholinergic toxicity, 154
Anticholinergics, 177, 181, 300
Anticoagulation, 52, 124
Antidepressant drugs, iii
Antidepressants, v, xvi, 94, 97
Anti-Hu
    ANNA-1, 241, 264, 277
Anti-NMDA-receptor encephalitis, 264
Antiphospholipid (aPL) antibody syndrome, 51, 73
Antistreptolysin O (ASO), vii, 202
Anti-Ta
    anti-Ma2, 264, 277
Anton syndrome, 215, 236
Anxiety disorders, vi
Apnea test, 100
Apperceptive visual agnosia, 212, 215
Apraxia, 155, 190, 194, 216
Arachnoid cyst, 276, 297
    Posterior fossa CSF collection, 276
Aromatic amino acid decarboxylase (AADC) deficiency, 174
Arsenic poisoning, 141
Arteritic AION, 233
Arylsulfatase A, 41
Ascending reticular activating system, vii, 98, 99
Aseptic meningitis, 73, 115
Aspergillus, 131
Associative visual agnosia, 215

Ataxia, v, vii, 13, 40, 47, 138, 140, 159, 160, 161, 162, 167, 175, 324
    Wernicke encephalopathy, v, 40, 140, 159, 160, 162, 167, 175
Ataxia-ocular motor apraxia 1, vii, 155, 161
Ataxia-ocular motor apraxia 2, vii, 161
Ataxia-telangiectasia, vii, 161, 175
Atlantoaxial instability, 14, 34, 175, 280, 297, 298
Atlantoaxial subluxation and instability, 43, 298
Attentional or sensory neglect, 219
Atypical absence seizures, 76
Auditory agnosia, 212, 215
Autism, 6, 29
Autoimmune channelopathies, 263
Autoimmune encephalopathies, 264, 277
Autosomal dominant nocturnal frontal lobe epilepsy, 26
Axonal polyneuropathies, 301
Azathioprine, 260

Baclofen, 27, 93, 177
Balint syndrome, 63, 212, 229, 236
Baltic myoclonus (Unverricht-Lundborg disease), 90
Baroreflex failure, 304
Becker muscular dystrophy, 313, 329
Beevor's sign, 318
Behavioral variant of frontotemporal dementia, 227
Behçet disease, 44, 115, 258
Benedikt syndrome, 63
Benign childhood epilepsy with centrotemporal spikes (benign rolandic epilepsy), 76, 91
Benign familial neonatal seizures, 26
Benign myoclonic epilepsy of infancy, 91
Benign paroxysmal positional vertigo, vii, 247, 248
Benzodiazepines, vii, 27, 97, 220
Bielschowsky head tilt test, 240
Bilateral INO, 244
Bilateral ventral pontine syndrome (Locked-in syndrome), 63
Biotinidase deficiency, 37, 43, 156
Bipolar disorder, v
Bismuth encephalopathy, 129, 141
Blastomycosis, 131
Bloch-Sulzberger syndrome (Incontinentia Pigmenti), 47
Bobble-head doll syndrome, 205
Body dysmorphic disorder (dysmorphobia), xvi
Botulism, 136, 192
Brachial neuropathies, 285

Brachial plexopathies, 284
Brachial plexus, 88, 305
Brain death, 100
Brainstem auditory evoked potentials, 87
Branching enzyme deficiency (Andersen disease, glycogenosis type IV), 324
Brevetoxin, 144
Bromocriptine, 154
Bruns nystagmus, 243
Buckthorn poisoning, 138
Bulimia nervosa, x
Buprenorphine, 152
Buspirone, vi, 18
Butorphanol, 102, 103

CADASIL, vii, 48, 70, 71, 258
Call-Fleming syndrome, 105
Calpain, 314
Canavan's disease, 35, 41, 43, 44
Candida, 131
Capgras syndrome, xiii
Carbamazepine, v, vii, 106, 240, 327
Carbohydrate-deficient glycoprotein syndromes, 167
Carbon disulfide, 143
Carbon monoxide, viii, 44, 134, 142, 166, 167
Cardiomyopathy, 5, 311, 313, 324
Carnitine palmitoyl transferase deficiency, 5
Carnitine palmitoyl transferase II deficiency, 321, 322
Carotid endarterectomy, vii, 56
Carpal tunnel syndrome, viii
Cataplexy, 95
Catecholamine deficiency, 16
Celiac disease, 168, 207
Central core disease, 25, 328, 329
Central neurocytoma, 270
Central nystagmus, 242
Central pontine myelinolysis, viii, 19, 148, 208
Central retinal artery occlusion, viii, 233
Cerebellar ataxia with bilateral vestibulopathy, 251
Cerebral amyloid angiopathy, vii, 49, 59, 201, 222, 225
Cerebral autoregulation, 304
Cerebral autosomal dominant arteriopathy with subcortical infarcts and leukoencephalopathy, vii, 48, 70, 71, 258
Cerebral Malaria, 123, 132
Cerebral neuroblastoma, 270
Cerebrotendinous xanthomatosis, 163
Ceruloplasmin, viii
Chagas Disease, 124
Channelopathies, 25, 26, 159

Charcot-Marie-Tooth, vii, 306, 307
Charles Bonnet syndrome, xiii
Chediak-Higashi syndrome, 161
Chédiak-Higashi syndrome, 47
Chiari malformation, 35, 105, 107, 166, 175, 242, 280
Childhood absence epilepsy, 76
Childhood ataxia with diffuse central nervous system hypomyelination, 160, 163
Childhood epilepsy with occipital paroxysms, 76
Chorea, 6, 142, 165, 170, 200
Chorea-acanthocytosis (neuroacanthocytosis), 170, 175
Choroid plexus carcinoma, 269
Chronic inflammatory demyelinating polyneuropathy, vii, 187, 292, 302, 305, 308, 309
Chronic progressive external ophthalmoplegia, viii, 38, 39, 317, 318
Ciguatera, 144
Cladribine, 260
Claude syndrome, 63
Clonazepam, vii, viii, 96, 177, 205
Clonidine, 17, 152, 191, 193, 209
Cluster headache, 105
CNS Paraneoplastic disorders, 44, 168, 325
  Anti-Hu, 277, 278
  Anti-recoverin, 277
  Anti-Ri, 277
  Anti-Yo, 277
  CRMP-5, 44, 264, 277
  Hypoventilation, 325
  Opsoclonus-myoclonus, 277
  Paraneoplastic cerebellar degeneration, 168, 277
  Paraneoplastic encephalomyelitis, 277
  Psychosis, i, xi, 134
  Rhomboencephalitis, 277
Cobalamin
  Vitamin B12, vii, 1, 2, 8, 9, 44, 51, 55, 141, 142, 156, 235, 258, 278, 301, 302
Cocaine, 17, 145, 150
Coccidioidomycosis, 131
cock walk, 135
Cockayne syndrome, 43, 162
Colloid cyst, 276
Colpocephaly, 280
Complex regional pain syndrome, 303
Conduction aphasia, 212, 217
Congenital ataxic disorders, 166
Congenital disorders of glycosylation, 167
Congenital muscular dystrophies, 315
Congenital myopathies, 31, 316, 328, 330
Congenital myotonic dystrophy, 317

Conversion disorder, xv
Corticobasal degeneration, 194, 198, 228
Corticobasal syndrome, 190
Cowden syndrome, 270
Cowdry type A, 111, 130
Cowdry type B, 130, 198
Coxibs, 104
Cramps, 321, 323
Craniolacunia, 280
Craniopharyngioma, 275
Creatine kinase, vii, 5, 21, 154, 161, 170, 313, 314, 315, 316, 319, 320, 321, 322, 330
Creutzfeldt-Jakob disease, vii, 44, 72, 128, 133, 141, 175, 209, 229, 236, 264, 294
Critical illness myopathy, 330
Critical illness polyneuropathy, 330
Cryoglobulinemia, 73, 310
Cryptococcal meningitis, 117
Cryptococcus, 131
CSF hypotension, 105
Curare, 137
Cyclophosphamide, 260
Cyclothymic disorder, ii
Cytochrome oxidase, viii, 4, 40, 44, 223
Cytomegalovirus, vii, 33, 109, 110, 111, 117, 129, 130, 234, 255, 282, 298
Cytotoxic edema, 60, 261

Dandy-Walker malformation, 35, 166, 280, 281, 282
Dantrolene, 329
Deafness, 14, 33, 156, 175
Debrancher deficiency (Cori-Forbes disease), 324
Deep dyslexia, 218
Delirium (a.k.a., acute confusional state, toxic-metabolic encephalopathy), v, 220
Delusional disorder, xiii
Dementia with Lewy bodies, viii, 129, 184, 191, 193, 196, 199, 221, 226, 228, 229
Demyelinating transverse myelitis, 298
Depersonalization disorder, xvii
Depression, ii, x, 151, 173
Dermatomyositis, 319
DeSanctis-Cacchione syndrome, 162
Desmin distal myopathy, 316, 328
Desmin-related myopathies, 328
Desmoplastic infantile ganglioglioma, 271
Detrusor areflexia, 299
Detrusor hyperreflexia, 299, 300
Detrusor-sphincter dyssynergia, 299
Dexamethasone, 102, 103, 115

Dialysis encephalopathy, 92
Diazepam, vii
Diffuse astrocytomas, 267
Dihydroergotamine, 102, 103, 105
Disseminated intravascular coagulation, viii, 33, 74, 75
Dissociative amnesia, xvii
Dissociative disorder, xvii
Dissociative fugue (Poriomania), xvii
Dissociative identity disorder (multiple personality disorder), xvii
Distal Acquired Demyelinating Symmetric neuropathy (DADS), 292
Distal myopathies, 316
Dix-Hallpike test, 248
Dizziness, iii, 247
DMSA (Meso-2,3-dimercaptosuccinic acid), viii, 139, 140
Domoic acid poisoning, 144
Dopamine deficiency, 16, 178
Dopamine depletors, 176, 177
Dopamine receptor blocking agents, viii, xiv, 175, 176
Dopa-responsive dystonia-parkinsonism (Segawa syndrome), 174, 185
Dorsal midbrain syndrome (Parinaud syndrome), 63, 244
Doublecortin, 282
Down syndrome, 34, 298
    Atlantoaxial instability, 34
Downbeat nystagmus, 242
Drug-induced lymphocytic pleocytosis, 115
Drug-induced parkinsonism, xiv, 197
Dry beriberi, 148
Duane retraction syndrome, 240
Duchenne muscular dystrophy, viii, 313, 329
Dysautonomia, 307, 311
Dysembryoplastic neuroepithelial tumor, 271
Dystonia, 157, 171, 173, 195
Dystonic tremor, 188
DYT1 (Oppenheim's dystonia, generalized primary torsion dystonia), 172, 314
DYT13, 172, 184
DYT2, 172
DYT4 (Whispering dysphonia), 172
DYT6, 172
DYT7 (familial cervical dystonia), 172

Early infantile myoclonic encephalopathy (Ohtahara syndrome), 93
Early onset cerebellar ataxia of Holmes' type, 160
Early onset cerebellar ataxia with retained tendon reflexes, 155, 160
Eastern equine encephalitis, 110, 116
Electrolyte derangements, 19

Emerin, 313
Emery-Dreifuss syndrome, 313
Encephalopathy, 3, 19, 73, 139, 156
Enhanced physiologic tremor, 188
Envenomations, 138
Ependymal tumors, 269
Ependymoma, 297
Epidural abscess, 297, 298
Epileptic encephalopathies, 93
Episodic Ataxia type 1, 159
Episodic Ataxia type 2, 159
Episodic ataxias, 159
Epley maneuver, 248
Epstein Barr virus, viii, 73, 110, 111, 115, 118, 234, 255, 256, 274, 298
Epstein-Barr virus, 110, 117
Essential palatal tremor, 188
Essential tremor, viii, 180, 187, 188
Ethyl mercury, 140
Ethylene glycol, 143
Evans ratio, 197

Fabry disease (Anderson-Fabry disease), 12, 44, 47, 301, 302
Facial synkinesis, 206
Facioscapulohumeral dystrophy, viii, 316, 318
Factitious disorder (Munchausen syndrome), xv
Familial amyloidotic polyneuropathy, 311
Familial hemiplegic migraine, 48, 101
Familial infantile myasthenia, 31
Familial periodic paralysis, 323
FAPED (autosomal dominant familial acanthocytosis with paroxysmal exertion-induced dyskinesias and epilepsy), 170
Fatal familial insomnia, 128
Fatty acid oxidation disorder
    Very-long-chain acyl-CoA dehydrogenase deficiency, 322
Febrile seizures, 78
Femoral neuropathy, 288
Ferritin, 169
Fetal alcohol syndrome, viii, 33, 149
Fibrillary astrocytoma, 267
Fludrocortisone, 191, 304
FMR1, 187
Foix-Chavany-Marie syndrome (opercular syndrome), 111
Fosphenytoin, 83
Fragile X syndrome, 35
Fragile X-associated tremor/ataxia syndrome, viii, 187
Fregoli syndrome, xiii
Friedreich Ataxia, 160
Frontal Assessment Battery, viii, 230

Frontotemporal dementia and Parkinsonism linked to chromosome 17, 198, 227, 228
Frontotemporal lobar degeneration, 227
Fukuyama congenital muscular dystrophy, 315
Fukuyama muscular dystrophy, 31, 282, 315

$GABA_A$ receptors, 27
$GABA_B$ receptors, 27
$GABA_C$ receptors, 27
Galactosialidosis, 13
Galloway–Mowat syndrome, 92
Gamma-aminobutyric acid, 27, 34, 80, 93, 97, 137, 147, 178, 279, 327
Gamma-aminobutyric acid (GABA), 27
Gamma-hydroxybutyric acid, viii, 147
Gangliocytoma, 270
Ganglioglioma, 271
Gaucher disease, 12, 91, 184, 185, 186, 241
Gaze-evoked nystagmus, 243
Gemistocytic astrocytoma, 267
Generalized anxiety disorder, vi
Generalized epilepsy with febrile seizures plus, viii, 26
Generalized epilepsy with febrile seizures plus (GEFS+), viii, 26
Gephyrin, 279
Germinoma, 275
Gerstmann-Sträussler-Scheinker disease, 128
Giant-cell arteritis, viii, 233, 245
Glasgow coma scale, 59, 98
Glatiramer acetate (Copaxone), 259
Glucocerebrosidase, 12, 184
Glucocorticoids, 260
Glutamate antagonists, 21, 191
  Ketamine, 134
  Magnesium, 21
  MK801, 28
  PCP, x, 28, 117, 134, 151
  Phencyclidine, x, 151
  Zinc, 141, 208
Glutamate receptor, viii, 3, 263
Glutamate receptors, 28, 80, 134, 146, 147, 151, 178, 181, 183, 225, 263, 264, 277
  AMPA, 28, 80, 134, 137, 263, 277
  Kainate, 28, 134
  NMDA, 178, 181, 183
Glutaric acid, 4, 11, 35, 36, 43, 44, 175
Glutaric aciduria type I, 4, 11, 36, 44
Glutaric aciduria type II, 11, 44
Glycine encephalopathy, 10
Glycogenosis, 44, 322, 324
Glycogenosis type V (McArdle disease, myophosphorylase deficiency), 322

GM_1 gangliosidosis, 12
GM_2 Gangliosidosis, 12, 44, 163
Gorlin syndrome, 272
Guillain-Barré syndrome, 15, 19, 73, 138, 143, 192, 291, 302, 307, 330
Guillain-Mollaret triangle, 111, 188
Gyromitrin mushroom poisoning, 138

Hallucinogens, 151
Hemangioblastoma, 273, 297
Hemangiopericytoma, 273
Hemifacial spasm, 205
Hemolytic uremic syndrome, 74
Hepatic encephalopathy, 149
Hereditary geniospasm, 187
Hereditary hemorrhagic telangiectasia, 47
Hereditary inclusion body myopathy, 316
Hereditary neuropathy with liability to pressure palsies (HNPP), 305
Hereditary spastic paraparesis, ix, 42, 73, 134, 258, 295, 296
Hereditary spastic paraplegia, ix, 42, 73, 134, 258, 295, 296
Heroin, 152
Herpes encephalitis, ix, 213, 214
Herpes simplex virus, ix, 111
Herpes virus, ix, 33, 111, 130, 213, 298
Heterotopias, 282
Histoplasmosis, 117, 131
Holmes-Adie syndrome, 192, 238
Holoprosencephaly, ix, 281
Homer Wright rosettes, 270
Homocystinuria, 2, 8, 175
Horizontal diplopia, 239
Horizontal gaze palsy, 231, 244
Horner syndrome, 62, 192, 233, 237, 240, 248, 284
Human herpes virus type 6, 110, 115, 255, 258
Huntington disease, 129, 134, 170, 201
Huntington disease-like 2, 170, 201
Hurler, 12, 14, 41, 43
Hurler phenotype, 14
Hydrocephalus, 14, 35, 269, 280
Hydroxykynurenuria, 10
Hyperammonemia, 7, 37, 149
Hypercalcemia, 22, 107
Hyperekplexia, 205
Hyperhomocysteinemia, 1, 51
Hyperkalemia, 21
Hyperkalemic periodic paralysis, ix, 25, 323, 326
Hypermagnesemia, 23
Hypermetric saccades, 241
Hypernatremia, 19
Hyperphenylalaninemia, 8, 174

Hyperphosphatemia, 23
Hypertryptophanemia, 10
Hyperventilation, 7, 165, 247
Hypnagogic hallucinations, 95
Hypocalcemia, 22
Hypocalcemic tetany, 327
Hypoceruloplasminemia, 169
Hypochondriasis, xvi
Hypoglycorrhachia, 109, 122
Hypokalemia, x, 21
Hypokalemic periodic paralysis type ix, 1,
      25, 323
Hypomagnesemia, 23, 101
Hypomelanosis of Ito, 47
Hypometric saccades, 241
Hyponatremia, 20, 81
Hypoparathyroidism, 196
Hypophosphatemia, 23
Hypoprebetalipoproteinemia,
      acanthocytosis, retinitis pigmentosa
      and pallidal degeneration, viii,
      169, 170
Hypoventilation, 325
Hypoxia, 213
      Amnesia, 213

Ideational or conceptual apraxia, 216
Ideomotor apraxia, 212, 216
Idiopathic intracranial hypertension
      (pseudotumor cerebri), 35, 106
IgM-MGUS neuropathy, 309
Inclusion body myositis, 294, 316, 320, 326
Incontinentia pigmenti, 47
Infantile botulism, 31
Infectious transverse myelitis, 298
Inflammatory myopathies, 316, 319
Intentional or motor neglect, 219
Interferon beta (IFNβ), 259
Internuclear ophthalmoplegia, ix, 244
Interstitial nucleus of Cajal, 243, 244
Intracerebral hemorrhage, ix, 19, 47, 49, 52,
      53, 59, 225, 258
Intracerebral hemorrhage (ICH), ix, 49, 59
Intravascular lymphomatosis, 72
Intravenous immunoglobulin, ix, 260, 295,
      319
Inverse Marcus Gunn phenomenon
      (Marin Amat syndrome), 206
Iron deficiency, 135, 203
Isopropyl alcohol, 143
Isotope cisternography, 197
Isovaleric acidemia, 9

JC virus, 117, 122, 130
Joubert syndrome, 166, 167, 282
      Posterior fossa CSF collection, 166, 167

Juvenile absence epilepsy, 76
Juvenile myoclonic epilepsy, ix, 76, 90, 91,
      325

KCNQ2, 26
KCNQ3, 26
Ketotic hyperglycinemia, 10
Kinsbourne syndrome, 241
Kleine-Levin syndrome, 95
Klinefelter, 165
Klippel-Feil anomaly, 14, 175, 280, 297, 298
      Atlantoaxial instability, 175
Korsakoff amnestic syndrome, ix, 129, 141,
      148, 213
Korsakoff syndrome
      Thiamine
            Wernicke encephalopathy, 213
Krabbe disease, 13, 41, 43, 305

L-5-hydroxytryptophan, 93
Lactate, 3, 40, 156, 321
Lafora bodies, 90
Lafora disease, 90
Laforin, 90
Laing distal myopathy, 316
Lambert-Brody syndrome, 326
Lambert-Eaton myasthenic syndrome, ix, 23,
      136, 263, 278
Lamin A/C, 313, 314
Landau-Kleffner syndrome, 93
Large-fiber axonal sensory polyneuropathy,
      301
Late-life migraine accompaniments, 72
Lateral medullary syndrome (Wallenberg
      syndrome), 63
Lathyrism, 137, 295
Latrotoxins, 138
Lead poisoning, 139
Leber hereditary optic neuropathy, ix, 4, 38,
      39, 175, 235
Leigh syndrome, ix, 36, 39, 40, 43, 44, 134,
      148, 165, 175, 203, 294, 295
Lennox-Gastaut syndrome, 45, 93
Leptomeningeal carcinomatosis, 115
Lesch-Nyhan syndrome, 6, 175
Levodopa, 177, 181, 183, 203, 226
Levodopa-induced dyskinesias, 183
Lewis-Sumner syndrome, 292
Lhermitte syndrome, xiii
LHON
      Leber hereditary optic neuropathy, 39, 235
Light-near dissociation, 238
Limb-girdle muscular dystrophies, 314
Limb-kinetic apraxia, 216
Lipoma, 276, 297
LIS1 gene, 282

Lissencephaly, 282
Lisuride, 93
Locked-in syndrome, 63, 148
Lorazepam, vii, 83
Lower plexus paralysis (Dejerine-Klumpke),
    284
LS
    Leigh syndrome, 36, 39, 40, 43, 44, 165,
        175
Lyme disease (neuroborreliosis), 73, 109, 121,
    206, 234, 258, 302
Lysine, 10
Lysosomal disorders, 12, 14, 35, 41, 44, 91
Lytico-Bodig, 137

Machado-Joseph disease (SCA 3), 195
Macrocephaly, 35
Magnesium, 21
Maintenance of wakefulness test, 96
Malignant hyperthermia, 25, 154, 329
Malignant peripheral nerve sheath tumor, 312
Malingering, xv, xvi
Mania, v
Mannitol, 60, 139, 144
Maple syrup urine disease, ix, 41, 44, 156
Marchiafava-Bignami disease, 148
Marcus Gunn jaw winking, 206
Marijuana, 145, 151
Marine biotoxins, 144
Marinesco-Sjögren Syndrome, 160, 162
Markesbery-Griggs/Udd distal myopathy, 316
Martin-Gruber anastomosis, 285
May and White syndrome, 92
McArdle disease (myophosphorylase
        deficiency), 31, 322
MCP sign, 187
MeCP2, 34, 165
    Rett syndrome, 34, 165
Medial inferior pontine syndrome, 63
Medial medullary syndrome, 63
Medial midpontine syndrome, 63
Median neuropathy, 190, 284, 285
Mediterranean myoclonus (Ramsay-Hunt
        Syndrome), 90
Medulloblastoma, 272
Medulloepithelioma, 272
Megaloblastic anemia, 2, 156
MELAS
    Mitochondrial encephalomyopathy, lactic
        acidosis, and stroke-like episodes,
        325
Melatonin-receptor agonists, 97
Meningioma, 273, 297
Menkes kinky hair disease
        (trichopoliodystrophy), 4, 43,
        164, 166

Meperidine, 102, 103, 152
Mercury vapor, 140
MERRF
    Myoclonus epilepsy with ragged-red fibers,
        39, 325
Metachromatic leukodystrophy, ix, 13, 41, 43,
        44, 160, 175, 305
Methadone, 103, 152
Methotrexate, 260
Methyl bromide toxicity, 142
3,4-methylenedioxy-meth-amphetamine
        (MDMA, Ecstasy), ix, 150, 154
Methyl mercury, 140
Methylcobalamin, ix
Methylmalonic academia, 9, 10, 44
Methylmalonic aciduria, 2
Methylphenidate, 150, 209
Metoclopramide, 102
Midazolam, vii, 83
Middle cerebral artery, ix, 52, 59, 62, 211,
        212, 217, 235
Middle cerebral artery (MCA) syndrome, 62
Migraine
    Stroke mimickers, 48, 72, 101, 104, 232, 248
Migraine equivalent of middle age, 72
Migraine Prophylaxis, 104
Migraine with aura, 101
Migraine without aura, 101
Mild cognitive impairment, 224
Miller-Dieker syndrome, 34, 282
Miller-Fisher syndrome, 155, 168, 291
Mitochondrial DNA, ix, 4, 38, 39, 40, 325
Mitochondrial encephalomyopathy, lactic
        acidosis, and stroke-like episodes,
        ix, 4, 38, 39, 43, 44, 48, 175, 258,
        325
Mitoxantrone (Novantrone), 259
Mixed ganglioneuronal tumors, 271
Mixed transcortical aphasia, 217
Miyoshi distal myopathy, 314, 316
MLD
    Metachromatic leukodystrophy, 175
Modafinil, 95
Monoclonal gammopathy of unknown
        significance, ix, 292, 309, 310
Monoclonal gammopathy of unknown
        significance (MGUS), ix, 309
Monomelic amyotrophy, 295
Morquio syndrome, 14, 298
Morvan syndrome, 263, 264
Motor axonal polyneuropathy, 301
Motor neuron disease, ix, 190
Motor neuron syndrome, 278
Moyamoya disease, 44, 46
MSUD
    Maple syrup urine disease, 44

mtDNA
  Mitochondrial DNA, 4, 38, 39, 40, 325
Mucopolysaccharidoses, 14, 35
Mucopolysaccharidosis type III (Sanfilippo
    Syndrome), 14
Mucopolysaccharidosis type IV, 14
  Morquio syndrome
    Klippel-Feil anomaly
      Atlantoaxial instability, 14
Mucopolysaccharidosis type IV (Morquio
    Syndrome), 14
Mucopolysaccharidosis type VI (Maroteaux-
    Lamy Syndrome), 14
Mucormycosis, 131
Multifocal Acquired Demyelinating Sensory
    and Motor neuropathy (MADSAM),
    292
Multifocal motor neuropathy, 294, 295
Multiple carboxylase deficiency, 156
Multiple myeloma, 308, 310
Multiple sclerosis, ix, 1, 41, 95, 115, 122, 154,
    175, 188, 234, 236, 252, 253, 255,
    256, 258, 259, 260, 294, 295, 297,
    298, 299, 327
Multiple sleep latency test, 95, 96
Multiple system atrophy, 191, 192, 199
Muscle-specific kinase, ix, 263, 293
Muscular dystrophies, 31, 313
Myasthenia gravis, 134, 293, 330
Myasthenic crisis, 293
Mycophenolate mofetil, 260
Mydriasis, 154, 192
Myelopathy, 304
Myoclonic encephalopathies, 90, 207
Myoclonus, ix, 38, 39, 92, 157, 173, 207, 325
Myoclonus epilepsy with ragged-red fibers,
    ix, 4, 38, 39, 43, 90, 175, 325
Myoclonus-dystonia, 173
Myophosphorylase deficiency, 3, 321
Myotonia, 25, 323, 326, 329
Myotonia congenital, 25, 326, 329
Myotonic dystrophy, 35, 316, 317, 329, 330
Myotubular myopathy, 328
Myxopapillary ependymoma, 269, 300

N-acetylcysteine, 93, 135
Naloxone, 152
Narcolepsy, 95
NARP
  Neuropathy, ataxia, and retinitis
    pigmentosa, 39, 40
nDNA
  Nuclear DNA, 4
Neglect, 212, 218, 219
Neglect dyslexia, 218
Negri bodies, 111, 130

Nemaline rod myopathy, 328
Neurocysticercosis, 123
Neurodegeneration with brain iron
    accumulation type 1, ix, 91, 169,
    191, 199, 201
Neurodegeneration with brain iron
    accumulation type 2, ix, 169
Neuroferritinopathy, ix, 169, 175
Neurofibrillary tangles, x, 128, 189, 198, 221,
    222, 225, 228
Neurofibroma, 297, 312
Neurofibromatosis, 46
Neuroleptic drugs, x, xiv, 154
Neuroleptic malignant syndrome, iv, x, xiv,
    154
Neuromyelitis optica, x, 252, 256
Neuromyotonia (Isaac's syndrome), 278, 327
Neuronal ceroid lipofuscinosis, ix, 34, 44,
    90, 175
Neuronal tumors, 270
Neuropathy, ataxia, and retinitis pigmentosa,
    ix, 4, 38, 39, 40
Neurosarcoidosis, 115, 125
Neurosyphilis, 117, 120, 258
n-Hexane, 134, 143
Nicotinic channel, 26
Niemann-Pick disease, 13, 189
Nitrous oxide, x, 142, 244, 329
NKH
  Nonketotic hyperglycinemia, 10
NMDA receptors, 28, 80, 134, 146, 147, 151,
    178, 181, 183, 225, 264, 277
NMO-IgG, 256
Nodular heterotopias, 282
Nonaka distal myopathy, 316
Non-arteritic AION, 233
Nonbenzodiazepine benzodiazepine-receptor
    agonists, 97
Nonketotic hyperglycinemia, x, 41
Norepinephrine, 16, 17, iii, iv
Normal pressure hydrocephalus, 197
Normeperidine, 145
Notch3 gene, 48, 70, 71
Nuclear DNA, ix, 4
Nucleotide metabolism defects
  Myoadenylate deaminase deficiency, 321,
    322
Nucleus raphe interpositus, x, 241
Nystagmus, 42, 160, 169, 242, 248

Object agnosia, 236
Obstructive sleep apnea, 96
Obturator neuropathy, 288
Ocular bobbing, 244
Ocular dipping, 244
Ocular neuromyotonia, 240

Oculocerebrorenal syndrome (Lowe syndrome), 31, 41
Oculomasticatory myorhythmia, 126, 129
Oculomotor (third nerve), viii, 63, 120, 231, 244
Oculomotor nerve palsy, 240
Oculopalatal tremor, 188
Oculopharyngeal muscular dystrophy, 316, 318
Oligoclonal bands, x, 125, 253, 256, 258, 298
Oligodendrogliomas, 268
One-and-a-half syndrome, 244
Optic neuritis, x, 234, 256
Organic acidurias, 5, 9, 10, 34, 37, 44
Organophosphate poisoning, 142
Orthostatic hypotension, x, 134, 192, 193, 247, 304, iii
Orthostatic tremor, x, 188, 212, 291
Oscillopsia, 251
Osler-Weber-Rendu disease (hereditary hemorrhagic telangiectasia), 47
Osteosclerotic myeloma, 308, 310
Overgrowth syndromes, 35

Paired helical filaments, x, 189, 221
Palatal tremor, 158
Panic disorder, vi, 248
Pappenheimer bodies, 164
Paramedian pontine reticular formation, x, 241
Paramyotonia congenita, x, 25, 299, 323, 326
Paraneoplastic limbic encephalitis, x, 44, 129, 263, 264
Paraproteinemic neuropathies, 308
Parinaud syndrome, 63, 244
PARK1, 184, 185
PARK2, 184
PARK3, 185
PARK5, 185
PARK6, 184
PARK7, 172, 184
PARK8, 184, 185
PARK9, 184
Parkinsonism, 16, 114, 116, 126, 129, 157, 158, 173, 184, 195, 227
Paroxysmal hypnogenic dystonia, 204
Paroxysmal kinesigenic dyskinesia, x, 173, 204, 205
Paroxysmal nocturnal hemoglobinuria, 107
Paroxysmal nonkinesigenic dyskinesia, x, 173, 204
Paroxysmal nonkinesigenic dyskinesia with episodic ataxia and spasticity, 173, 204
Patent foramen ovale, 61

Pediatric Autoimmune Neuropsychiatric Disorders Associated with Streptococci (PANDAS), 202, 209
Peduncular hallucinosis, xiii
Pelizaeus-Merzbacher disease, 34, 42, 44, 296, 305, 316
Pendular nystagmus, 243
Pentobarbital, 83
PEO
    Progressive external ophthalmoplegia, 325
Periodic alternating nystagmus, 243
Periodic limb movements of sleep, x, 95, 203
Periodic limb movements while awake, x, 203
Peripheral nerve tumors, 312
Peripheral nystagmus, 242
Perry syndrome, 185
Persistent vegetative state, 99
Personal neglect, 219
Personality disorders, ix
Phentolamine, 151, 154
Pheochromocytoma, 107
Phonological dyslexia, 218
Phosphofructokinase deficiency
    Tarui's disease, 322
Phosphoglycerate kinase deficiency, 322
Phytanic acid, 11, 156, 162, 307
Pigmentary retinopathy, 170
Pilocytic astrocytomas, 266
Pineal tumors, 275
Piracetam, 93
Piriformis syndrome, 290
Pituitary adenoma, 276
PLA2G6-associated neurodegeneration (Karak syndrome), 169
Plasmapharesis, 260
Platelet activating factor, vii, 191, 192, 193, 199, 282
Pleomorphic xanthoastrocytomas, 266
POEMS syndrome, 292, 310
Polymicrogyria, 282
Polymyalgia rheumatica, 73, 245, 326
Polymyositis, 320
Polysomnography, x, 95, 96
Porphyria, 302
Postencephalitic parkinsonism, 108, 116
Posterior cerebral artery, x, 59, 63, 64, 212, 213, 215, 217, 218, 235, 236
Posterior cortical atrophy, 229
Posterior fossa CSF collection, 166, 167, 276, 282, 297
Posterior inferior cerebellar artery (PICA) syndrome, 62
Posterior reversible encephalopathy syndrome, x, 73, 74, 236, 261
Postpolio muscular atrophy, 295

Post-streptococcal acute disseminated encephalomyelitis (PSADEM), 202
Potassium-aggravated myotonia, 25
Prader-Willi syndrome, 31, 45
Presenilin 1, x, 221
Presenilin 2, x, 221
Primary angiitis of the central nervous system, 73
Primary central nervous system lymphoma, 274
Primary CNS lymphoma, 117
Primary lateral sclerosis, x, 295
Primary progressive aphasia, 194, 227
Primitive neuroectodermal tumors, 272
Prion Diseases, 128
Prochlorperazine, 102, 103
Progesterone, 84
Progressive external ophthalmoplegia, x, 325
Progressive multifocal leukoencephalopathy, x, 117, 122, 130, 207, 258
Progressive muscular atrophy, 295
Progressive myoclonic encephalopathies, x
Progressive myoclonic epilepsy, x, 90, 91, 93, 159, 207
Progressive non-fluent aphasia, 190, 194, 227, 228, 229
Progressive supranuclear palsy, x, 116, 126, 180, 183, 189, 190, 194, 198, 221, 228, 229, 230, 241
Propionic academia, 9, 37, 44
Propofol, 83
Prosopagnosia, 211, 212, 236
Proximal myotonic myopathy, 317
PRPP synthetase superactivity, 6
Pyridostigmine, 193, 304
Pyruvate, x, 3, 37, 44, 156
Pyruvate dehydrogenase complex, x, 3, 4, 40, 41, 165, 325
    X-linked intermittent ataxia with lactic acidosis, 3, 4, 40, 41, 165, 325

Rabies, 108, 111, 130
Ramsay Hunt syndrome, 206
Rapid onset dystonia-parkinsonism, 173, 185
Rasmussen syndrome, 93
Rathke Cleft cyst, 276
Rebound nystagmus, 243
Refsum disease, 11, 156, 305
Relative afferent pupillary defect, x, 234
REM sleep behavior disorder, x, 96
Renal failure, 74
Representational neglect, 219
Restless leg syndrome, x, 203
Retinal degeneration, 170
Retinitis pigmentosa, 170
Rett syndrome, 33, 34, 45, 165, 175

Rhizomelic chondrodysplasia punctata, 11
Ribosomal RNA, x, 4
Rigid spine muscular dystrophy, 315
Rippling muscle disease, 326
Rituximab, 260
Ross syndrome, 238
Rostral interstitial nucleus of the medial longitudinal fasciculus, x, 241, 244
Roussy-Lévy syndrome, 187, 307
rRNA
    Ribosomal RNA, 4
Rubella, 33
Rubinstein-Taybi syndrome, 34

Sandifer syndrome, 175, 205
Satoyoshi syndrome, 175, 327, 329
Saxitoxin, 144
Scapuloperoneal dystrophy, 316, 318
Schistosomiasis, 124
Schizencephaly, 33, 281
Schwannoma, 297, 312
Schwartz-Jampel syndrome, 175, 326, 329
Scorpion stings, 138
Seesaw nystagmus, 243
Selective serotonin reuptake inhibitors, iii, viii, xi, xvi, 154
Semantic dementia, 227
Senior-Löken syndrome, 282
Septo-optic dysplasia, 281
Septo-optic dysplasia (de Morsier syndrome), 281
Serotonin, iii, iv, vi, vii, xi, xii 16, 18, 27, 102, 147, 154, 174, 181, 183
Serotonin norepinephrine reuptake inhibitors, xi
Serotonin syndrome, 154, 181
Severe myoclonic epilepsy in infancy (Dravet syndrome), 26
Sialidosis, 90
Silberstein ER protocol, 102
Simpson-Golabi syndrome, 35
Sleep terrors, 94
Sleepwalking, 94
Small-fiber axonal sensory polyneuropathy, 301
Smith-Lemli-Opitz syndrome, 34
Snake envenomation, 138
Sodium oxybate, 95
somatization disorder, xv
Somatoform disorder, xv, xvi
Somatoform pain disorder, xvi
Somatosensory evoked potentials, 88
Sotos syndrome, 35
Spasmus nutans, 205, 243
Spastic ataxia of Charlevoix-Saguenay, 155, 162
Spatial neglect, 219

Sphingolipidoses, 12, 91
Spider envenomation, 138
Spinal muscular atrophy, 32
St. Louis encephalitis, x, 109, 110, 114, 116
Staphylococcus aureus, 298
Steinert disease (Classical myotonic
    dystrophy), 317
Stereotypies, 165
Steroid-responsive encephalopathy associated
    with autoimmune thyroiditis
    (Hashimoto encephalopathy), 129,
    264, 327
Stiff person syndrome, 327
Stiff-person syndrome, 175, 279
Stroke mimickers, 72
Strongyloidiasis, 124
Strychnine poisoning, 134, 137, 327
Sturge-Weber syndrome, 35, 47
Subacute combined degeneration, 2
    Megaloblastic anemia
        Cobalamin
            Vitamin B12, 2
Subacute sclerosing panencephalitis, 91, 127,
    236
Subacute sensory neuronopathy, 278
Subarachnoid hemorrhage, x, 49, 58
Subependymal giant cell astrocytoma, 266
Substance abuse, 145
Substance dependence, 145
Superior cerebellar artery (SCA) syndrome,
    62
Superior oblique myokymia, 240
Surface dyslexia, 218
Susac syndrome, 258
Sydenham disease, 44, 202, 209
Symptomatic palatal tremor, 188
Syndrome of inappropriate secretion of
    antidiuretic hormone (SIADH), iii,
    20, 81, 114
Syphilis, 33, 120, 234
Syphilitic meningitis, 109
Syringomyelia, 280, 297

Tabes dorsalis, 108, 120
Tardive dyskinesia, iv, xiv, 176
Tardive dystonia, xiv 176
Tardive syndromes, xiv
Tay-Sachs disease, 12, 43, 163, 166, 294
Tetanus poisoning, 134, 137, 327
Tetany, 21, 23
Tetrodotoxin poisoning, 24, 144
Thalamic syndromes, 64
Thalidomide, 240
Thallium, 141
Thiamine, 82, 148, 156, 165, 213
Thrombolysis, 52, 53

Thrombotic microangiopathies, 74
Thyrotropin releasing hormone, 93
Tick paralysis, 138
Tics, 209
Tolosa-Hunt syndrome, 246
Toluene (methylbenzene), 143, 153
Tonic spasm, 205, 327
Top-of-the-basilar syndrome, 63
TORCH, 33, 43
torsinA, 172
Torsional (rotary) nystagmus, 243
Total parenteral nutrition, xi
Tourette syndrome, viii, 209
Toxic leukoencephalopathies, 153
Toxic mushroom poisoning, 138
Toxoplasmosis, 33, 117, 132
Transcortical motor aphasia, 217
Transcortical sensory aphasia, 217
Transependymal flow, 197
Transfer RNA, xi, 4, 48, 320
Transient binocular visual loss, 235
Transient global amnesia, vii, 72, 213, 214
Transient ischemic attack, xi, 49, 53, 56, 57,
    232
Transient monocular visual loss, 232
Transient visual obscurations, 232
Transverse myelitis, xi, 256, 298
Tricyclic antidepressants, xi, 97, 104, 279
Trigeminal neuralgia, 106
tRNA
    Transfer RNA, 4, 320
Trochlear (fourth nerve), viii, 231
Trochlear (fourth nerve) palsy, 239
Tropical spastic paraparesis, 258, 295
Tryptophan disorders, 10, 16, 154, 156
Tuberculous meningitis, 115
Turcot syndrome, 267, 272
Tyramine cheese reaction, 154
Tyrosine hydroxylase deficiency, 16, 174
Tyrosinemia (Tyrosinosis I), 8

Ubiquitin-proteasomal system, 179
Ullrich congenital muscular dystrophy, 315
Ulnar neuropathy, 284, 285
Upbeat nystagmus, 242
Upper plexus paralysis (Erb-Duchenne), 284
Urea cycle defects, 4, 7, 156
Uremic encephalopathy, 92
Uric acid, 6

Valproate, 5, 27, 104
Varicella zoster virus, 111
Vascular dementia, xi, 225
Vascular parkinsonism, 196
Vasculitides, 73
Vasogenic edema, 60, 74

Vasovagal presyncope, 247
Ventral posterior lateral thalamic nucleus, 64
Ventral posterior medial thalamic nucleus, 64
Ventrolateral thalamic nucleus, 64
Vertical diplopia, 231, 239
Vertigo, 247
Very-long-chain fatty acids, xi, 31, 41, 164
Vesicle-associated membrane protein, xi, 136, 137, 177
Vestibular neuritis, 247
Vestibular nystagmus, 242
Vestibular paroxysmia, 247
Vestibulo-ocular reflex, 251
Viral encephalitis, 111
Virchow-Robin spaces, 14, 117
Visual agnosias, 215
Visual evoked potentials, 88
Vitamin B12, 2, 156
Vitamin E deficiency, 156, 160
Voltage-gated calcium channels, xi, 24, 263, 278
Voltage-gated potassium channel antibodies, 263
   VGKC antibodies, 263, 264
Voltage-gated potassium channels, xi, 24, 263, 264, 277, 278, 327
von Hippel-Lindau syndrome, 273

Walker-Warburg syndrome, 35, 167, 282, 315
Wallenberg syndrome, 63, 248

Watson-Schwartz test, 15
Weaver syndrome, 35
Weber syndrome, 35, 47, 63
Wegener granulomatosis, 73, 115, 234
Welander distal myopathy, 32, 316
Werdnig-Hoffmann disease, 32, 330
Wernicke encephalopathy, 40, 64, 142, 148, 213
Wernicke-Korsakoff syndrome, 129, 148
West Nile virus encephalitis, xi, 114
West syndrome, 47, 76, 78, 93
Wet beriberi, 148
Withdrawal syndrome, 146

Xeroderma pigmentosum, 160, 162
X-linked adrenoleukodystrophy, 5, 11, 164
X-linked bulbospinal neuronopathy (Kennedy's disease), 295
X-linked dystonia-parkinsonism, 171, 173, 185, 186
X-linked dystrophinopathies, 313
X-linked intermittent ataxia with lactic acidosis, x, 3, 4, 40, 41, 165, 325
X-linked McLeod syndrome, 170, 201
X-linked sideroblastic anemia with ataxia, 164

Zellweger syndrome, 11, 31, 282
Zinc toxicity, 141